D0267985

Parenteral and Enteral Nutrition for the Hospitalized Patient

Howard Silberman, M.D.
Associate Professor of Surgery
University of Southern California School of Medicine and the
Los Angeles County-University of Southern California Medical Center
Los Angeles, California

Daniel Eisenberg, M.D.
Clinical Instructor of Medicine
University of Southern California School of Medicine and the
Los Angeles County-University of Southern California Medical Center
Los Angeles, California

With a Foreword by Jonathan E. Rhoads, M.D.

APPLETON-CENTURY-CROFTS/Norwalk, Connecticut

Copyright © 1982 by APPLETON-CENTURY-CROFTS
A Publishing Division of Prentice-Hall, Inc.

82 83 84 85 86 / 10 9 8 7 6 5 4 3 2 1

Prentice-Hall International, Inc., London
Prentice-Hall of Australia, Pty. Ltd., Sydney
Prentice-Hall of India Private Limited, New Delhi
Prentice-Hall of Japan, Inc., Tokyo
Prentice-Hall of Southeast Asia (Pte.) Ltd., Singapore
Whitehall Books Ltd., Wellington, New Zealand

Library of Congress Cataloging in Publication Data
Silberman, Howard.
    Parenteral and enteral nutrition for the hospitalized patient.
    Includes index.
    1. Parenteral feeding. 2. Diet therapy.   I. Eisenberg, Daniel.   II.
Title. [DNLM: 1. Enteral feeding. 2. Infusions, Parenteral. 3. Nutrition
disorders. WB 410 P228]
RM224.S54   1982   615.8'55   82-8837
ISBN 0-8385-7728-8   AACR2

Text design: Gloria J. Moyer
Cover design: Jean M. Sabato
Production: Carol Pierce

PRINTED IN THE UNITED STATES OF AMERICA

To our parents

CONTENTS

FOREWORD

Dr. Silberman and Dr. Eisenberg have written a very succinct book on therapeutic nutrition as it is needed for the care of hospitalized patients. Therapeutic nutrition is of relatively recent origin. In 1943, I was asked to serve on a subcommittee of the Food and Nutrition Board which was to concern itself with nutritional needs of sick and injured patients. This was during World War II, when there was a sharp focus on military casualties and what could be done to enhance their chance of recovery and to expedite it. It was surprising how little information there was on the subject and when the report of the Committee was finally written and submitted to the Food and Nutrition Board, it was published and then more or less taken out of circulation by the National Research Council. I believe this was done because of the thinness of the data base.

In the decade prior to this, attention had been called by Jones and Eaton in Boston and by Ravdin and a number of co-workers in Philadelphia to a complication of gastroenterostomy which seemed to be associated with protein deficits and sodium chloride excesses. The occurrence of edema in patients with food deficits has been observed through the centuries and was known as famine edema in some areas and as prison edema in others. Methods for actually measuring the serum protein, however, developed much later and came into use principally in the present century. Jones and Eaton observed that in patients undergoing gastroenterostomy it was not infrequent to see gross edema in the abdominal organs, and Jones, Eaton and White produced this in cats, partly by increasing the sodium chloride intake.

A highly significant observation had been made at the clinical level during World War I by Dr. Martin Tinker of Ithaca. It was during 1918 that the great influenza epidemic occurred which had a very high mortality among young people congregated together as in military camps. While some of these patients died early, others developed pneumonia and then empyema. Open drainage of these empyemas proved disastrous as many were due to strepto-cocci with very little attachment of the lung to the parietal pleura. In another group of cases, however, drainage was accomplished and yet the patients continued to go downhill and expired later. Tinker conceived the idea that the large quantities of pus draining from these empyema cavities carried so much protein away from the body as to weaken the individual and his resistance. He set about feeding high-protein diets to a group of such patients and demonstrated a greatly improved survival.

During the 1920's, Dr. George Whipple and his colleagues in Rochester, New York added a great deal of basic information to our knowledge of protein nutrition. They worked largely with dogs, removing blood five days a week and each time centrifuging it and returning the cells so that the animals did not become very anemic. The plasma was retained and protein in it measured. The dogs were kept on a 1 percent protein diet and gradually developed low-serum protein. The amounts of protein formed were higher during the early weeks of the experiment and gradually leveled off at about three weeks to a constant amount. Certain animals were then given additional protein. This amount would increase the yield and by relating the increment in plasma protein formed to the grams of protein added to the diet, they could determine the efficacy of a particular protein for the formation of plasma proteins. This was known as the biologic value of the protein. For plasma protein itself, given orally, it was about three to one as contrasted with hemoglobin where it took ten grams of hemoglobin to form one gram of plasma protein. Most common food proteins lay between these two extremes. They also showed that if a dog were given ample calories in the form of carbohydrates and fat, he could be kept in equilibrium by giving him plasma protein intravenously. Thus, the plasma seemed to contain all of the necessary proteins and/or protein derivatives necessary for survival. Going one step beyond this, they were able to demonstrate that even in the phlorhizinized dog, with the glucose derived from protein constantly draining out through the kidney, plasma protein administered intravenously seemed to be retained for use in the body economy. They interpreted this experiment as meaning that plasma protein could be converted to other proteins without being broken down all the way to amino acids. The excess of plasma protein recovered by plasmapheresis in the first three weeks over that in the subsequent weeks—when the production became constant—was referred to as the labile protein reserve, and they showed that this could be broken down to a large extent by inducing an infection or even a sterile inflammation.

In the 1930's, Dr. I. S. Ravdin and a group of collaborators showed that protein deficits in dogs would delay gastric emptying in dogs with fresh gastroenterostomies, in dogs with year-old gastroenterostomies, and in dogs with unoperated stomachs. They also showed that the transit time of a water barium meal from the pylorus to the cecum was delayed by hypoproteinemia.

Counterparts of these experimental models were found in clinical settings among patients. In the course of these experiments, they observed frequent dehiscence of abdominal wounds and showed the defect to be a failure of fibroplasia. Other workers in the laboratory showed a delay in callus formation after experimental fractures in the dog in the presence of hypoproteinemia. A further paper showed that the hypoproteinemic animals were much more susceptible to hemorrhagic shock. During the same decade Dr. Paul Cannon, Professor of Pathology at the University of Chicago, showed a profound interference with mechanisms of resistance to infection in rodents, and Dr. Matthew Wohl demonstrated a similar retardation of the formation of antibody to the typhoid H antigen in patients at the Philadelphia General Hospital who were hypoproteinemic.

By 1940, most of the vitamins were recognized and many of them were isolated. The essential amino acids were identified by Dr. W. C. Rose at the University of Illinois and the necessity for their simultaneous presentation to the body, if they were to be utilized, had been demonstrated. In England, Dr. D.P. Cuthbertson had carried out his notable studies on the injured patient, particularly those with fractures of the femur, which showed that such injuries initiated a catabolic state in which much more nitrogen was broken down and excreted as urea than seemed to be represented by the injured tissue.

Thus, by 1945, there was a fairly good understanding of many of the dangers of hypoproteinemia in surgical patients. There was a considerable body of data showing the amount of food nitrogen and the number of calories needed per kilogram of body weight after a variety of surgical procedures and after burns of varying extent. There was a good knowledge of which amino acids were essential and approximately in what proportions, and a fair amount of knowledge of the vitamins and minerals required for complete nutrition. All of these materials could be given intravenously to some extent. There remained the problem of developing the means of giving them in sufficient amounts to meet the needs of the injured or operated patient, and there remained the very intriguing problem of what might be accomplished if, instead of aiming for nitrogen equilibrium, one aimed for a much higher intake of calories and protein components. Both problems were confronted by four difficult facts: one, the fixed caloric value per gram of the various food components—carbohydrate, fat and protein; two, the fact that hypertonic solutions caused thrombosis of peripheral veins; three, the limitation on volume due to the fact that sick persons given over 3.0 or 3.5 liters a day occasionally develop pulmonary edema; and four, thrombosis which had been observed at autopsy along catheters introduced from the forearm or elbow into the central veins.

In our clinic, effort was directed first in using intravenous fats. They provided a helpful boost to the caloric intake but caused too much fever and other side effects to permit satisfactory use with the preparations then available to us. It is to be noted that the Swedish scientists and physicians did develop a quite satisfactory preparation of fat for intravenous use and they tended to solve the problem using that. The next solution which occurred to us was to take advantage of the diuretics which had been developed for the treatment of hypertension and were being used chronically without apparent harm to the kidney. This permitted us to increase the daily ration of fluid from three to five and, even, seven liters per day. We obtained some of our first equilibrium data in a patient with inoperable gastric carcinoma who was nourished in our Clinical Research Center by peripheral infusions of these large volumes. We found, however, that diuretic responses were irregular and that they occasioned major losses of electrolytes. We were able to compensate for the electrolyte loss satisfactorily but adjustment of the rate of fluid adminstration had to be carried on constantly in relation to the response to the diuretics. This fine degree of regulation sometimes was not accomplished within the schedules of our busy residents and we did, indeed, produce pulmonary edema on one occasion. The plan of giving more concentrated solutions into larger veins was carried out in dogs and was reported by Dr. Harry Vars, Dr. C. Martin Rhode, Dr. Dee Tourtellotte and Dr. William Parkins in 1949. They developed an apparatus by which they could give a dog continuous intravenous solutions for over four months. This plan was adapted to the study of 12-week-old puppies by Dr. Stanley Dudrick and associates, and the animals were compared with litter mates fed isocalorically by mouth. The results were that the puppies grew equally well on the intravenous ration and, emboldened by this, the method was applied in man. Dr. Dudrick learned of the subclavian route from a paper published by Dr. Dominic DeLaurentis who had adapted it for central venous pressure measurements from the original paper by a French investigator named Aubaniac. In infants, in which the subclavian vein was small, the internal jugular was often chosen as the site of injection, making the setup very similar to that used by Vars and Rhode in the dog.

    The sum total of these advances was that we have a method of substituting for the digestive tract in man and not only providing sufficient nutrients for maintenance but an abundance of additional nutrients for restoration of deficits. The results were often striking. Many small-bowel fistulas closed spontaneously; newborn infants with ruptured omphaloceles could be nourished until they grew sufficiently to permit satisfactory closure of the abdominal defect; patients with inflammatory bowel disease could have the bowel put at rest while their nourishment was being improved, and a significant percent of them went into long remissions. Patients with acute renal failure could be given still higher concentrations with minimal amounts of fluid. The nitrogen intake was balanced among the essential amino acids and the volume of solutions kept very low. In this way, the need for renal dialysis was decreased and many of these patients lived to regenerate their renal tubules and recover urinary function.

It is to update and complete this fascinating panorama that the following book has evolved. Success with intravenous hyperalimentation has been dependent on careful attention to details which required an extensive team. All of this will be emphasized and clarified in the following chapters which do, indeed, provide the nitty gritty of the methodology, a description of the complications encountered, and the ways of avoiding them and of treating them if they occur. The authors also discuss the alternatives of enteral feeding and the use of peripheral veins with larger amounts of fats. They have been successful in preparing a very lucid treatise on the methods which, although they are beset with obstacles, are enormously rewarding when properly carried out.

Jonathan E. Rhoads, M.D.
Professor of Surgery
School of Medicine
University of Pennsylvania
Philadelphia, Pennsylvania

PREFACE

Intensive nutrition therapy as a adjuvant in the management of a wide range of primarily nonnutritional medical conditions has received increasing attention in recent years. This ground swell of interest is substantially related to several recent developments.

The first of these was the development of an effective and safe method of parenteral nutrition by Dudrick and Rhoads and their associates in the mid-1960s. Prior to the advent of intravenous feeding, adequate nutrition was dependent on a normal alimentary tract, a requirement that is frequently not met by seriously ill hospitalized patients.

More recently, numerous liquid formula diets of varying composition for specific purposes have been produced. These preparations allow many patients even with severe impairment of gastrointestinal function to be nourished through the alimentary tract using a variety of feeding tubes.

The last factor accounting for an upsurge in interest in nutrition is the perception that a surprisingly high proportion of hospitalized patients has one or more nutritional deficits, that these deficits are frequently not apparent on routine physical examination, and, further, that these deficits are often associated with adverse clinical consequences which can develop after remarkably short periods of nutritional deprivation.

In preparing this volume, our objectives have been to review the morphologic and physiologic consequences of malnutrition, to outline presently available methods to evaluate nutritional status, emphasizing the limitations of present techniques, and to bring together in a single reference source the current principles and procedures of enteral and parenteral nutrition as they apply to the hospitalized patient.

Our goal has been to be concise and practical yet rigorous. Thus, we have attempted to summarize the scientific basis for current recommendations by reviewing the pertinent literature on each issue, and, where controversy exists, we have sought to present a fair balance between the pros and cons. In addition, we hope we have presented the methods of therapy in sufficient detail and with sufficient clarity to allow practitioners to prescribe treatment without requiring reference to other sources.

Undertaking this project was a more arduous task than we anticipated and could never have been accomplished without the support of many friends and colleagues. Consequently, we gratefully acknowledge the encouragement and interest of Dr. Arthur J. Donovan, Chairman, Department of Surgery, University of Southern California, and the guidance and assistance of Robert E. McGrath and Carol Pierce, our editors at Appleton-Century-Crofts. We are grateful to Dr. Allan Silberman for his constructive review of the manuscript and to Ms. Patti Eisenberg for her support and patience. Finally, this book has been brought to completion only through the devoted and extraordinary efforts of our secretary and research assistant, Ms. Linda Freehauf to whom we are greatly indebted.

Consequences of Malnutrition

The clinical manifestations of protein–calorie malnutrition are multivaried, and their severity is related to the magnitude and duration of nutritional deprivation (Fig. 1-1). In addition, the prognosis of concurrent clinical conditions tends to be adversely affected by the presence of malnutrition.

The extent and rapidity of weight loss relates to the degree of nutritional deprivation (Table 1-1). Most previously healthy adults can tolerate a weight loss of 5 to 10 percent with relatively little functional disorganization. In contrast, survival is unusual when weight loss exceeds 35 to 40 percent. The length of survival during starvation correlates with the quantity of fat stores present at the onset of the fast. After metabolic adaption to starvation, the proportion of calories obtained from protein becomes quite constant, 15 to 18 percent, until fat stores are depleted. After adipose reserves have been exhausted, protein catabolism increases.[1]

The overall changes in body composition associated with protein–calorie deprivation are illustrated in Figure 1-2. There is a relative increase in the extracellular water compartment, a disproportionate loss of fat, and a lesser loss of metabolically "active" tissue (lean body mass).[1,2]

Although loss of body weight is the most obvious manifestation of protein–calorie malnutrition, detailed laboratory studies disclose that starvation is associated with morphologic and physiologic alterations in nearly every organ and system of the body (Table 1-2). Much of the current knowledge about the effects of starvation derives from the classic studies of Keys and associates[2]

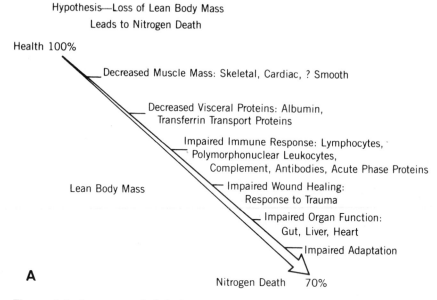

Figure 1-1. Sequence of clinical and laboratory events in the natural history of starvation. Creatinine–height index is a measure of skeletal muscle mass (see Chapter 2). (A: From Heymsfield SB, et al: Ann Intern Med 90:63–71, 1979; B: From Steffee WP: JAMA 244: 2630–2635, 1980. Copyright 1980, American Medical Association)

and the observations of the Jewish physicians in the Warsaw ghetto.[3] In 1944, Keys and associates began the "Minnesota Experiment," in which the natural history of semistarvation was studied in 32 male volunteers.[2] The subjects completed a 6 month period of semistarvation, during which time the average daily intake was 1570 kcal, including about 50 gm of protein and 30 gm of fat. In the second study, conducted between 1940 and 1942, 28 physicians confined to the Warsaw ghetto undertook a careful medical investigation of the clinical, metabolic, and pathologic consequences of starvation in their fellow inmates.[3] The residents of the Warsaw ghetto were permitted 800 kcal/day, consisting of 3 gm of fat, 20 to 30 gm of low quality vegetable protein, and the remainder carbohydrate.

EFFECTS OF MALNUTRITION ON THE CARDIOVASCULAR SYSTEM

Early workers assumed that the vital organs were protected from the ravages of malnutrition. Thus Starling stated in 1912 that in starvation "the organs which are most necessary for life (brain, heart, respiratory muscles, dia-

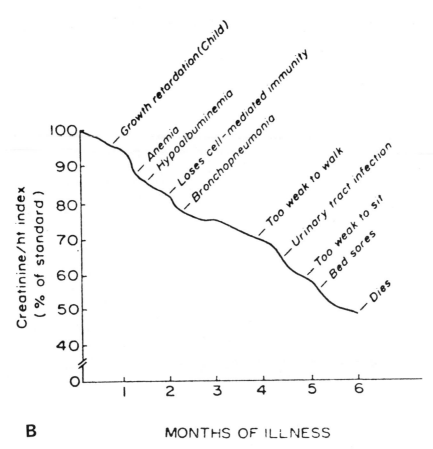

B   MONTHS OF ILLNESS

Figure 1-1 (Cont.)

TABLE 1-1
Percentage Weight Loss as a Function of Caloric Intake

Caloric Intake (% of Maintenance Requirements)	Percentage Weight Loss		
	AT 3 MONTHS	AT 6 MONTHS	AT 12 OR MORE MONTHS
90	5	8	10
80	8	12	15
70	10	15	20
60	12	20	25
50	15	25	30
40	20	30	35
30	25	35	40
20	30	45	—

Adapted from Keys A, et al: The Biology of Human Starvation, Vol 1, Minneapolis, University of Minnesota Press, 1950 p 129.

3

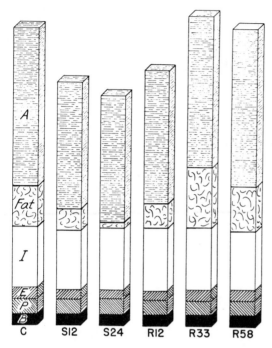

Figure 1-2. The major compartments, as weight, of the bodies of young men in the normal state of nutrition, in semistarvation, and in subsequent rehabilitation. Columns: C—control (prestarvation); S 12 and S24—12 and 24 weeks of semistarvation; R12, R33, and R58—12, 33, and 58 weeks of rehabilitation. Compartments: B—bone mineral; P—blood plasma; E—erythrocytes; I—interstitial fluid; A—active tissue (lean body mass). *(From Keys A, et al: The Biology of Human Starvation. Minneapolis, University of Minnesota Press, 1950)*

TABLE 1-2
Relative Losses of Protein from Various
Organs and Tissues of Rats After a 7 Day Fast

Organ or Tissue	Percentage Loss
Liver	40
Prostate	29
Seminal vesicles	29
Gastrointestinal tract	28
Kidneys	20
Blood	20
Heart	18
Muscle, skin, and skeleton	8
Brain	5
Eyes	0
Testicles	0
Adrenals	0

From Addis T, et al: J Biol Chem 115: 111–116, 1936.

phragm) undergo very little loss of weight" and in 1924 Vasquez stated that "inanition has no harmful effect on the heart."[4] Unfortunately, these conclusions were erroneous, and many studies have disclosed the adverse effects of malnutrition on the structure and function of the heart.

The Minnesota experiment revealed that semistarvation producing a 24 percent loss of body weight was associated with a 17 percent decrease in heart volume.[2] In addition, malnutrition of this magnitude was associated with bradycardia, mild arterial hypotension, reduced venous pressure, decreased oxygen consumption, low stroke volume, and reduced cardiac output (Table 1-3, Fig. 1-3). The reduction in cardiac output was somewhat greater than the absolute reduction in the basal metabolic rate, resulting in a relative as well as an absolute depression of total resting circulation. Heart work decreased and venous oxygen saturation and arterial oxygen content fell (Fig. 1-3).

Electrocardiographic changes included a sinus bradycardia, increased QT interval, decreased voltage of all deflections (P-wave, QRS-complex, T-wave), and a marked right shift of the QRS-axis and the T-axis.

Although in this study semistarvation was not associated with serious clinical manifestations of heart disease, cardiac reserve was reduced. Thus the adverse effects of malnutrition may be manifest during rapid nutritional repletion when incipient cardiac failure has been observed. The increased metabolic rate associated with refeeding may produce demands beyond the functional capacity of the slowly recovering heart.[2,4]

Observations in the Warsaw ghetto confirmed many of the findings of

TABLE 1-3
Cardiovascular Parameters in Malnutrition (Minnesota Experiment)

	Control Value	After Semistarvation*	Percentage of Control Value
Body weight (kg)	70.0	53.2	76%
Heart volume (ml)	620.4	514.1	84%
Pulse rate (beats/min)	56.1	37.8	67.4%
Systolic blood pressure (mmHg)	105.3	92.7	88%
Venous pressure (cm saline)	9.7	4.8	49.5%
Stroke volume (ml)	66.9	54.8	81.9%
Cardiac output (liters/min)	3.75	2.07	55.2%
Cardiac index (liters/min/M²)	2.02	1.25	61.9%

*After 24 weeks of semistarvation.
Data from Keys A, et al: The Biology of Human Starvation, Vol 1, Minneapolis, University of Minnesota Press, 1950, pp 607–634.

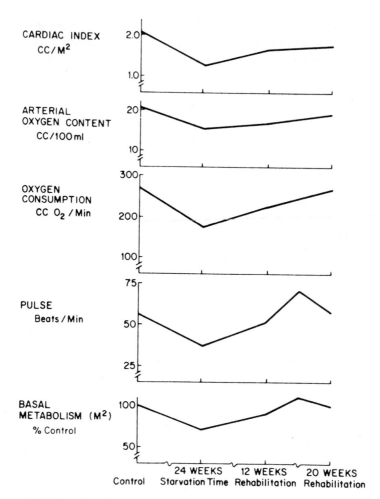

Figure 1-3. Alterations in oxygen transport parameters during semistarvation and nutritional rehabilitation observed in volunteers in the Minnesota experiment. *(From Sheldon GF, Peterson SR: JPEN 4:376–383, 1980 based on data from Keys et al, The Biology of Human Starvation)*

the Minnesota experiment.[3] Thus ghetto residents also had reduced cardiac output and stroke volume and similar electrocardiographic changes. In addition, these severely malnourished persons had a markedly increased circulation time and a greater reduction in arterial blood pressure than was observed by Keys and associates. The hypotension observed by the ghetto physicians was unaltered by exercise.

Abel and associates studied hemodynamic and morphologic parameters in malnourished dogs.[5] The animals studied had lost 40 percent of their body weight after 7 weeks of a hypocaloric, nitrogen-poor diet. Myocardial contractility was assessed acutely by obtaining isovolumetric left ventricular contractions on cardiopulmonary bypass at constant heart rate, at constant mean aortic pressure, and at a wide range of end-diastolic volumes. Results obtained from the malnourished animals were compared to those obtained from a matched group of animals which were fed normally. There was a consistent decrease in left ventricular compliance in the malnourished animals; indices of ventricular contractility (left ventricular dp/dt, force–velocity relations, and peak left ventricular pressure) were also diminished. Myocardial concentration of glycogen was decreased in the malnourished animals, and light and electron microscopy confirmed the presence of myofibrillar atrophy in the presence of interstitial edema. The authors concluded that severe protein–calorie malnutrition seriously interferes with normal left ventricular function in the experimental animal by reducing myocardial contractility and compliance.

The data reviewed above concern alterations in cardiovascular function which occur when malnutrition is the major sole pathologic condition. However, in clinical practice, malnutrition generally is due to or associated with another underlying primary disease which also may affect cardiovascular function. Thus Heymsfield and associates studied 10 severely malnourished patients in whom other diagnoses included cancer, cirrhosis, inflammatory bowel disease, and anemia.[6] Heart volume, cardiac mass, and cardiac output were decreased, but, in contrast to the findings of Keys and associates, cardiac index was elevated, since the reduction in cardiac output was less than the reduction in lean body mass. Furthermore, indices of ventricular function were normal or enhanced, suggesting that a relative hyperdynamic circulatory state was present. Five of these patients were also studied during rapid nutritional repletion. Ventricular volume and cardiac output corrected more rapidly than left ventricular mass. This combination plus excessive sodium retention was apparently responsible for the cardiac decompensation that occurred in 2 of the 5 patients.

EFFECTS OF MALNUTRITION ON THE LUNGS AND RESPIRATION

Morphologic changes in the lung are minimal in malnutrition. However, 13.8 percent of autopsied Warsaw ghetto residents had emphysema.[3] This finding is particularly striking since 14 of the 50 patients studied were under 30 years of age. Despite the limited anatomic findings, bronchitis, tuberculosis, and pneumonia are common, and pneumonia is the most common cause of death in protein–calorie malnutrition.[2-4] Increased susceptibility to pneumonia may be due to atrophy and weakness of the muscles of respiration, impairing the ability of the patient to clear secretions. In addition, impaired host defenses in

TABLE 1-4
Pulmonary Function in Malnutrition (Minnesota Experiment)

	Control	After Semistarvation*
Vital capacity (liters)	5.17	4.78
Respiratory rate (per min)	11.45	9.86
Minute volume (liters/min)	4.82	3.35
Tidal volume (ml)	421	340

*After 24 weeks of semistarvation.
Data from Keys A, et al: The Biology of Human Starvation, Vol 1, Minneapolis, University of Minnesota Press, 1950, p 603.

malnutrition (discussed later in this chapter) decrease resistance to infection in general.

Abnormalities in the mechanics of ventilation are the most striking respiratory effects of malnutrition. In the Minnesota experiment, vital capacity, respiratory rate, minute ventilation, and tidal volume progressively diminished during semistarvation (Table 1-4) and slowly returned to normal with resumption of a normal diet.[2] Decreased vital capacity was attributed to substantial loss of strength of the respiratory musculature.

Doekel and associates studied ventilatory responses in 7 normal volunteers initially and after a 10 day period during which the only nutrient intake consisted of a 2 liter liquid diet providing 500 kcal of glucose daily.[7] The experimental protocol was designed to simulate the semistarvation to which hospitalized patients receiving only intravenous crystalloid solutions are routinely subjected. After 10 days of this regimen, progressive isocapnic hypoxia failed to stimulate the anticipated increase in minute ventilation; a 42 percent decrease in the hypoxic ventilatory response was observed. In 2 of the 7 subjects, the hypoxic stimulus of an end-tidal oxygen tension of 40 mmHg produced virtually no increase in ventilation. The subjects in this study also developed a significantly reduced metabolic rate. Since this reduction is known to influence the ventilatory response to hypoxia, Doekel and associates suggested that the effect of semistarvation may be mediated through its effects on metabolic rate.[7]

EFFECTS OF MALNUTRITION
ON THE GASTROINTESTINAL TRACT

Severe malnutrition is associated with decreased gastric acid secretion and slowed gastric motility.[1-3] Gastric acidity was studied in 10 volunteers in the Minnesota experiment.[2] Five had fasting achlorhydria, but all responded to histamine stimulation. The findings were similar among Warsaw ghetto victims.[3] However, these latter subjects failed to respond to stimulation of acid output with caffeine or alcohol.

The mucous membranes throughout the gastrointestinal tract become congested and edematous.[2] In the small intestine, mucosal atrophy eventually ensues, resulting in a reduction in intestinal mass.[8,9] The enteric mucosa becomes flat without villi, and the surface epithelial cells are flattened and infiltrated with lymphocytes. Epithelial cell renewal, mitotic index, and disaccharidase activity are decreased. In addition, both starvation and protein deprivation result in a reduced rate of amino acid absorption.[10]

These changes in the gastrointestinal tract are discussed in relation to enteral and parenteral nutrition in Chapters 4 and 8, respectively.

EFFECTS OF MALNUTRITION ON THE PANCREAS

Pancreatic acinar atrophy and fibrosis resulting in exocrine pancreatic insufficiency are commonly associated with severe malnutrition. The pancreatic islets, however, are generally spared.[1] Pancreatic insufficiency and disaccharide intolerance combine to produce a malabsorption syndrome which contributes to the diarrhea characteristic of advanced malnutrition.[8]

EFFECTS OF MALNUTRITION ON THE LIVER

The effect of malnutrition on the liver is dependent on the duration of nutritional deprivation and the substrates withheld. In patients deprived of both calories and protein (marasmus), glycogen is rapidly lost from the liver and fat accumulates initially. As starvation proceeds, the liver becomes smaller,[3] liver fat decreases, and liver protein is lost, but the number of hepatocytes seems to go unchanged for prolonged periods.[1] There is no specific associated histologic abnormality in the liver,[11] but Drenick and associates found that prolonged fasts were associated with sulfobromophthalein (BSP) retention while other liver function tests remained normal or showed inconsistent changes.[12]

In contrast, patients with isolated protein malnutrition (kwashiorkor) have enlarged livers, large amounts of glycogen are present, and fatty infiltration, predominantly due to triglyceride accumulation, is a prominent feature.[11,13,14] Electron microscopy reveals a marked proliferation of smooth endoplasmic reticulum and a reduction in the amount of rough endoplasmic reticulum. The mechanism of these last changes is unknown.[11]

EFFECTS OF MALNUTRITION ON THE KIDNEY

Nearly normal renal function is maintained during starvation despite the high metabolic requirements of the kidneys.[1] However, polyuria and nocturia routinely develop and were observed early in the course of semistarvation in the Minnesota experiment.[2] In the latter study, polyuria was most marked after 6 weeks of nutritional repletion. Urinalysis usually reveals low specific gravity, little sediment, and no white cells, red cells, casts, or protein.[2] It has been suggested that the impaired concentrating ability of the kidney may be due to decreased amounts of urea in the renal medulla with lowering of the medullary osmolar gradient.[1] No significant histologic changes have been observed.[2]

HEMATOLOGIC EFFECTS OF MALNUTRITION

Malnutrition is associated with a mild normochromic, normocytic anemia which is unaccompanied by reticulocytosis in the presence of adequate iron stores.[1,4,15] Sanders and associates suggested that patients receiving some dietary protein, but in inadequate amounts, develop an anemia which is due to decreased synthesis of erythropoietin.[16] In contrast, starved patients receiving no dietary protein develop an anemia which is due to developmental failure of bone marrow stem cells as well as decreased erythropoietin synthesis.

Severe malnutrition is associated with a leukopenia and normal differential white cell count.[1-3] Neutrophils appear normal morphologically, and there is usually, but not always, an increase in neutrophils in response to infection even late in starvation.[1,3] There are, however, abnormalities in neutrophil function. In vitro studies disclose impaired chemotaxis and defective Candidacidal and bactericidal activity. Phagocytic function is preserved.[17]

A reduced platelet count was also observed among Warsaw ghetto residents.[3]

EFFECTS OF MALNUTRITION ON
IMMUNE FUNCTIONS

A variety of immunologic parameters are altered in malnourished patients.

Immunologic responses may be categorized as cell-mediated, involving thymus-derived (T) lymphocytes, or antibody-mediated (humoral immunity), involving bone marrow-derived (B) lymphocytes. T-cells play a major role in protection against intracellular parasites, most notably Myobacterium tuberculosis, and viral and fungal infections. B-cells produce specific antibodies and have a major role in resistance to encapsulated or pyogenic bacteria.[18]

Assays of cell-mediated immunity are frequently abnormal in protein-calorie malnutrition. Thus reactivity to common recall skin test antigens (such as tuberculin, Candida, and Trichophyton) is depressed during both acute and chronic malnutrition.[1,19-23] Response to dinitrochlorobenzene is similarly depressed,[20] and decreased lymphocyte responsiveness to immunogenic (blastogenic) stimuli, such as phytohemagglutinin or poke weed mitogens, is also a feature of protein–calorie malnutrition. Low peripheral blood lymphocyte counts have been observed in some studies,[20,21,24-26] and the percentage of T-cells is likewise reduced.[21] In addition, marked thymic and lymphoid tissue atrophy is found in malnourished children.[21]

Whereas cell-mediated immune functions are consistently impaired, the effect of malnutrition on humoral immunity is less clear. Data on specific serum antibody responses in human malnutrition are conflicting.[27] Antibody formation is adequate to many antigens, including tetanus and diphtheria toxoids, poliovirus, measles, pneumococcal polysaccharide, and keyhole limpet hemocyanin. In contrast, impaired antibody response has been reported to yellow fever vaccine, killed influenza A Hong Kong, flagellin, tobacco mosaic virus, and avian red cells. In addition, antibody responses have been compared in malnourished children given different levels of protein intake. For example, those on high protein intakes had significantly higher antibody response to typhoid vaccine.[27]

In addition to these changes in cellular and humoral immunity, malnourished patients have a depressed level of total serum hemolytic complement and individual serum complement components, with the exception of C4. The low levels of complement may be the result of decreased synthesis or increased consumption.[28]

EFFECTS OF MALNUTRITION ON SUSCEPTIBILITY TO INFECTION

The synergistic interaction of infection and malnutrition is well recognized on the basis of clinical observations and epidemiologic data.[20,29] Although the mechanism by which malnutrition reduces host resistance is not completely defined, it is known that various host defenses are impaired in malnutrition. The effects on neutrophil function and immunologic responses have already been discussed. In addition, there are a variety of nonspecific host defense factors which may be adversely affected by protein–calorie deprivation. These include the anatomic barriers to invasive microorganisms and plasma factors, such as interferon, lysozyme, properidin, acute-phase reactant proteins, and carrier proteins.[30]

Severe protein deficiency is associated with changes in the body's anatomic barriers. These effects include atrophic changes of the skin with extensive desquamation, atrophy of the gastrointestinal mucosa, and tissue edema.

Such changes may facilitate entry and proliferation of infectious organisms. In addition, the ability to wall off initially localized infection may be impaired, leading to dissemination and systemic sepsis.[31]

Many of the nonspecific plasma factors are proteins and therefore should be adversely affected by protein malnutrition.[31]

EFFECTS OF MALNUTRITION ON WOUND HEALING

Clinical evidence supports the concept that during periods of catabolism the wound is a favored tissue which has a high biologic priority. Early wound healing proceeds in the total absence of external intake, and the nitrogen substrates required for fibroblastic synthesis of collagen generally can be derived from endogenous sources. Most surgical wounds heal to the point of tensile integrity during a period of negative nitrogen balance.[32] Nevertheless, *marked* protein deficiency delays almost all aspects of healing, including neovascularization, fibroblast proliferation, collagen synthesis, and wound remodeling.[33] In addition, if serum albumin falls, edema may follow, which itself further interferes with healing. This is of special importance in the healing of gastrointestinal anastomoses.[33,34]

Irvin studied the healing of colonic anastomoses and surgical incisions of the skin and abdominal wall in rats who had received protein-free diets.[35] Significant changes in wound healing occurred only when weight loss exceeded one-third of the normal body weight. Such a severe degree of malnutrition was associated with a profound reduction in the mechanical strength of the abdominal and skin wounds, but the changes in the tensile strength of colonic anastomoses were much less pronounced. Evidently, malnutrition has different effects on visceral and parietal tissues, and Irvin concluded that visceral collagen is preserved to a much greater extent than the collagen of skin or parietal tissues.

EFFECTS OF STARVATION ON INTERMEDIARY METABOLISM

Potential energy sources for fasting man include glycogen, protein, and fat. Glycogen stores are limited and are totally dissipated within the first 1 to 3 days of fasting. Body protein represents a large potential energy source, but since each molecule of protein serves a specific nonfuel function as an enzyme or for structural or functional purposes, prolonged survival is dependent upon protein conservation. Thus adaption to starvation involves mechanisms by which fat and fat-derived fuels become the major energy sources, glucose utilization is reduced, and protein is conserved.

The initial adaptive response to fasting is directed primarily at providing glucose for the brain and the glycolytic tissues, including erythrocytes, bone marrow, renal medulla, and peripheral nerve. Ongoing glucose utilization, particularly by the brain, results in a slight decline in blood glucose concentration (10 to 15 mg/dl), which leads, in turn, to decreased insulin levels and increased glucagon levels. These changes in hormonal milieu facilitate an outpouring of amino acids, especially alanine, from muscle and favor lipolysis, leading to free fatty acid mobilization. At this stage, gluconeogenesis supports the central nervous system and the glycolytic tissues, and oxidation of the mobilized fatty acids provides the fuel for the remaining tissues (Fig. 1-4). Insulin participates in this scheme as the major regulator of peripheral lipolysis and proteolysis, whereas the role of glucogon is at the level of hepatic glycogenolysis and gluconeogenesis, stimulating glycogen release and hepatic uptake of alanine.[36] Alanine released from muscle is the major substrate used by the liver for gluconeogenesis. Most of the alanine is synthesized in muscle by transamination of glucose-derived pyruvate, and the branched-chain ami-

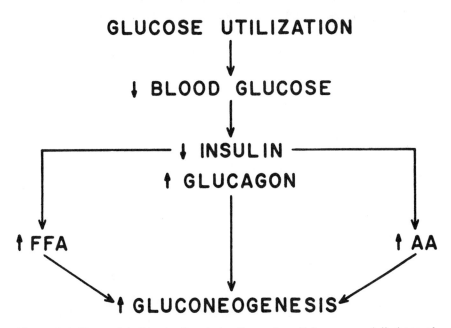

Figure 1-4. The metabolic adaption during the early or "gluconeogenic" phase of starvation. Ongoing glucose utilization results in lowered blood glucose, leading to a decrease in insulin and an increase in glucagon. As a consequence, free fatty acids are mobilized from adipose stores, and amino acids, especially alanine, are released from muscle. Gluconeogenesis is enhanced and fatty acid oxidation provides energy for conversion of lactate to glucose. Fatty acids also serve as the energy source for most tissues. *(From Saudek CD, Felig P: Am J Med 60:117–126, 1976)*

no acids (valine, leucine, and isoleucine) are the major source of nitrogen for this reaction[36,37] (Fig. 1-5). Additional gluconeogenic substrates include lactate and glycerol (Fig. 1-6). Glucose may be synthesized from the end-glycolytic product, lactate, utilizing energy derived from oxidation of free fatty acids (Cori cycle). In addition, the glycerol skeleton of triglyceride is readily converted to glucose.[36]

This sequence of events, involving primarily gluconeogenesis, characterizes the first 5 to 10 days of fasting and is achieved at the expense of rapid proteolysis. Since death occurs when one-third to one-half of the body protein is lost, survival in prolonged starvation necessitates a reduction in the rate of protein dissolution and, therefore, a reduction in glucose utilization.[36] As starvation proceeds, progressively less fatty acid is fully oxidized and progressively more goes into ketone body formation.[38] Thus, in this later phase of adaption to starvation, ketones become the major energy-yielding substrate for the brain, thereby reducing the demand for glucose and hence gluconeogenesis.

It is postulated that the elevated ketone levels provide a signal to muscle, resulting in decreased amino acid catabolism and reduced output of alanine. The resulting hypoalaninemia is in turn responsible for the reduction in he-

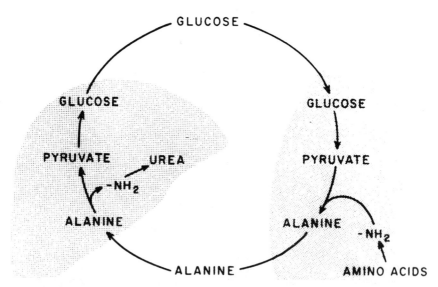

Figure 1-5. The glucose–alanine cycle. From 60 to 70 percent of the alanine coming from muscle tissue is synthesized by transamination of glucose-derived pyruvate. The alanine released from muscle is taken up by the liver, where its carbon skeleton is reconverted to glucose. *(From Felig P: Metabolism 22:179–207, 1973)*

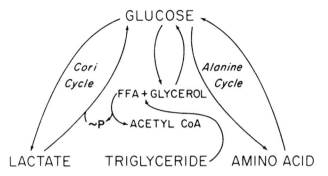

Figure 1-6. Major gluconeogenic substrates. In the Cori cycle, glucose is synthesized from lactate with energy derived from oxidation of free fatty acids. The glycerol moiety of triglyceride enters directly into gluconeogenesis. *(From Saudek CD, Felig P: Am J Med 60:117–126, 1976)*

patic gluconeogenesis (Fig. 1-7).[36] Thus glucose utilization is reduced and protein conservation is enhanced. Nevertheless, an ongoing demand for some glucose continues, and during prolonged starvation the kidney becomes a significant source. After 30 days of fasting, renal gluconeogenesis provides nearly half of the body glucose.[39] The substrate for this glucose is primarily glutamine.

Finally, when all lipid stores are depleted, the body again turns to the protein compartment, and eventually even the essential proteins of the heart, lungs, blood cells, and other vital tissues are consumed.[40]

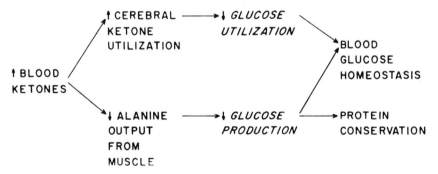

Figure 1-7. The metabolic adaption during the late or "protein conservation" phase of starvation. Ketones replace glucose as substrate for the brain and signal a reduction in protein catabolism. Consequently, protein conservation is achieved and glucose homeostasis is maintained. *(From Saudek CD, Felig P: Am J Med 60:117–126, 1976)*

SUMMARY

Nutritional deprivation has adverse effects on the structure and function of nearly all the organs and systems of the body. These changes in themselves may produce clinical disease, but in addition, they may have a detrimental effect on concurrent illness.

The problems of malnutrition are not restricted to persons in underdeveloped parts of the world but are encountered daily in western society.[36] Moreover, prolonged starvation is not a prerequisite for the development of nutritional deficits. Such deficits have been observed in patients in whom well-balanced diets have been withheld for a few as 10 days.

An appreciation of the multivaried, often subtle consequences of malnutrition has stimulated considerable interest in the diagnosis and treatment of nutritional deficits. These latter topics are considered in the following chapters.

REFERENCES

1. Levenson SM, Crowley LV, Seifter E: Starvation, in Ballinger WF, Collins JA, Drucker WR, et al (eds): Manual of Surgical Nutrition. Philadelphia: WB Saunders, 1975, pp 236–264.
2. Keys A, Brozek J, Henschel A, et al: The Biology of Human Starvation, vols 1, 2. Minneapolis, University of Minnesota Press, 1950.
3. Winick M (ed): Hunger Disease: Studies by the Jewish Physicians in the Warsaw Ghetto. New York, John Wiley and Sons, 1979.
4. Sheldon GF, Petersen SR: Malnutrition and cardiopulmonary function: Relation to oxygen transport. JPEN 4:376–383, 1980.
5. Abel RM, Grimes JB, Alonso D, et al: Adverse hemodynamic and ultrastructural changes in dog hearts subjected to protein–calorie malnutrition. Am Heart J 97:733–744, 1979.
6. Heymsfield SB, Bethel RA, Ansley JD, et al: Cardiac abnormalities in cachectic patients before and during nutritional repletion. Am Heart J 95:584–594, 1978.
7. Doekel RC, Zwillich CW, Scoggin CH, et al: Clinical semi-starvation: Depression of hypoxic ventilatory response. N Engl J Med 295:358–361, 1976.
8. Herskovic T: Protein malnutrition and the small intestine. Am J Clin Nutr 22:300–304, 1969.
9. Levine GM, Deren JJ, Steiger E, Zinno R: Role of oral intake in maintenance of gut mass and disacchride activity. Gastroenterology 67:975–982, 1974.
10. Adibi SA, Allen ER: Impaired jejunal absorption rates of essential amino acids induced by either dietary caloric or protein deprivation in man. Gastroenterology 59:404–413, 1970.
11. Blanchard J, Steiger E, O'Neil M, et al: Effect of protein depletion and repletion on liver structures, nitrogen content and serum proteins. Ann Surg 190:144–150, 1979.

12. Drenick EJ, Swendseid ME, Blahd WH, Tuttle SG: Prolonged starvation as treatment for severe obesity. JAMA 187:100–105, 1964.
13. Steiger E, Daly JM, Allen TR, et al: Post-operative intravenous nutrition: Effect on body weight, protein regeneration, wound healing, and liver morphology. Surgery 73:686–691, 1973.
14. Madi K, Jervis HR, Anderson PR, Zimmerman MR: A protein deficient diet: Effect on liver, pancreas, stomach, and small intestine of the rat. Arch Pathol 89:38–52, 1970.
15. Adams EB: Anemia associated with protein deficiency. Semin Hematol 7:55–66, 1970.
16. Sanders R, Sheldon GF, Garcia J, et al: Erythropoietin synthesis in rats during total parenteral nutrition. J Surg Res 22:649–653, 1977.
17. Douglas SD, Schopfer K: The phagocyte in protein–calorie malnutrition: A review, in Suskind RM (ed): Malnutrition and the Immune Response. New York, Raven Press, 1977, pp 231–243.
18. Dionigi R, Gnes F, Bonera A, Dominioni L: Nutrition and infection. JPEN 3:62–68, 1979.
19. Bistrian BR, Sherman M, Blackburn GL, et al: Cellular immunity in adult marasmus. Arch Intern Med 137:1408–1411, 1977.
20. Chandra RK: Immunocompetence in undernutrition. J Pediatr 81:1194–1200, 1972.
21. Edelman R: Cell-mediated immune response in protein–calorie malnutrition: A review, in Suskind RM (ed): Malnutrition and the Immune Response. New York, Raven Press, 1977, pp 47–75.
22. Law DK, Dudrick SJ, Abdou NI: Immunocompetence of patients with protein–calorie malnutrition: The effects of nutritional repletion. Ann Intern Med 79:545–550, 1973.
23. Law DK, Dudrick SJ, Abdou NI: The effect of protein–calorie malnutrition on immune competence of the surgical patient. Surg Gynecol Obstet 139:257–266, 1974.
24. Baker CC, Hohn DC: Sepsis in trauma patients (trauma rounds—San Francisco General Hospital). West J Med 130:378–383, 1979.
25. Lewis RT, Klein H: Risk factors in postoperative sepsis: Significance of preoperative lymphocytopenia. J Surg Res 26:365–371, 1979.
26. Smythe PM, Schonland M, Brereton-Stiles GG, et al: Thymolymphatic deficiency and depression of cell-mediated immunity in protein–calorie malnutrition. Lancet 2:939–944, 1971.
27. Chandra RK: Immunoglobulin and antibody response in protein–calorie malnutrition: A review, in Suskind RM (ed): Malnutrition and the Immune Response. New York, Raven Press, 1977, pp 155–168.
28. Sirisinha S, Suskind RM, Edelman R, et al: The complement system in protein–calorie malnutrition: A review, in Suskind RM (ed): Malnutrition and the Immune Response. New York, Raven Press, 1977, pp 309–320.
29. Scrimshaw NS, Taylor CE, Gordon JE: Interactions of Nutrition and Infection. WHO Monograph Series, No 57. Geneva, World Health Organization, 1968.
30. Beisel WR: Nonspecific host factors: A review, in Suskind RM (ed): Malnutrition and the Immune Response. New York, Raven Press, 1977, pp 341–374.

31. Neumann CG: Non-specific host factors and infection in malnutrition: A review, in Suskind RM (ed): Malnutrition and the Immune Response. New York, Raven Press, 1977, pp 355–374.
32. Moore FD, Brennan MF: Surgical injury: Body composition, protein metabolism, and neuroendocrinology, in Ballinger WF, Collins JA, Drucker WR, et al (eds): Manual of Surgical Nutrition. Philadelphia, WB Saunders Co, 1975, pp 169–222.
33. Levenson S, Seifter E, Van Winkle W Jr: Nutrition, in Hunt TK, Dunphy JE (eds): Fundamentals of Wound Management. New York, Appleton–Century–Crofts, 1979, pp 286–363.
34. Thompson WD, Ravdin IS, Frank IL: Effect of hypoproteinemia on wound disruption. Arch Surg 36:500–508, 1938.
35. Irvin TT: Effects of malnutrition and hyperalimentation on wound healing. Surg Gynecol Obstet 146:33–37, 1978.
36. Saudek CD, Felig P: The metabolic events of starvation. Am J Med 60:117–126, 1976.
37. Felig P: The glucose–alanine cycle. Metabolism 22:179–207, 1973.
38. Dietze G, Wicklmayer M, Mehnert H: Physiology of metabolism during starvation, in Ahnefeld FW, Burri C, Dick W, Halmagyi M (eds): Parenteral Nutrition. New York, Springer–Verlag, 1976, pp 17–30.
39. Wilmore DW: The Metabolic Management of the Critically Ill. New York, Plenum Medical Book Co, 1977.
40. McMurray WC: Essentials of Human Metabolism. Hagerstown, Md, Harper and Row, 1977.

2

Evaluation of Nutritional Status

It is commonly assumed that malnutrition is rare in industrialized societies with high standards of living, such as the United States. However, surveys of nutritional status among affluent as well as indigent patients hospitalized in the United States indicate that a surprising number— one-third to one-half or more—have significant deficits in one or more of the nutritional indices discussed below.[1-7] Such deficits often remain undetected when physical examination is the sole diagnostic tool.[8] Thus approximately 50 percent of general surgical patients,[1] 44 percent of general medical patients,[2] 48 percent of orthopedic patients,[4] and 32 percent of patients admitted to a family practice service[6] have been found to have abnormalities. Moreover, a prospective analysis of 134 consecutive admissions to a general medicine service revealed that putative nutritional parameters deteriorated during hospitalization in 75 percent of patients admitted with normal values.[9]

This high incidence of nutritional deficits plus the advent of effective therapy has stimulated considerable interest in developing sensitive methods of identifying patients who would benefit from intensive nutritional support. At the present time, however, the diagnosis of abnormalities in body composition that would be amenable to nutrition therapy is more elusive than was anticipated. Presently available nutritional indices may be significantly influenced by nonnutritional factors, and standards of normal derived from epidemiologic studies may not always be applicable to the evaluation of a given individual.

Thus the ideal diagnostic test is still being sought. Such a test should be specific for deficits of nutritional origin, deviations from normal should imply the presence of abnormalities of clinical or prognostic significance, and changes in nutritional status, either deterioration or improvement, should be promptly reflected by appropriate changes in the test value.

At present, nutritional assessment should not be dependent upon a single parameter but should involve the determination of multiple parameters, the interpretation of which must always take into account the entire medical status of the patient. When viewed in this context, nutritional indices form an important part of a patient's total evaluation and may serve as sensitive harbingers of the increased morbidity and mortality associated with malnutrition.

MEDICAL HISTORY AND BODY WEIGHT

The initial step in evaluating nutritional status is to obtain the patient's medical and dietary history. Past dietary intake, number of meals usually eaten, types of food consumed, recent changes in dietary patterns, and any food allergies or intolerances are recorded, and usual weight, present weight, and height are likewise noted. From the weight and height data, the percentage weight loss can be calculated, and present weight can be compared with "ideal" values based on actuarial studies of "desirable" weight as related to height and body build (Table 2-1). However, such standard tables give values which are only approximations, since no scientific or standard definition of "body frame" is available, and increases in body weight associated with advancing age are not taken into account. In fact, available data are probably inadequate to describe the actual weight of "average" members of the population or to specify what weight would be most conducive to health.[10] Given an appreciation of the shortcomings of presently available "standard" or "desirable" weight data, measurements of body weight can still provide valuable information. A patient's weight can be calculated as a percentage of ideal body weight (%IBW) as follows:

$$\%IBW = \frac{\text{Actual weight}}{\text{IBW}} \times 100$$

According to Blackburn and associates, [11] actual body weight less than 80 percent of IBW may be considered significant. Although %IBW is a valuable parameter, there are certain potential problems in its interpretation. Thus if a patient who is usually markedly obese experiences a significant weight loss due to nutritional depletion (including visceral and skeletal protein loss), such a deficit may go unobserved, since the %IBW may well remain normal or high. In order to circumvent this problem, the patient's present or actual weight can be compared to his usual weight. The percent usual body weight (%UBW) or percent weight loss can be calculated as follows:

$$\%UBW = \frac{\text{Actual weight}}{\text{Usual weight}} \times 100$$

$$\%\text{ Weight Loss} = \frac{\text{UBW} - \text{Actual body weight}}{\text{UBW}} \times 100$$

The significance of weight loss has been emphasized by many investigators. Garrow and associates reported significant mortality among otherwise healthy infants who had lost 40 percent or more of their body weight.[12] When malnutrition was accompanied by significant illness or injury, Kinney and associates observed an increased rate of mortality after loss of only 25 percent of body weight.[13] In an analysis of surgical patients, Studley reported a nearly 10 -fold increase in operative mortality among patients who had sustained a weight loss of 20 percent or more.[14] The significance of weight loss can also be correlated with the rapidity with which it occurred (Table 2-2).[11]

Parameters based on body weight may be misleading indices of nutritional status in patients with fluid overload, since these patients may increase or maintain body weight despite severe protein depletion. Such patients may include those with congestive heart failure, liver disease, and renal failure. In addition, increased extracellular fluid volume during starvation may maintain weight to some extent despite severe loss of energy stores and metabolically active tissues.[15,16]

The sensitivity of nutritional analysis can be augmented by evaluating each of the body's basic fuel compartments.

Table 2-3 outlines the fuel composition of a normally proportioned 70 kg man. It is apparent that fat is the main fuel or caloric reserve and protein is the other major potential energy source. In contrast, stored glucose, in the form of glycogen, would provide less than 2000 calories if it were completely combusted for fuel. During starvation, then, the body relies on two major sources: muscle protein and adipose triglycerides. As starvation proceeds, the adipose stores and the protein compartments, both skeletal and visceral, become depleted. Since protein is not stored and each molecule of protein serves some nonfuel function, either as an enzyme or as a contractile or structural protein, compromise of vital body function occurs as protein–fuel conversion continues.[17]

Each of the body's basic fuel reserves can be evaluated using anthropometric, biochemical, and immunologic parameters (Table 2-4).

TABLE 2-1
Ideal Body Weights for Men and Women Ages 25 and Over*

Height (FT AND IN)	(CM)	Small Frame (LB)	(KG)	Medium Frame (LB)	(KG)	Large Frame (LB)	(KG)
Men							
5'1"	155	105–113	48–51	111–122	50–55	119–134	54–61
2"	157	108–116	49–53	114–126	52–57	122–137	55–62
3"	160	111–119	50–54	117–129	53–59	125–141	57–64
4"	163	114–122	52–55	120–132	55–60	128–145	58–66
5"	165	117–126	53–57	123–136	56–62	131–149	60–68
6"	168	121–130	55–59	127–140	58–64	135–154	61–70
7"	170	125–134	57–61	131–145	60–66	140–159	64–72
8"	173	129–138	59–63	135–149	61–68	144–163	65–74
9"	175	133–143	60–65	139–153	63–70	148–167	67–76
10"	178	137–147	62–67	143–158	65–72	152–172	69–78
11"	180	141–151	64–69	147–163	67–74	157–177	71–80
6'0"	183	145–155	66–70	151–168	69–76	161–182	73–83
1"	185	149–160	68–73	155–173	70–79	166–187	75–85
2"	188	153–164	70–75	160–178	73–81	171–192	78–87
3"	191	157–168	71–76	165–183	75–83	175–197	80–90

Women

Height							
4'8"	142	88–94	40–43	92–103	42–47	100–115	45–52
9"	145	90–97	41–44	94–106	43–48	102–118	46–54
10"	147	92–100	42–45	97–109	44–50	105–121	48–55
11"	150	95–103	43–47	100–112	45–51	108–124	49–56
5'0"	151	98–106	45–48	103–115	47–52	111–127	50–58
1"	155	101–109	46–50	106–118	48–54	114–130	52–59
2"	157	104–112	47–51	109–122	50–55	117–134	53–61
3"	160	107–115	49–52	112–126	51–57	121–138	55–63
4"	163	110–119	46–54	116–131	53–60	125–142	57–65
5"	165	114–123	52–56	121–135	55–61	129–146	59–66
6"	168	118–127	54–58	124–139	56–63	133–151	60–69
7"	170	122–131	55–60	128–143	58–65	137–154	62–70
8"	173	126–136	57–62	132–147	60–67	141–159	64–72
9"	175	130–140	59–64	136–151	62–69	145–164	66–75
10"	178	134–144	61–65	140–155	64–70	149–169	68–77

*Nude weights, adapted from the table of desirable weights (the weights associated with lowest mortality) developed by the statistical bureau of the Metropolitan Life Insurance Company, based on data from the 1959 Build and Blood Pressure Study of the Society of Actuaries. Adapted from Metropolitan Life Insurance Company Statistical Bulletin, Vol 58, October, 1977, p 5.

TABLE 2-2
Evaluation of Weight Change

Time	Significant Weight Loss (%)*	Severe Weight Loss (%)*
1 Week	1–2	> 2
1 Month	5	> 5
3 Months	7.5	> 7.5
6 Months	10	> 10

*Percentage of usual body weight lost. From Blackburn GL, et al: JPEN 1:11–22, 1977.

TABLE 2-3
Fuel Composition of Normal Man

Fuel	Amount (kg)	Calories (kcal)
Tissue		
Fat (adipose triglyceride)	15	141,000
Protein (mainly muscle)	6	24,000
Glycogen (muscle)	0.150	600
Glycogen (liver)	0.075	300
Total		165,900
Circulating fuels		
Glucose (extracellular fluid)	0.020	80
Free fatty acids (plasma)	0.0003	3
Triglycerides (plasma)	0.003	30
Total		113

From Cahill GF Jr: N Engl J Med 282:668–675, 1970.
(Reprinted with permission of the New England Journal of Medicine).

TABLE 2-4
Nutritional Status Parameters

Compartment	Test or Measurement
Fat	Triceps skin fold
Visceral protein	Plasma proteins: albumin, transferrin, prealbumin, retinol-binding protein
	Immune function: lymphocyte count, skin tests
Skeletal muscle	Arm muscle circumference, creatinine–height index

ANTHROPOMETRIC MEASURES

Parameters derived directly from the patient's body are called *anthropometric measures.* These include triceps skin fold (TSF), mid-arm circumference (AC), and mid-arm muscle circumference (AMC). The triceps skin fold provides an estimate of fat stores, and the mid-arm muscle circumference is thought to reflect skeletal muscle mass.[18]

The mid-arm circumference and the triceps skin fold are measured at a site located at the midpoint between the acromion and the olecranon of the nondominant arm (Fig. 2-1). The triceps skin fold is determined by grasping the skin and adipose tissue overlying the triceps muscle; the thickness of the pinched tissue is measured with the Lange skin-fold calipers* (Figs. 2-2, 2-3). The measurement is repeated three times, and the average value is recorded. The mid-arm muscle circumference is calculated from the mid-arm circumference, determined with a tape measure (Fig. 2-4), and the triceps skin fold from the following formula:

$$\text{AMC (cm)} = \text{AC (cm)} - [0.314 \times \text{TSF (mm)}]$$

AMC values derived from this formula are approximations, since the equation assumes that the upper arm is cylindrical and does not take into account the humeral diameter, which may vary from person to person.[19]

The interpretation of anthropometric data derived from a given individual is confounded by the variability of "normal" values obtained from different populations (Tables 2-5, 2-6). In addition, the magnitude of deviation from a given normal standard which constitutes "malnutrition" is ill-defined, and suggested criteria have not been rigorously validated. Blackburn and associates have adopted Jelliffe's standards (Table 2-6) and have defined mild to moderate nutritional depletion as 60 to 90 percent of standard and severe depletion as less than 60 percent of standard (Table 2-7).[11,22] However, application of these criteria to urban Americans may produce errors of interpretation, since Jelliffe's data were intended for use in nonindustrialized societies.[23] Thus, Jelliffe's values differ significantly from those obtained from more recent studies of American populations (Table 2-6). For example, deficiencies in TSF in males would be overestimated using the Jelliffe standard. In addition, Jelliffe's standards do not take into account variation of anthropometric parameters with age. Interpretation of anthropometric measurements is further confused because normal variation for some parameters is greater than for others. Thus some patients may appear deficient in one parameter and normal in another.

It has been suggested that many of these problems of interpretation can

---

Available from Cambridge Scientific Instruments, Cambridge, Maryland.

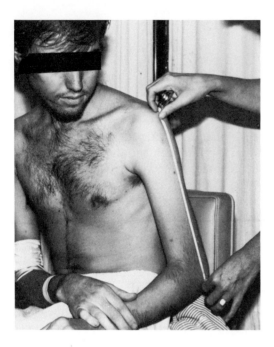

Figure 2-1. Arm circumference and triceps skin fold are determined from the nondominant arm at the midpoint between the acromion and olecranon processes.

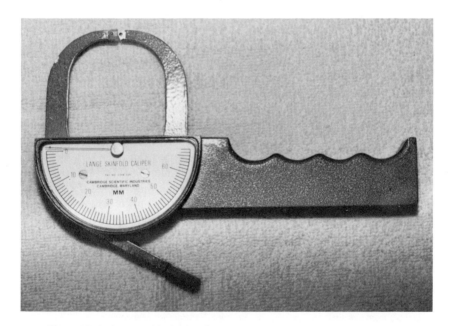

Figure 2-2. Lange skin fold caliper for measuring the triceps skin fold.

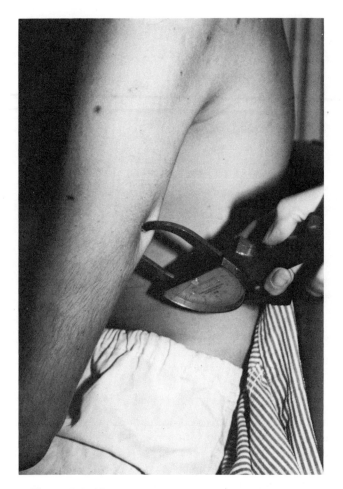

Figure 2-3. Measurement of triceps skin fold thickness.

be avoided by using data derived from American populations and by comparing measurements to percentiles rather than to percentages of a standard value.[23] Thus Gray and Gray[23] and Burgert and Anderson[18] suggested that values for TSF thickness and arm circumference be related to the age- and sex-specific population percentiles presented in the report of the National Health Survey (Tables 2-8, 2-9).[20] Because the National Health Survey did not report population percentiles for mid-arm muscle circumference, Burgert and Anderson[18] suggested using the arm muscle circumference percentiles presented in the United States Ten-State Nutrition Survey[19] (Table 2-10). Gray and Gray suggested that anthropometric values falling below the 5th percentile be

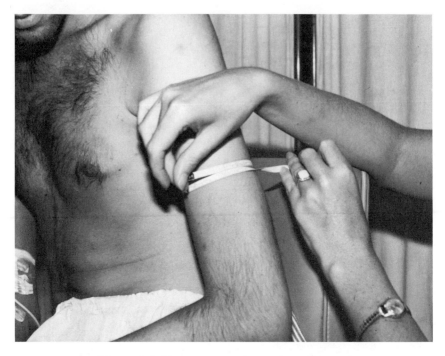

Figure 2-4. Measurement of arm circumference.

considered as evidence of nutritional depletion, while measurements between the 5th and 10th, or the 5th and 15th percentiles be considered as evidence of marginal depletion.[23]

Thus anthropometric measurements, so valuable in epidemiologic studies, *may* reflect the nutritional status of individuals, but standards of normal with which to compare the measurements from a given patient are not well defined.

Collins and associates recently evaluated the use of anthropometric measurements to assess protein malnutrition in surgical patients.[24] They used an in vivo neutron activation analyzer for the measurement of total body nitrogen as an index of protein stores. Studying 10 normal persons and 82 surgical patients, they found anthropometric measurements very weak indicators of protein depletion when studied over a period of 2 weeks or less.

Mullen and associates prospectively evaluated the nutritional status of 64 consecutive elective surgical patients.[25] Anthropometric data were abnormal in the majority of patients, but the measurements were not of value in identifying a high-risk patient population—that is, the anthropometric data did not correlate with postoperative morbidity or mortality. However, in a

TABLE 2-5
Standard Right Arm Measurements (Median)

Reference	Population Studied	Men			Women		
		TSF (mm)	AC (cm)	AMC (cm)	TSF (mm)	AC (cm)	AMC (cm)
Burgert and Anderson[18]	American men, 22–60 years (median, 25 years); American women, 21–56 years (median, 27 years)	10.6	30.0	26.6	21.1	26.3	19.9
Frisancho[19]	Americans, 17–44 years, mostly low income	10–12	29.2–31.2	24.5–27.0	17–22	26.0–28.6	19.6–21.6
Stoudt et al[20]	Americans, random population, ages 18–79	11	30.7	—	22	28.2	—

TABLE 2-6
Standard Left Arm Measurements (Median)

Reference	Population Studied	Men				Women			
		TSF (mm)	AC (cm)	AMC (cm)		TSF (mm)	AC (cm)	AMC (cm)	
Burgert and Anderson[18]	American men, 22–60 years (median, 25 years) American women, 21–56 years (median, 27 years)	10.1	30.2	26.9		19.9	26.4	20.1	
Jelliffe[21]	AC from low income American women and military men from Italy, Greece, Turkey. Source of TSF unknown	12.5	29.3	25.3		16.5	28.5	23.2	
		(P < 0.01)*	(P < 0.05)*	(P < 0.01)*		(P < 0.05)*	(P < 0.01)*	(P < 0.01)*	

*Levels of significance for values of Burgert vs. values of Jelliffe for each parameter
Adapted from Burgert SL, Anderson CF: Am J Clin Nutr 32:2136–2142, 1979.

TABLE 2-7
Adult Standards for Anthropometric Measurements and Nutritional Depletion

	Standard	Not Depleted (90% of Standard)	Mildly Depleted (80% of Standard)	Moderately Depleted (70% of Standard)	(60% of Standard)	Severely Depleted (<60% of Standard)
Triceps skin fold (mm)						
Male	12.5	11.3	10.0	8.8	7.5	< 7.5
Female	16.5	14.9	13.2	11.6	9.9	< 9.9
Arm muscle circumference (cm)						
Male	25.3	28.8	20.2	17.7	15.2	<15.2
Female	23.2	20.9	18.6	16.2	13.9	<13.9

Adapted from Blackburn GL, Thornton PA: Med Clin North Am 63:1103–1115, 1979.

TABLE 2-8
Right Triceps Skin Fold: Average Values and Selected Percentiles for Adults by Age and Sex, United States, 1960–1962

Sex, Average, and Percentile	TOTAL, 18–79 YEARS	Measurement in Centimeters						
		18–24 YEARS	25–34 YEARS	35–44 YEARS	45–54 YEARS	55–64 YEARS	65–74 YEARS	75–79 YEARS
Men								
Average right triceps skin fold	1.3	1.1	1.4	1.4	1.3	1.2	1.2	1.1
Percentile*								
99	4.1	3.7	4.5	4.0	3.8	3.3	3.2	3.0
95	2.8	2.6	3.3	2.9	2.8	2.4	2.7	2.0
90	2.3	2.4	2.6	2.4	2.2	2.0	2.2	1.7
80	1.8	1.7	2.0	1.9	1.8	1.6	1.7	1.5
70	1.5	1.3	1.6	1.6	1.5	1.4	1.4	1.3
60	1.3	1.1	1.4	1.4	1.3	1.3	1.3	1.1
50	1.1	0.9	1.2	1.2	1.1	1.2	1.1	1.0
40	1.0	0.8	1.0	1.1	1.0	1.0	1.0	0.9
30	0.8	0.7	0.8	1.0	0.9	0.9	0.8	0.8
20	0.7	0.6	0.7	0.8	0.7	0.8	0.7	0.7
10	0.6	0.5	0.5	0.6	0.6	0.6	0.6	0.6
5	0.5	0.5	0.5	0.5	0.5	0.5	0.5	0.5
1	0.4	0.4	0.4	0.4	0.4	0.4	0.3	0.4

Women

Average right triceps skin fold

Percentile*	2.2	1.8	2.1	2.3	2.4	2.5	2.4	2.0
99	4.6	4.3	4.7	4.6	4.8	4.7	4.7	3.9
95	3.8	3.2	3.7	3.9	4.0	4.0	3.6	3.3
90	3.4	2.8	3.2	3.5	3.6	3.7	3.4	3.1
80	3.0	2.4	2.8	3.0	3.2	3.2	3.0	2.7
70	2.6	2.1	2.4	2.7	2.8	2.9	2.7	2.5
60	2.4	2.0	2.2	2.5	2.6	2.7	2.5	2.3
50	2.2	1.7	2.0	2.3	2.4	2.5	2.4	2.2
40	2.0	1.6	1.9	2.1	2.2	2.3	2.2	2.0
30	1.8	1.5	1.7	1.8	2.0	2.1	2.0	1.7
20	1.6	1.3	1.5	1.6	1.8	1.9	1.7	1.4
10	1.3	1.1	1.2	1.4	1.5	1.6	1.5	1.0
5	1.1	0.9	1.0	1.2	1.2	1.4	1.2	0.7
1	0.8	0.6	0.7	1.0	0.8	1.0	0.8	0.3

*Measurement below which the indicated percent of persons in the given age group fall.

From Stoudt HW, et al: Skin Folds, Body Girths, Biacromical Diameters, and Selected Anthropometric Indices of Adults: United States, 1960–1962. Vital and Health Statistics Series 11, National Health Survey No 35. Washington, DC, HEW, Public Health Service, 1970.

TABLE 2-9
Right Arm Circumference: Average Values and Selected Percentiles for Adults by Age and Sex, United States, 1960–1962

Sex, Average, and Percentile	Measurement in Centimeters							
	TOTAL, 18–79 YEARS	18–24 YEARS	25–34 YEARS	35–44 YEARS	45–54 YEARS	55–64 YEARS	65–74 YEARS	75–79 YEARS
Men								
Average right arm circumference	30.7	30.0	31.2	31.5	31.2	30.2	29.5	27.7
Percentile*								
99	39.1	38.1	39.6	39.6	38.9	38.1	36.8	34.3
95	36.1	36.3	36.8	36.8	36.1	35.6	34.8	32.3
90	35.1	35.1	35.6	35.1	35.3	34.3	33.5	31.8
80	33.5	32.8	34.0	33.8	33.8	33.3	32.0	30.0
70	32.5	31.8	32.8	33.0	33.0	32.0	31.5	29.7
60	31.8	30.7	32.0	32.3	32.0	31.2	30.5	29.0
50	30.7	29.7	31.2	31.8	31.2	30.5	29.7	28.2
40	30.0	29.0	30.5	31.0	30.5	29.5	29.0	27.2
30	29.0	28.2	29.7	30.2	29.7	28.4	27.9	26.2
20	28.2	27.4	28.4	29.2	28.7	27.7	26.9	25.1
10	26.9	26.4	27.2	27.2	27.7	26.7	25.4	24.1
5	25.7	25.9	26.2	26.9	26.7	25.4	23.6	23.1
1	23.4	23.9	24.4	24.9	24.1	22.9	20.3	20.3

Women

Average right arm circumference	28.4	25.9	27.4	29.0	29.7	30.2	29.2	27.9
Percentile*								
99	40.1	38.6	39.4	40.6	41.7	41.4	38.9	37.1
95	36.6	32.5	34.8	37.1	37.3	37.6	35.6	35.1
90	34.3	30.2	33.0	34.8	35.1	35.6	34.3	33.8
80	31.8	28.7	30.0	32.0	32.8	33.5	32.3	31.8
70	30.2	27.2	28.4	30.7	31.5	31.8	31.5	30.7
60	29.2	26.4	27.7	29.2	30.2	31.0	30.1	29.0
50	28.2	25.7	26.9	28.4	29.2	30.0	29.2	28.0
40	27.2	24.9	26.4	27.4	28.4	29.0	28.4	26.9
30	26.4	24.1	25.7	26.7	27.7	28.2	27.7	25.7
20	25.1	23.4	24.6	25.7	26.7	27.2	26.7	24.1
10	23.9	22.6	23.4	24.4	25.1	26.2	24.9	22.6
5	22.9	21.8	22.6	23.9	23.6	24.6	23.4	21.3
1	21.1	20.6	21.3	22.1	21.6	21.1	20.8	20.1

*Measurement below which the indicated percent of persons in the given age group fall.

Adapted from Stoudt HW, et al: Skin Folds, Body Girths, Biacromical Diameters, and Selected Anthropometric Indices of Adults: United States, 1960–1962. Vital and Health Statistics Series 11, National Health Survey No 35. Washington, DC, HEW, Public Health Service, 1970, p 42.

TABLE 2-10
Percentiles for Right Arm Muscle Circumference from the United States Ten-State Nutrition Survey*

	Age (years)	Arm Muscle Circumference Percentiles (cm)				
		5TH	15TH	50TH	85TH	95TH
Males	16.5–17.4	20.6	21.7	24.5	27.1	29.0
	17.5–24.4	21.7	23.2	25.8	28.6	30.5
	24.5–34.4	22.0	24.1	27.0	29.5	31.5
	34.4–44.4	22.2	23.9	27.0	30.0	31.8
Females	16.5–17.4	17.1	17.7	19.6	22.3	24.1
	17.5–24.4	17.0	18.3	20.5	22.9	25.3
	24.5–34.4	17.7	18.9	21.3	24.5	27.2
	34.5–44.4	18.0	19.2	21.6	25.0	27.9

*Based on a cross-sectional sample of 5046 white subjects derived from the United States Ten-State Nutrition Survey of 1968–70.
Adapted from Frisancho RA: Am J Clin Nutr 27:1052–1058, 1974.

subsequent study of a larger group of patients from the same institution, triceps skin fold was found to have prognostic significance.[26] Patients who died or sustained postoperative complications had TSF values which were significantly lower than patients who survived without complications.

BIOCHEMICAL MEASUREMENTS

Various biochemical parameters reflect nutritional status. These include plasma protein levels, creatinine–height index, and hemoglobin concentration.

Plasma Proteins

The plasma proteins are constituents of the visceral protein compartment, which is vital for maintaining tissue function, oncotic pressure, enzymatic processes, and immune function. Measurements of albumin, transferrin, thyroxine-binding prealbumin, and retinol-binding protein are useful in evaluating nutritional status, and in malnutrition low levels reflect a decrease in liver protein synthesis due to a limiting supply of substrate (Table 2-11).[27]

However, a variety of nonnutritional factors may affect the concentration of the plasma proteins. For example, expansion of the extracellular fluid compartment will result in a reduction in albumin concentration. Thus, hypoalbuminemia is observed in acutely injured patients after intensive crystalloid fluid resuscitation.[28,29] In addition, concentration measurements do not

TABLE 2-11
Visceral Proteins Useful in Nutritional Assessment

	Half-life	*Normal levels*
Albumin	18 days	3.5–5.5 gm/dl
Transferrin	8 days	200–400 mg/dl
Thyroxine-binding prealbumin	2 days	15.7–29.6 mg/dl
Retinol-binding protein	12 hours	2.6–7.6 mg/dl

reflect turnover. In certain acutely ill patients (for example, those with sepsis), albumin production may actually be elevated, but because the albumin compartment is expanded and the rate of breakdown is also increased, the concentration is reduced.[30] Liver failure and renal failure may also affect levels of plasma proteins.

In the absence of these nonnutritional factors, serum albumin and transferrin levels are of value in assessing the severity of malnutrition (Tables 2-11, 2-12). Albumin levels of less than 3.0 gm/dl due to malnutrition have been found to be indicative of kwashiorkor, [31] and persistently low transferrin levels in children with kwashiorkor were found to be associated with poor prognosis.[32] Kaminski and associates found that serum transferrin levels of less than 170 mg/dl correlated with an increased rate of mortality among 55 patients assessed before aggressive nutritional support was initiated.[33] Mullen and associates observed that depressed visceral protein levels were predictive of postoperative morbidity and mortality among a series of elective surgical patients.[25] They found that albumin concentrations of less than 3 gm/dl and transferrin levels less than 220 mg/dl were associated with a 2.5-fold and a 5-fold increase in complications, respectively.

Studies by Eisenberg and associates, however, disclosed that significant deficits in the serum concentrations of albumin and transferrin occurring in

TABLE 2-12
Visceral Proteins and Malnutrition

	Serum Albumin (gm/dl)	*Serum Transferrin (mg/dl)**
Mild malnutrition	3.0–3.5	150–175
Moderate malnutrition	2.1–3.0	100–150
Severe malnutrition	<2.1	<100

Values derived from total iron-binding capacity.
From Blackburn GL, Thornton PA: Med Clin North Am 63:1103–1115,1979.

acutely injured postoperative patients were not predictive of outcome, evidently reflecting the influence of nonnutritional factors in this subset of patients.[34]

Albumin has a long half-life—approximately 18 days—compared to transferrin, which has a half-life of approximately 8 days (Table 2-11).[35,36] Depending on albumin values alone to monitor the visceral protein compartment may lead to delays in recognizing and treating deficits, since albumin levels can be maintained for long periods despite marked deterioration in nutritional status. Transferrin levels more accurately reflect rapidly changing nutritional status because of transferrin's shorter half-life. Transferrin levels are most accurately determined using direct assay, for example by single radial immunodiffusion. If direct measurement is not available, approximate values can be derived from the total iron binding capacity (TIBC) by applying the following formula[22]:

$$\text{Serum transferrin} = (0.8 \times \text{TIBC}) - 43$$

Transferrin values calculated from the TIBC may be useful in the serial assessment of an individual patient, but such values should not be compared with those determined directly. Miller and associates found that values derived from the above formula were substantially lower than those obtained directly by radial immunodiffusion.[37] In addition, the interpretation of transferrin values should take into account the fact that elevated levels are observed in patients with severe iron deficiency anemia.[36]

Recently, attempts have been made to measure visceral proteins with shorter half-lives in order to determine abnormalities of visceral protein status sooner than was previously possible (Table 2-11). Thyroxine-binding prealbumin, with a halflife of 2 days, was found to be the first visceral protein to decrease in children who were apparently healthy but who were consuming only marginal amounts of protein.[38] Infection and trauma also may depress prealbumin. Shetty and associates[39] found that prealbumin and retinol-binding protein, with a half-life of 12 hours, were much more sensitive than albumin and transferrin to short-term restrictions in protein and total caloric intake, and therefore the former parameters could be used to detect subclinical malnutrition as well as to monitor the effectiveness of treatment. It should be noted that kidney disease may confound the interpretation of retinol-binding protein levels, since this protein is filtered by the glomeruli and metabolized by the kidney and, therefore, could be elevated in kidney disease despite deficiencies in the visceral protein compartment.[40,41]

Creatinine–Height Index

In most individuals, creatinine production from creatine is directly related to the skeletal muscle mass, provided there is no very rapid loss of skeletal muscle, as in severe sepsis or trauma. Therefore, an estimate of lean body mass can be based on urinary excretion of creatinine.[42] The creatinine–height index (CHI) is defined as the 24 hour urinary creatinine excretion by a given patient divided by the expected 24 hour urinary creatinine excretion of a normal person of the same sex and height with an "ideal" body weight (IBW) [22]:

$$CHI(\%) = \frac{\text{Measured urinary creatinine}}{\text{Ideal urinary creatinine}} \times 100$$

The ideal urinary creatinine has been found to be 23 mg/kg IBW/24 hours for men and 18 mg for women.[22,43] For this assessment to be of value, renal function must be normal, and accurate urine collections are required.[42]

According to Blackburn and associates, CHI values of 60 to 80 percent represent moderate skeletal muscle depletion, whereas values of 40 to 50 percent signify severe depletion.[11] Since the calculation of CHI is in part dependent upon ideal body weight, CHI is subject to the same errors of interpretation as is the latter. Although arm muscle circumference and creatinine–height index are both thought to reflect skeletal muscle protein stores, Shenkin and Steel reported a lack of correlation between these two parameters.[42]

Hemoglobin

In addition to the vitamin-specific and mineral-related anemias occurring in malnutrition, prolonged protein starvation may also lead to a normochromic, normocytic anemia (see Chapter 1).[44] Sanders and associates found that an anemia associated with decreased erythropoietin synthesis developed in rats receiving a protein-restricted diet but in which normal serum vitamin B_{12} and folic acid levels had been maintained.[45] Thus hemoglobin levels in combination with other parameters discussed may be useful in the assessment of nutritional status.[29]

IMMUNOLOGIC FUNCTIONS

Immune functions are influenced by many factors, including nutritional status, and therefore, evaluation of these parameters constitute an important part of nutritional assessment. Total lymphocyte count and reactivity to recall skin test antigens are the immune functions most commonly evaluated.

Lymphocyte Count

Various investigators have found that total lymphocyte count correlates with cellular immune status,[46] and low counts reflect the degree of visceral protein depletion.[47] However, the utility of total lymphocyte count as a nutritional parameter is dependent upon excluding the influence of many possible nonnutritional factors. For example, lymphocytopenia has been observed in well nourished patients following anesthesia and operation; such depressed counts usually return to normal within 48 hours. This change has been attributed in part to the cortisol-induced immunosuppressive effect of surgery.[47,48] In the absence of other factors influencing the lymphocyte count, Blackburn and associates suggested that cell counts of 1200 to 1500/mm³ reflect a mild nutritional deficiency; a count of 800 to 1200, moderate deficiency; and counts less than 800, severe deficiency.[11]

Lewis and Klein found that preoperative lymphocytopenia was significantly associated with depressed albumin levels, and when both parameters were depressed, increased rates of postoperative sepsis were observed.[47] Seltzer and associates found that 30.2 percent of 500 patients admitted to a medical or surgical service had a lymphocyte count of less than 1500 cells/mm³.[49] Depressed lymphocyte count was associated with a 4-fold increase in mortality. When both the lymphocyte count and serum albumin were abnormal, a 4-fold increase in morbidity and a 20-fold increase in mortality were observed. In contrast, Mullen and associates were unable to confirm any relationship between preoperative total lymphocyte count and outcome among elective surgical patients.[25,26]

Skin Tests

Cellular immunity can also be evaluated by observing a patient's reaction to a series of delayed hypersensitivity recall antigens. The skin test antigens chosen are those to which normal persons in a given geographical area commonly would have had prior exposure and, therefore, would be expected to develop an immunologic response upon re-exposure.

The antigens frequently used in the United States include Candida, mumps, Trichophyton, streptokinase–streptodornase (SKSD), and purified protein derivative (PPD).

The utility of this method of immunologic examination is compromised to some extent by variation in the concentration of antigens used and in the

TABLE 2-13
Skin Test Antigens Used in Nutritional Assessment

Antigen	Distributor	Concentration
PPD	Parke, Davis, Detroit	5 TU/0.1 ml*
Mumps	Eli Lilly, Indianapolis	0.1 ml, undiluted
Streptokinase– streptodornase	Lederle, Pearl River, N.Y.	10 U SK + 2.5 U SD/0.1 ml*
Candida albicans	Hollister–Stier, Spokane	100 PNU/0.1 ml*
"Trichophyton"	Hollister–Stier, Spokane	100 PNU/0.1 ml

*TU, U.S. tuberculin unit; U, unit; PNU, protein–nitrogen units.

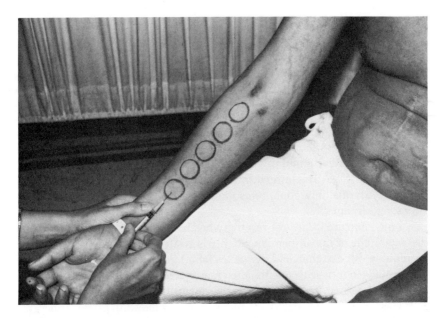

Figure 2-5. Skin test antigens are injected intradermally on the volar surface of the forearm.

measurement and interpretation of responses, and by the potential booster effect of repeated antigen administration.[50,51] Hypersensitivity to a given antigen is usually manifest by both erythema and induration around the intradermal injection site. A "positive" response is usually defined as 5 mm or more of cutaneous induration at 24 to 48 hours, but 15 mm of erythema without induration is considered a positive response to mumps antigens by the distributor of the antigen, Eli Lilly Company.[52] At the Los Angeles County–University of Southern California Medical Center, skin testing is carried out using the five antigens previously mentioned. The appropriate amount of each antigen is prepared in a volume of 0.1 ml which is injected intradermally on the volar surface of the forearm (Table 2-13, Fig. 2-5). The diameters of both the areas of erythema and induration are recorded at 24 and 48 hours, but, at present, a positive reaction is defined as 5 mm of induration at either time of observation. Patients' reactivity to the five skin tests are then classified as normal (two or more positive responses), relatively anergic (one positive response), or anergic (no positive responses).[53]

Instead of defining the response to a given skin test antigen as an all-or-none (positive/negative) phenomenon, Bates and associates suggested grading the response as follows[50]:

- 1+: Induration, 1 to 5 mm; or erythema, 10 mm or more without induration.

- 2+: Induration, 7 to 10 mm.
- 3+: Induration, 11 to 20 mm.
- 4+: Induration, more than 20 mm.

Depression of cellular immunity has been consistently documented in malnourished patients,[54-58] and nutritional repletion is associated with improved immunocompetence.[54,58-61] However, the interpretation of skin test reactivity requires careful consideration since many conditions in addition to malnutrition affect the immune response.[52,62-68] Nonnutritional factors which may depress cellular immunity include anesthesia, burns, certain drugs (eg., corticosteroids), gastrointestinal hemorrhage, infections, liver disease, malignancy, myocardial infarction, renal failure, sarcoidosis, shock, surgical operations, and trauma.

Thus, impaired skin test reactivity has been observed after trauma, and the magnitude of impairment apparently is related to the severity of injury.[66] In addition, McLoughlin and associates found that anergy developed in 13 of 31 normally nourished patients after major elective cardiovascular surgery and was associated with a circulating immunosuppressive factor in 11 of the 13.[67] Gastrointestinal hemorrhage and malignancy may also produce anergy.[68]

Studies of surgical patients by Meakins et al.,[53] Pietsch et al.,[65] and Johnson et al.,[69] disclosed a striking relationship between impaired skin test reactivity and the subsequent incidence of morbidity and mortality (Table 2-14). Johnson and associates found that anergic patients had a 3-fold greater risk of postoperative complications and an 8-fold greater risk of mortal-

TABLE 2-14
Morbidity and Mortality Related to Initial Skin Test Reactivity

Group	Response	Patients		Sepsis		Death	
		NO.	%	NO.	%	NO.	%
Preoperative	Anergy	21	6.5	4	19.0	7	33.3
	Relative anergy	21	6.5	5	23.8	7	33.3
	Normal	280	87.0	13	4.6	12	4.3
Total		322					
Postoperative/	Anergy	71	61.8	44	62.0	24	33.8
posttrauma	Relative anergy	25	21.7	15	60.0	6	24.0
	Normal	19	16.5	5	26.3	1	5.3
Total		115					
Nonoperative	Anergy	23	27.7	5	21.7	11	47.8
	Relative anergy	4	4.8	1	25.0	1	25.0
	Normal	56	67.5	0	0.0	1	1.8
Total		83					

Adapted from Pietsch JB, et al: Surgery 82:349–355, 1977.

TABLE 2-15
Morbidity and Mortality Related to Sequential Skin Test Responses

Responses	Patients	Sepsis		Deaths	
		NO.	%	NO.	%
Anergy→anergy	30	19	63.3	20	66.7
Anergy→relative anergy	8	3	37.5	1	12.5
Anergy→normal	30	14	46.7	2	6.7
Relative anergy→anergy	7	4	57.1	7	100
Relative anergy→relative anergy	3	2	66.7	2	66.7
Relative anergy→normal	21	8	38.1	0	0
Normal→anergy	3	3	100	3	100
Normal→relative anergy	0	0	0	0	0
Normal→normal	76	5	6.6	0	0

From Meakins JL, et al: Ann Surg 186:241–250, 1977.

ity.[69] Sequential testing is of even greater prognostic value. Among 135 surgical patients studied by Meakins and associates who remained normal or improved their skin test reactivity, the sepsis rate was 21 percent and mortality rate 2.1 percent.[53] By contrast, in 43 patients who were abnormal and did not improve, the sepsis rate was 65 percent and mortality 74 percent (Table 2-15).

The impaired skin test reactivity observed by these investigators occurred in patients in whom nonnutritional as well as nutritional factors were present. Therefore, these studies suggest but do not prove that abnormalities in delayed hypersensitivity responses due exclusively to malnutrition would have the same prognostic significance. Thus it appears from the studies of Meakins et al.,[53] Pietsch et al.,[65] Johnson et al., [69], and Christou et al.,[68] that impaired responses, regardless of cause, are associated with a poor prognosis in surgical patients.

In contrast, Eisenberg and associates found that anergy, though frequently present, was not predictive of mortality in their study of critically ill postoperative patients who had sustained acute traumatic injuries.[34]

PROGNOSTIC NUTRITIONAL INDEX

Mullen and Buzby and associates have developed a multiparameter index of nutritional status which relates the risk of postoperative morbidity and mortality to an individual's baseline nutritional status.[26,70,71] Initially, nutritional assessment parameters were determined in a series of patients scheduled to undergo an elective surgical procedure. Discriminant analysis and a computer-based stepwise regression procedure were used to identify the most important predictive variables. The significant factors were serum albumin concentration, serum transferrin level, triceps skin fold, and delayed hypersensitivity skin test reactivity. These variables were assigned coefficients appropriately weighting their impact on clinical outcome. The resulting Prognostic Nutritional Index (PNI), representing the risk of operative complications in an individual patient, is given by the expression:

$$PNI (\%) = 158 - 16.6 (ALB) - 0.78 (TSF) - 0.20 (TFN) - 5.8 (DH),$$

where ALB is the serum albumin concentration (gm/dl); TSF is the triceps skin fold thickness (mm); TFN is the serum transferrin level (mg/dl); and DH is the delayed hypersensitivity skin test reactivity to any one of three recall antigens (mumps, Candida, streptokinase–streptodornase) graded 0 (nonreactive), 1 (< 5 mm induration), or 2 (≥ 5 mm induration).

When the PNI was subsequently applied prospectively to additional series of elective preoperative patients, the actual incidence of morbidity and mortality increased as the predicted risk (PNI) increased (Table 2-16).[70] While the PNI appears to be of significant value in the assessment of patients scheduled to undergo *elective* surgery, its applicability to other groups of patients requires further study. Thus, Eisenberg and associates found that the PNI was not predictive of survival in critically ill postoperative surgical patients, presumably because of the influence of nonnutritional factors, such as anesthesia, fluid resuscitation, and operation, upon the individual parameters

TABLE 2-16
Comparison of Actual and Predicted Outcome Based on the Prognostic Nutritional Index

Predicted Risk of Complications	No. of Patients	Actual Incidence of Complications— No. of Patients (%)			
		ALL COMPLICATIONS	SEPSIS	MAJOR SEPSIS	DEATH
Low risk (PNI < 40%)	38	3 (8%)	2 (5%)	1 (3%)	1 (3%)
Intermediate risk (PNI=40-49%)	23	7 (30%)	5 (22%)	2 (9%)	1 (4.3%)
High risk (PNI ≥ 50%)	39	18 (46%)	11 (28%)	10 (26%)	13 (33%)
Total	100	28 (28%)	18 (18%)	13 (13%)	15 (15%)
P-value (chi-square analysis)		<0.0005	<0.025	<0.005	<0.0005

From Buzby GP, et al: Am J Surg 139:160–167, 1980.

used in the calculation of the PNI.[72] Similarly, Jones and associates found that the PNI was relatively ineffective in predicting complications following acute abdominal trauma.[73]

BODY COMPOSITION MEASUREMENTS

The body is composed of the extracellular supporting component and the body cell mass. The latter is the living portion of body composition consisting of the mitotically active, work-performing cells.[15,74] The extracellular supporting component can be assessed by measuring the extracellular water volume and the total exchangeable sodium (Na_e). The size of the body cell mass is linearly related to the intracellular water volume and the total exchangeable potassium (K_e).[15] Determination of the latter has been used as an index of body cell mass. Total exchangeable potassium can be measured directly by an isotope dilution technique using K-42 or indirectly using a method developed by Edelman et al[75] and Shizgal et al[76] which is based on a constant relationship among total exchangeable potassium, total exchangeable sodium, and total body water. The latter two parameters are determined by isotope dilution using Na-22 and tritiated water. In addition, whole body counters have been used to determine total body potassium by counting the subject's naturally occurring radioactive K-40, which has a fixed ratio with K-39 in body tissues.[74]

In the normally nourished individual, the body cell mass and the extracellular mass are approximately equal in size, and therefore the Na_e/K_e ratio approximates unity. Malnutrition, however, results in a loss of body cell mass, is accompanied by an expansion of the extracellular mass, and consequently is associated with an increase in the Na_e/K_e ratio.[77] Data obtained by Shizgal and Forse from a study of patients receiving parenteral nutrition indicate that malnutrition can be defined by the presence of a Na_e/K_e ratio of greater than 1.22.[77] In this study the Na_e/K_e ratio accurately differentiated the malnourished from the normally nourished individual.

Body composition also can be evaluated by using in vivo neutron activation analysis for the measurement of total body nitrogen. The latter value can be used to determine total body protein.[24]

At present, body composition measurements are usually research procedures and are not widely available. They require expensive equipment and complex techniques.

CLASSIFICATION OF MALNUTRITION

Recently, the terms *marasmus* and *kwashiorkor* have been popularized in the United States to denote two forms of protein–calorie malnutrition.

Marasmus. Marasmus, or simple starvation, is a chronic disease developing over months or years due to marked caloric deprivation. The physical examination is striking and reveals evidence of substantial weight loss, including marked fat and muscle wasting.[78] In affected patients, fat is mobilized and combusted for energy, and skeletal muscle is broken down to provide energy and to maintain visceral protein levels.[21,79] This sequence of compensatory metabolic events explains the relative preservation of the visceral protein compartment and the depressed anthropometric measures and low creatinine–height index characteristic of marasmus (Table 2-17).[80]

Kwashiorkor. Kwashiorkor, or visceral protein depletion, is a more acute process which develops over weeks to months. It is due to poor protein intake with some but inadequate carbohydrate ingestion against a background of acute illness or major surgery.[78] Affected patients often *appear* well nourished on physical examination, but further evaluation reveals major deficits in immune function and in the visceral protein compartment (Table 2-17). This condition may develop during hospitalization in patients receiving only isotonic infusions of glucose. The constant 5 percent glucose infusion induces a tonic stimulation to insulin secretion. The antilipolytic and antiproteolytic properties of insulin prevent the compensatory mobilization of fat and skeletal muscle seen in marasmus. These features explain the relative preservation of the anthropometric measures and creatinine–height index in the face of severe visceral protein attrition. A similar mechanism occurs in stress states associated with insulin resistance and hyperinsulinemia.[81,82]

TABLE 2-17
Nutritional Assessment in Marasmus and Kwashiorkor

	Marasmus	*Kwashiorkor*
Clinical setting	Decreased caloric intake	Decreased protein intake plus stress
Time course to develop	Months to years	Weeks to months
Physical examination	Cachectic; fat depletion, muscle wasting	May look well nourished
Anthropometrics		
TSF	Depressed	Relatively preserved
AMC	Depressed	Relatively preserved
Weight for height	Depressed	Relatively preserved
Creatinine–height index	Depressed	Relatively preserved
Skin test responses	Normal or depressed	Depressed
Visceral proteins		
Albumin	Relatively normal	Low
Transferrin	Relatively normal	Low
Lymphocyte count	Relatively normal	Low

ASSESSING RESPONSE TO NUTRITION THERAPY

Determination of 24 hour nitrogen balance is the most useful clinical study to assess whether the anabolic state has been achieved in response to nutrition therapy. Nitrogen balance is determined by calculating the difference between the amount of nitrogen consumed and the amount of nitrogen excreted. The latter can be estimated from measurements of urinary nitrogen plus 1.5 gm to account for nonurinary losses.[83] When direct measurements of urinary nitrogen are unavailable, urinary nitrogen losses can be estimated by adding an additional 20 percent to urinary urea measurements, since urinary urea accounts for 80 to 90 percent of the urinary nitrogen excreted.[84] Nitrogen balance can be calculated from the following expressions:

1. Nitrogen intake (gm)   = Protein intake (gm) ÷ 6.25
2. Nitrogen balance (gm) = 24 hour nitrogen intake − (24 hour urinary nitrogen + 1.5)

or

3. Nitrogen balance (gm) = 24 hour nitrogen intake − (1.2 × 24 hour urinary urea nitrogen + 1.5)

The progress of nutritional repletion can be evaluated by serial determinations of body weight, albumin and transferrin concentrations, anthropometric parameters, creatinine–height index, immune function, and body composition. Such serial measurements from an individual patient obviate many of the problems which complicate the use of these tests for initial nutritional evaluation. Each patient serves as his own control; successive measurements are compared with the previous values, and comparison with standards for a given population are less important.

REFERENCES

1. Bistrian BR, Blackburn GL, Hallowell E, Heddle R: Protein status of general surgical patients. JAMA 230:858–860, 1974.
2. Bistrian RB, Blackburn GL, Vitale J, et al: Prevalence of malnutrition in general medical patients. JAMA 235:1567–1570, 1976.
3. Apelgren KN, Rombeau JE, Miller RA, et al: Malnutrition in Veterans Administration surgical patients. Arch Surg 116:1059–1061, 1981.
4. Dreblow DM, Anderson CF, Moxness K: Nutritional assessment of orthopedic patients. Mayo Clin Proc 56:51–54, 1981.
5. Hill GL, Pickford I, Young GA, et al: Malnutrition in surgical patients: An unrecognized problem. Lancet 1:689–692, 1977.
6. Willard MD, Gilsdorf RB, Price RA: Protein–calorie malnutrition in a community hospital. JAMA 243:1720–1722, 1980.
7. Willcutts HD: Nutritional assessment of 1000 surgical patients in an affluent suburban community hospital. JPEN 1:25, 1977.

8. Blackburn GL: Hospital malnutrition: A diagnostic challenge. Arch Intern Med 139:278–279, 1979.

9. Weinsier RL, Hunker EM, Krumdieck CL, Butterworth CE Jr: Hospital malnutrition: A prospective evaluation of general medical patients during the course of hospitalization. Am J Clin Nutr 32:418–426, 1979.

10. Seltzer CC, Mayer J: How representative are the weights of insured men and women? JAMA 201:221–224, 1967.

11. Blackburn GL, Bistrian BR, Maini BS, et al: Nutritional and metabolic assessment of the hospitalized patient. JPEN 1:11–22, 1977.

12. Garrows JS, Fletcher J, Halliday D: Body composition in severe infantile malnutrition. J Clin Invest 44:417–425, 1965.

13. Kinney JM, Duke JH Jr, Long CL, et al: Tissue fuel and weight loss after injury. J Clin Pathol 23 Suppl 4:65–72, 1970.

14. Studley HO: Percentage of weight loss: A basic indicator of surgical risk in patients with chronic peptic ulcer. JAMA 106:458–460, 1936.

15. Shizgal HM, Spanier AH, Kurtz RS: Effect of parenteral nutrition on body composition in the critically ill patient. Am J Surg 131:156–161, 1976.

16. Elwyn DH, Bryan-Brown CW, Shoemaker WC: Nutritional aspects of body water dislocations in postoperative and depleted patients. Ann Surg 182:76–85, 1975.

17. Cahill GF Jr: Starvation in man. N Engl J Med 282:668–675, 1970.

18. Burgert SL, Anderson CF: An evaluation of upper arm measurements used in nutritional assessment. Am J Clin Nutr 32:2136–2142, 1979.

19. Frisancho RA: Triceps skin fold and upper arm muscle size norms for assessment of nutritional status. Am J Clin Nutr 27:1052–1058, 1974.

20. Stoudt HW, Damon A, McFarland RA, Roberts J: Skin Folds, Body Girths, Biacromical Diameters, and Selected Anthropometric Indices of Adults: United States, 1960–1962. Vital and Health Statistics Series 11, National Health Survey No. 35. Washington, DC, United States Department of Health, Education and Welfare, Public Health Service, 1970.

21. Jelliffe DB: The Assessment of the Nutritional Status of the Community; with Special Reference to Field Surveys in Developing Regions of the World. WHO Monograph 53. Geneva, World Health Organization, 1966.

22. Blackburn GL, Thornton PA: Nutritional assessment of the hospitalized patient. Med Clin North Am 63:1103–1115, 1979.

23. Gray GE, Gray LK: Validity of anthropometric norms used in the assessment of hospitalized patients. JPEN 3:366–368, 1979.

24. Collins JP, McCarthy ID, Hill GL: Assessment of protein nutrition in surgical patients: The value of anthropometrics. Am J Clin Nutr 32:1527–1530, 1979.

25. Mullen JL, Gertner MH, Buzby GP, et al: Implications of malnutrition in the surgical patient. Arch Surg 114:121–125, 1979.

26. Mullen JL, Buzby GP, Waldman MT, et al: Prediction of operative mortality by preoperative nutritional assessment. Surg Forum 30:80–82, 1979.

27. Tavill AS: The synthesis and degradation of liver-produced proteins. Gut 13:225–241, 1972.

28. Viriglio RW, Rice CL, Smith DE, et al: Crystalloid vs colloid resuscitation: Is one better? Surgery 85:129–139, 1979.

29. Young GA, Chem C, Hill GL: Assessment of protein–calorie malnutrition in sur-

gical patients from plasma proteins and anthropometric measurements. Am J Clin Nutr 31:429–435, 1978.

30. Wilmore DW, Editorial comment on Dahn M, Kirkpatrick JR, Bouwman D: Sepsis, glucose intolerance, and protein malnutrition. Arch Surg 115:1415–1418, 1980.
31. Whitehead RG, Coward WA, Lunn PG: Serum-albumin concentration and the onset of kwashiorkor. Lancet 1:63–66, 1973.
32. McFarlane H, Ogbeide MI, Reddy S, et al: Biochemical assessment of protein–calorie malnutrition. Lancet 1:392–394, 1969.
33. Kaminski MV, Fitzgerald MJ, Murphy RJ, et al: Correlation of mortality with serum transferrin and anergy. JPEN 1: 27, 1977.
34. Eisenberg D, Shofler R, Ryan J, et al: Nutrition-related factors in acutely injured patients. JPEN 4:583, 1980.
35. Beeken WL, Volwiler W, Goldsworthy PD, et al: Studies of I[131]-albumin catabolism and distribution in normal young male adults. J Clin Invest 41:1312–1333, 1962.
36. Awai M, Brown EB: Studies of the metabolism of I[131] labelled human transferrin. J Lab Clin Med 61:363–365, 1963.
37. Miller SF, Finley RK Jr, Morath MA: Derivation of serum transferrin. JAMA 246:39, 1981.
38. Ingenbleek Y, Van Den Schrieck HG, DeNayer P, DeVisscher M: Albumin, transferrin and the thyroxine-binding prealbumin/retinol-binding protein (TBPA-RBP) complex in assessment of malnutrition. Clin Chim Acta 63:61–67, 1975.
39. Shetty PS, Watrasiewicz KE, Jung RT, James WPT: Rapid-turnover transport proteins: An index of subclinical protein–energy malnutrition. Lancet 2:230–232, 1979.
40. VanLandingham S, Spiekerman AM, Newmark S: Retinol-binding protein and prealbumin levels in renal failure. JPEN 5:582, 1981.
41. Smith FR, Goodman DS: The effects of diseases of the liver, thyroid, and kidneys on the transport of vitamin A in human plasma. J Clin Invest 50:2426–2436, 1971.
42. Shenkin A, Steel LW: Clinical and laboratory assessment of nutritional status. Proc Nutr Soc 37:95–103, 1978.
43. Bistrian BR, Blackburn GL, Sherman M, Scrimshaw NS: Therapeutic index of nutritional depletion in hospitalized patients. Surg Gynecol Obstet 141:512–516, 1975.
44. Adams EB: Anemia associated with protein deficiency. Semin Hematol 7:55–66, 1970.
45. Sanders R, Sheldon GF, Garcia J, et al: Erythropoietin synthesis in rats during total parenteral nutrition. J Surg Res 22:649–653, 1977.
46. Lee YN, Sparks FC, Eilber FR, Morton DL: Delayed cutaneous hypersensitivity and peripheral lymphocyte counts in patients with advanced cancer. Cancer 35:748–755, 1975.
47. Lewis RT, Klein H: Risk factors in postoperative sepsis: Significance of preoperative lymphocytopenia. J Surg Res 26:365–371, 1979.
48. Slade MS, Simmons RL, Yunis E, Greenberg LJ: Immunodepression after major surgery in normal patients. Surgery 78:363–372, 1975.

49. Seltzer MH, Bastidas AJ, Cooper DM, et al: Instant nutritional assessment. JPEN 3:157–159, 1979.
50. Bates SE, Suen JY, Tranum BL: Immunological skin testing and interpretation: A plea for uniformity. Cancer 43:2306–2314, 1979.
51. Sokal JE: Measurement of delayed skin-test responses. N Engl J Med 293:501–502, 1975.
52. Eli Lilly and Company: Mumps skin-test antigens package insert, revised June 27, 1972.
53. Meakins JL, Pietsch JB, Bubenick O, et al: Delayed hypersensitivity: Indicator of acquired failure of host defenses in sepsis and trauma. Ann Surg 186:241–250, 1977.
54. Geefhuysen J, Rosen EU, Katz J, et al: Impaired cellular immunity in kwashiorkor with improvement after therapy. Br Med J 4:527–529, 1971.
55. Bistrian BR, Blackburn GL, Scrimshaw NS, Flatt JP: Cellular immunity in semi-starved states in hospitalized adults. Am J Clin Nutr 28:1148–1155, 1975.
56. Forse RA, Christou N, Meakins JL, et al: Reliability of skin testing as a measure of nutritional state. Arch Surg 116:1284–1288, 1981.
57. Smythe PM, Schonland M, Brereton-Stiles GG, et al: Thymolymphatic deficiency and depression of cell-mediated immunity in protein–calorie malnutrition. Lancet 2:939–944, 1971.
58. Spanier AH, Pietsch JB, Meakins JL, et al: The relationship between immune competence and nutrition. Surg Forum 27:332–336, 1976.
59. Law DK, Dudrick SJ, Abdou NI: Immunocompetence of patients with protein–calorie malnutrition: The effects of nutritional repletion. Ann Intern Med 79:545–550, 1973.
60. Daly JM, Dudrick SJ, Copeland EM: Effects of protein depletion and repletion to cell-mediated immunity in experimental animals. Ann Surg 188:791–796, 1978.
61. Copeland EM, MacFadyen BV Jr, Dudrick SJ: Effect of intravenous hyperalimentation on established delayed hypersensitivity in the cancer patient. Ann Surg 184:60–64, 1976.
62. Kantor FS: Infection, anergy and cell-mediated immunity. N Engl J Med 292:629–634, 1975.
63. MacLean LD, Meakins JL, Taguchi K, et al: Host resistance in sepsis and trauma. Ann Surg 182:207–217, 1975.
64. Walton B: Anaesthesia, surgery and immunology. Anaesthesia 33:322–348, 1978.
65. Pietsch JB, Meakins JL, MacLean LD: The delayed hypersensitivity response: Application in clinical surgery. Surgery 82:349–355, 1977.
66. Meakins JL, McLean APH, Kelly R, et al: Delayed hypersensitivity and neutrophil chemotaxis: Effect of trauma. J Trauma 18:240–247, 1978.
67. McLoughlin GA, Wu AV, Saporoschetz I, et al: Correlation between anergy and a circulating immunosuppressive factor following major surgical trauma. Ann Surg 190:297–304, 1979.
68. Christou NV, Meakins JL, MacLean LD: The predictive role of delayed hypersensitivity in preoperative patients. Surg Gynecol Obstet 152:297–301, 1981.
69. Johnson WC, Ulrich F, Meguid MM, et al: Role of delayed hypersensitivity in predicting postoperative morbidity and mortality. Am J Surg 137:536–542, 1979.
70. Buzby GP, Mullen JL, Matthews DC, et al: Prognostic nutritional index in gastrointestinal surgery. Am J Surg 139:160–167, 1980.

71. Mullen JL, Buzby GP: Nutritional assessment of the hospitalized patient—Why bother? Drug Therapy, August 1980, pp 33–42.
72. Eisenberg D, Silberman H, Maryniuk J, et al: Inapplicability of the prognostic nutritional index in critically ill patients. Surg Forum 32:109–111, 1981.
73. Jones, TN, Moore EE, VanWay CW III: Factors influencing nutritional assessment in trauma patients. JPEN 5:559, 1981.
74. Bocking JK, Holliday RL, Reid B, et al: Total exchangeable potassium in patients receiving total parenteral nutrition. Surgery 88:551–556, 1980.
75. Edelman IS, Liebman J, O'Meara MP, Birkenfeld LW: Interrelations between serum sodium concentration, serum osmolarity and total exchangeable sodium, total exchangeable potassium and total body water. J Clin Invest 37:1236–1256, 1958.
76. Shizgal HM, Kurtz RS, Wood CD: Total body potassium in surgical patients. Surgery 75:900–907, 1974.
77. Shizgal HM, Forse RA: Protein and calorie requirements with total parenteral nutrition. Ann Surg 192:562–569, 1980.
78. Butterworth CE Jr, Weinsier RL: Malnutrition in hospital patients: Assessment and treatment, in Goodhart RS, Shils ME (eds): Modern Nutrition in Health and Disease. Philadelphia, Lea and Febiger, 1980, pp 667–684.
79. Schlesinger L, Stekel A: Impaired cellular immunity in marasmic infants. Am J Clin Nutr 27:615–620, 1974.
80. Bistrian BR, Sherman M, Blackburn GL, et al: Cellular immunity in adult marasmus. Arch Intern Med 137:1408–1411, 1977.
81. Cahill GF Jr: Physiology of insulin in man. Diabetes 20:785–799, 1971.
82. Hoover HC Jr, Grant JP, Gorschboth C, Ketchum AS: Nitrogen-sparing intravenous fluids in postoperative patients. N Engl J Med 293:172–175, 1975.
83. Blackburn GL, Flatt JP, Hensle TW: Peripheral amino acid infusions, in Fischer JE (ed): Total Parenteral Nutrition. Boston, Little, Brown and Co., 1976, pp 363–394.
84. Wilmore DW: The Metabolic Management of the Critically Ill. New York, Plenum Medical Book Co., 1977.

3

Nutritional Requirements

ENERGY REQUIREMENTS

Individuals require energy for metabolic processes, growth or homeostasis, repair, maintenance of body temperature, and physical activity. Energy needs are met by the ingestion or intravenous infusion of organic nutrients, the oxidation of which produces the energy for physiologic work.

Nutrient energy values are generally expressed in kilocalories (kcal), the traditional unit of nutritionists. One kilocalorie is defined as the amount of heat necessary to raise the temperature of 1 kg of water from 15°C to 16°C. In the International System of Units, the unit of energy is the joule (J), which is the energy expended when 1 kg is moved 1 meter by 1 newton. The latter is the force which accelerates 1 kg by 1 meter per sec². The relationship between kilocalories (kcal), joules (J), kilojoules (KJ), and megajoules (MJ) is as follows:

$$1 \text{ kcal} = 4.184 \text{ KJ}$$
$$1000 \text{ kcal} = 4184 \text{ KJ}$$
$$1000 \text{ kcal} = 4.184 \text{ MJ}$$
$$1 \text{ KJ} = 0.239 \text{ kcal}$$
$$1000 \text{ KJ} = 239 \text{ kcal}$$
$$1 \text{ MJ} = 239 \text{ kcal}$$

The energy values for the various nutrients, based on the Atwater factors, are presented in Table 3-1.[1]

Basal metabolism, or the basal metabolic rate (BMR), comprises the major component of energy requirement for any given individual. BMR refers to energy production per unit time under "basal" conditions—i.e., at complete physical and mental rest, shortly after awakening, and in the postabsorptive state approximately 14 hours after taking food. BMR varies with body size, age, and sex. A table of standard metabolic rates has been adopted by the Joint FAO/WHO Ad Hoc Expert Committee on Energy and Protein Requirements (Table 3-2).[1] The values are based on measurements of 2200 persons by Talbot.[2] The values are not applicable to obese body weights.

The dominant factor leading to variability in energy requirements of the normal person is the proportion of time devoted to and the magnitude of physical activity.[3] In addition, the metabolism of nutrients results in increased heat production, a phenomenon referred to as the specific dynamic action of foods (SDA). The extent of this increased heat production above the basal level depends on the nature and quantity of the food. It is greatest for protein, less for carbohydrate, and least for fat. The increment is greater during the process of lipogenesis from glucose than from the oxidation of glucose to CO_2 and H_2O.[4]

The average energy requirements for healthy individuals have been determined by a Joint FAO/WHO Ad Hoc Expert Committee.[1] Estimates for a reference man and a reference woman have been adopted by the Committee, as follows:

Male	46 kcal/kg
Female	40 kcal/kg

The "reference man" is healthy and between 20 and 39 years of age and weighs 65 kg. On each working day he is employed for 8 hours in an occupation that usually involves moderate activity. When not at work he spends 8 hours in bed, 4 to 6 hours sitting or moving around in only very light activity, and 2 hours in walking, in active recreation, or in household duties.

TABLE 3-1
Energy Value of Body Fuels*

	kcal/gm	kJ/gm
Carbohydrate		
Monosaccharides	3.75	16
Polysaccharides	4.2	18
Protein	4	17
Fat	9	38
Ethanol	7.1	30

*These are average, rounded off values used clinically.

TABLE 3-2
Standard Basal Metabolic Rates

Body Weight (kg)	kcal per 24 Hours		MJ per 24 Hours	
	MALES	FEMALES	MALES	FEMALES
30.0	1140	1063	4.8	4.4
32.0	1190	1101	5.0	4.6
34.0	1230	1137	5.1	4.8
36.0	1270	1173	5.3	4.9
38.0	1305	1207	5.5	5.0
40.0	1340	1241	5.6	5.2
42.0	1370	1274	5.7	5.3
44.0	1400	1306	5.9	5.5
46.0	1430	1338	6.0	5.6
48.0	1460	1369	6.1	5.7
50.0	1485	1399	6.2	5.8
52.0	1505	1429	6.3	6.0
54.0	1555	1458	6.5	6.1
56.0	1580	1487	6.6	6.2
58.0	1600	1516	6.7	6.3
60.0	1630	1544	6.8	6.5
62.0	1660	1572	6.9	6.6
64.0	1690	1599	7.1	6.7
66.0	1725	1626	7.2	6.8
68.0	1765	1653	7.4	6.9
70.0	1785	1679	7.5	7.0
72.0	1815	1705	7.6	7.1
74.0	1845	1731	7.7	7.2
76.0	1870	1756	7.8	7.3
78.0	1900	1781	7.9	7.4
80.0	—	1805	—	7.5
82.0	—	1830	—	7.7
84.0	2000	1855	8.4	7.8

(From Talbot FB: Am J Dis Child 55: 455–459, 1938. Copyright 1938, American Medical Association)

The "reference woman" is similarly healthy and between 20 and 39 years of age and weighs 55 kg. She is engaged for 8 hours in general household work, in light industry, or in other moderately active work. Apart from 8 hours in bed, she spends 4 to 6 hours sitting or moving around in only very light activity and 2 hours in walking, in active recreation, or in household duties.

Energy requirements for an individual differing from the reference man or woman in age or physical activity are then determined by the application of correction factors as follows:

Energy Requirements for Healthy Adults: Adjustments for Age[1]

AGE RANGE (YR)	CORRECTION FACTOR (% AGE GROUP 20–39)
20–39	100
40–49	95
50–59	90
60–69	80
≥ 70	70

Energy Requirements for Healthy Adults: Adjustments for Physical Activity[1]

PHYSICAL ACTIVITY	CORRECTION FACTOR (% MODERATE ACTIVITY)
Light activity*	90
Moderate activity†	100
Very active‡	117
Exceptionally active¶	134

For example, a 50-year-old man weighing 70 kg and engaged in light activity has an energy requirement of 2608 kcal/day, as determined from the expression:

46 kcal/kg $\times$ 70 kg $\times$ 0.90 (age factor) $\times$ 0.90 (activity factor)

The energy requirements for normal persons estimated by these methods proposed by the FAO/WHO Committee very closely approximate the daily allowances recommended by the National Research Council.[5] The estimation of energy requirements for hospitalized patients must take into account additional factors, including fever, the severity of illness, and the energy demands of nutritional repletion and tissue repair.

---

*Light Activity: men—office workers, most professional men (such as lawyers, doctors, accountants, teachers, architects, etc.), shop workers; women—office workers, housewives in houses with mechanical household appliances, teachers, and most other professional women.

†Moderate activity: men—most men in light industry, students, building workers (excluding heavy laborers), many farm workers, fishermen; women—light industry, students, department store workers.

‡Very active: men—some agricultural workers, unskilled laborers, forestry workers, army recruits and soldiers on active service, mine workers, steel workers; women—some farm workers, dancers, athletes.

¶Exceptionally active: men—lumberjacks; women—construction workers.

Average values for caloric intake which will satisfy the needs of most patients have been estimated by Jeejeebhoy, as follows[6]:

CLINICAL STATUS	KCAL/KG IDEAL BODY WEIGHT
Basal state	25–30
Maintenance (ambulatory)	30–35
Mild stress and malnutrition	40
Severe injuries and sepsis	50–60
Extensive burns	80

Precise requirements can be determined using direct or indirect calorimetry. Data derived from series of normal and sick persons studied by indirect calorimetry allow accurate estimations of the energy demands of a given patient.

Direct Calorimetry

The human body oxidizes organic nutrients to produce energy for physiologic work, but ultimately such work is reflected largely in heat production.[3,4] Consequently, the amount of heat produced should be equivalent to the amount of energy required for equilibrium. Heat lost from the body may be measured by direct calorimetry. The patient is placed in an insulated chamber. Heat loss is computed from changes in the temperature of water and air which circulate through the chamber and by analysis of the water vapor.[4,7]

This method requires elaborate and expensive apparatus and is rarely used in clinical practice, since indirect calorimetry gives results which closely approximate those obtained by direct calorimetry.

Indirect Calorimetry

Energy expenditure can be determined indirectly from data on gas exchange. In the steady state, the amount of oxygen consumed and the amount of carbon dioxide produced are related quantitatively to the release of energy from the body. A constant amount of oxygen is consumed, a constant amount of carbon dioxide is produced, and a constant amount of energy is released for each mole of a specific carbohydrate, protein, or fat oxidized.[7]

Respiratory quotient. The respiratory quotient (RQ) is defined as the ratio of the volume of CO_2 produced to that of O_2 consumed during the course of oxidation of body fuels. Complete oxidation of glucose may be represented as follows[4]:

$$C_6H_{12}O_6 \; + \quad 6O_2 \longrightarrow 6CO_2 \; + \; 6H_2O \; + 673 \text{ kcal}$$

(1 mole) + (6 moles) ⟶ (6 moles) + (6 moles) + 673 kcal
(180 gm) + (134.4 liters)* ⟶ (134.4 liters) + (108 gm) + 673 kcal
(1.34 gm) + (1 liter) ⟶ (1 liter) + (8 gm) + 5.0 kcal

*One mole of gas occupies 22.4 liters at standard temperature and pressure.

TABLE 3-3
Caloric, O_2, and CO_2 Equivalents of Body Fuels

	Carbohydrate	Fat	Protein	Ethanol	Average Diet
kcal/gm	3.7 –4.3	9.3	4.2	7.1	—
CO_2 (liters/gm)	0.75–0.83	1.39	0.75	0.98	—
O_2 (liters/gm)	0.75–0.83	1.96	0.94	1.46	—
RQ	1.0	0.71	0.80	0.67	0.82
Calorie value per liter O_2	5.0	4.7	4.5	4.9	4.8

Adapted from Cantarow A, Trumper M: Clinical Biochemistry. Philadelphia, WB Saunders Co, 1955, p 364; Wilmore DW: The Metabolic Management of the Critically Ill. New York, Plenum Medical Book Co, 1977, p 10.

Thus the glucose RQ is 1.0 (134.4/134.4), and the caloric value of 1 liter of oxygen for glucose oxidation is 5.0 kcal. Similar calculations allow determination of RQ and caloric value per liter of oxygen for the other body fuels (Table 3-3).

On the basis of analytic data for the average protein, it is generally estimated that 1 gm of urinary nitrogen represents (1) the metabolism of 6.25 gm of protein; (2) utilization of 5.91 liters of oxygen; (3) production 4.76 liters of carbon dioxide; and (4) liberation of 26.51 kcal.[4]

Energy expenditure.   Energy expenditure can be determined from knowledge of (1) oxygen consumption (2) carbon dioxide production, and (3) urinary nitrogen excretion. These data allow calculation of nonprotein oxygen consumption, nonprotein carbon dioxide production, and hence the nonprotein RQ. From this latter value the caloric value per liter of oxygen consumed can be determined (Table 3-4). Energy expenditure is then calculated by multiplying the liters of oxygen consumed by the caloric value per liter. When oxygen consumption alone is measured (utilizing simpler apparatus than that required for determinations including carbon dioxide production), energy expenditure can be estimated by assuming an RQ of 0.82. According to Wilmore, such an estimate will be within 8 percent of the true value.[7]

The calculation of energy expenditure using indirect calorimetry is illustrated by the following example adapted from Cantarow and Trumper.[4] These data were obtained from a patient under basal conditions: (1) urinary nitrogen, 0.18 gm/hr; (2) oxygen consumption, 12.2 liters/hr; (3) carbon dioxide production, 9.2 liters/hr.

0.18 gm of urinary N represents:
0.18 × 5.91 = 1.06 liters of oxygen
0.18 × 4.76 = 0.85 liters of carbon dioxide
0.18 × 26.51 = 4.77 kcal

Nonprotein oxygen consumption $= 12.2 - 1.06 = 11.14$ liters
Nonprotein carbon dioxide production $= 9.2 - 0.85 = 8.35$ liters
Nonprotein RQ $= 0.75$, representing the liberation of 4.739 kcal per liter
of oxygen (Table 3-4)
Nonprotein energy expenditure $= 4.739 \times 11.14 = 52.79$ kcal/hr
Total energy expenditure $= 52.79 + 4.77 = 57.76$ kcal/hr

When indirect calorimetry is carried out under "basal" conditions, the BMR is determined. The resting metabolic expenditure (RME) is determined when indirect calorimetry is carried out in persons in a normal life situation while at rest and under conditions of thermal neutrality. The RME, thought to be approximately 10 percent above the BMR in normal persons, includes the specific dynamic action of food and reflects the average minimal metabolism for the night and periods of the day when there is no exercise or exposure to cold.[5] However, these two terms, BMR and RME, are frequently used interchangeably in clinical medicine.

By applying indirect calorimetry to series of normal persons and hospitalized patients, various investigators have determined the pattern of altered energy expenditure associated with a variety of diseases and injuries (Fig. 3-1).[8] These kinds of data can be tabulated to create a table of correction factors to account for the energy demands of various stresses (Table 3-5).[3,7-10]

For a given patient, the total energy requirement to achieve energy balance is taken to be the energy expenditure estimated from the product of the applicable correction factors and the BMR or RME of a healthy person matched for weight and sex. The BMR can be determined from standard Ta-

TABLE 3-4
Respiratory Quotient (RQ) and Calorie Equivalent of Oxygen for Different Mixtures of Fat and Carbohydrate

RQ*	Percentage of Total O_2 Consumed by:		Percentage of Heat Produced by:		Calories per Liter O_2
	CARBOHYDRATE	FAT	CARBOHYDRATE	FAT	
0.707	0	100	0	100	4.686
0.75	14.7	85.3	15.6	84.4	4.739
0.80	31.7	68.3	33.4	66.6	4.801
0.82	38.6	61.4	40.3	59.7	4.825
0.85	48.8	51.2	50.7	49.3	4.862
0.90	65.9	34.2	67.5	32.5	4.924
0.95	82.9	17.1	84.0	16.0	4.985
1.00	100	0	100	0	5.047

*Nonprotein RQ.
From Cantarow A, Trumper M: Clinical Biochemistry. Philadelphia, WB Saunders Co, 1955, p 367.

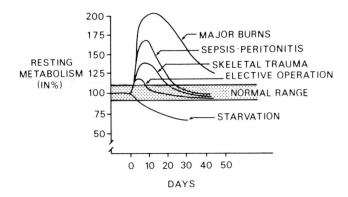

Figure 3-1. Changes in resting metabolic expenditure with time in various patient groups. Note that the peak metabolic response occurs about a week following the initial stress. *(From Long CL: Contemp Surg 16: 29–42, 1980. Reprinted with permission of Contemporary Surgery)*

bles (Table 3-2), and the RME can be calculated from the Harris–Benedict equations (HBE), as follows[11]:

For men: RME (kcal/day)* = 66.4730 + 13.7516 (W) + 5.0033 (H) − 6.7550 (A);

For women: RME (kcal/day)* = 655.095 + 9.563 (W) + 1.8496 (H) − 4.6756 (A),

where W = present weight in kg; H = height in cm; A = age in years.

Determination of energy requirements using RME rather than BMR may be more accurate since Long and associates found that values predicted from the Harris–Benedict equations very closely approximate (within 3 percent) the RME of healthy persons determined by indirect calorimetry.[8,9]

For example, the 24 hour caloric requirement of a patient 1 week after he sustained multiple fractures and who is confined to bed can be estimated from the following expression:

$$kcal/day = HBE \times 1.2 \times 1.35$$

It should be noted, however, that Kinney found that, for reasons that are unknown, stable weight and nitrogen equilibrium were not always achieved in patients with acute surgical conditions receiving parenteral nutrition when the caloric intake was exactly equal to the measured or estimated caloric expenditure. Consequently, Kinney recommended that such patients receive a caloric intake 50 percent above the measured or estimated value.[3]

Carbohydrate, fats, and protein can all act as sources of energy for the

---

These equations were originally thought to predict BMR,[11] but values were found to be slightly high[7]; Long et al found that HBE closely predicts RME.[9]

TABLE 3-5
Correction Factors for Predicting Energy Requirements
in Hospitalized Patients*

Clinical Condition	Correction Factor†	References
Physical activity		
Confined to bed	1.2	Long et al.[9]
Out of bed	1.3	Long et al.[9]
Fever	1.0 + 0.13 per °C	Kinney[3]
Elective surgery	1.0–1.2	Kinney,[3] Long[8]
Peritonitis	1.2–1.5	Kinney[3]
Soft tissue trauma	1.14–1.37	Duke et al.,[10] Long et al.[9]
Multiple fractures	1.2–1.35	Kinney,[3] Long et al.[9]
Major sepsis	1.4–1.8	Kinney,[3] Long et al.[9]
Thermal injury‡		Wilmore[7]
0–20%	1.0–1.5	
20–40%	1.5–1.85	
40–100%	1.85–2.05	
Starvation (adults)	0.70	Long et al.[9]

*Total energy requirement is predicted by product of correction factors × RME (or BMR).
†Correction factors apply to men and women; figures represent maximum increases and must be adjusted as recovery and convalescence proceeds (see Fig. 3-1).
‡Percent body surface burned.

body and in normal persons are interchangeable in terms of energy within wide limits. Ethanol may also contribute energy to a variable extent. However, at least 100 to 150 gm of carbohydrate are required to achieve maximal protein utilization.

Although protein can serve as a source of calories, the major function of administered protein is to provide the amino acids required for tissue synthesis. Consequently, in the nutritional support of hospitalized patients, the calculated energy requirements generally are provided from nonprotein sources, and the protein or nitrogen required for tissue synthesis is calculated separately.

PROTEIN REQUIREMENTS

Dietary protein provides the amino acids required for synthesis of the major functional components of the body. The human proteins derived from these amino acids are the essential elements of cell structure and are indispensable for growth; neuromuscular, enzymatic, and mental processes; and immunologic responses.[12]

Protein requirements are generally estimated from nitrogen balance studies, since the overall metabolism of proteins in the body can be summarized by calculating the difference between nitrogen intake and nitrogen output. The latter is the sum of nitrogen lost in the urine, feces, and from the skin plus the small amounts of nitrogen found in nasal secretions, hair cuttings, menstrual fluid, and semen. Positive nitrogen balance or nitrogen retention exists when intake exceeds output; this occurs during active growth or tissue repair. Nitrogen equilibrium or zero nitrogen balance describes the state in which nitrogen intake equals losses. Finally, negative nitrogen balance is present when losses exceed intake. Since the nitrogen content of the average food protein is about 16 percent, the excretion of 1 gm of nitrogen represents the metabolism of about 6.25 gm of protein. The validity of this calculation is based on the assumption that nearly all nitrogen lost is derived from protein metabolism. The protein requirement for normal adults is the amount of protein necessary to meet physiologic needs and maintain health and is taken to be the lowest protein intake at which nitrogen equilibrium can be achieved. The protein requirement for children is the lowest protein intake necessary for satisfactory growth and nitrogen retention. Nitrogen balance and hence protein requirements are significantly influenced by a variety of factors, including energy and nitrogen intake, nutritional and metabolic status of the patient, and the amino acid composition of dietary protein.

Energy Intake

Nonprotein calories significantly influence the impact of protein intake on nitrogen balance. Nitrogen equilibrium can never be achieved in patients receiving no protein, but the administration of nonprotein calories will reduce nitrogen excretion and therefore improve nitrogen balance. This protein-sparing effect is maximally achieved with about 100 to 150 gm of carbohydrate. No further benefit accrues with higher caloric intake in the absence of protein.[13-15]

At any given level of protein (or nitrogen) intake, nitrogen balance progressively improves to some maximum level as caloric intake increases from levels below requirements to levels exceeding requirements (Figs. 3-2, 3-3).[15,16]

The source of nonprotein calories also affects nitrogen balance. The protein-sparing effect observed with the administration of carbohydrate to patients receiving diets devoid of protein is not observed when an equal number of calories is supplied as fat.[17,18] Maximum protein-sparing and optimal utilization of dietary protein is achieved when the energy sources include at least 100 to 150 gm of carbohydrate daily.[13] The remaining energy requirements of most individuals can be met equally effectively by carbohydrate, fat, or a combination of these two. The efficacy of lipids as a caloric source in hypermetabolic and septic patients is uncertain and controversial (see Chapter 9). The specific effect of carbohydrate on nitrogen balance relates (1) to its ability to serve as an energy substrate for the glycolytic tissues and (2) to the insulin response which it evokes. When sufficient carbohydrate is supplied to meet the energy demands of the central nervous system, erythrocytes, leukocytes, active fibroblasts, and certain phagocytes, the need for gluconeogenesis from protein is diminished. In addition, the secretion of insulin, stimulated by carbohydrate consumption, results in nitrogen conservation, since insulin diminishes amino acid efflux from skeletal muscle, promotes amino acid uptake into muscle, and suppresses hepatic urea synthesis.[19]

Nitrogen Intake

At any given level of energy intake, nitrogen balance improves as nitrogen intake increases. The dose–response relationship is curvilinear, and the nitrogen balance plateaus at higher doses of nitrogen intake (Fig. 3-3).[15]

The interaction among calories, nitrogen, and nitrogen balance has been illustrated by Jeejeebhoy.[6] In patients receiving parenteral nutrition, positive nitrogen balance was achieved with infusions devoid of nonprotein calories when 1.7 to 2.0 gm/kg/day of amino acids were provided. In contrast, only 0.4 gm/kg/day of amino acids was required when total nonprotein calorie intake was increased to 55 kcal/kg/day.

To avoid the limiting effects of calories on nitrogen, or of nitrogen on calories, Calloway and Spector suggested that nitrogen intake be related or fixed to caloric intake.[14] In studies of normal, active young men, optimal efficiency was achieved at a calorie:nitrogen ratio of approximately 300 to 350 kcal to 1 gm of nitrogen.[14,15]

Nutritional and Metabolic Status

Healthy individuals do not store nitrogen, and therefore nitrogen balance curves plateau at or only slightly above the zero balance line when excess di-

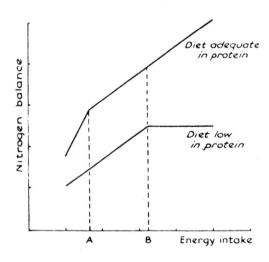

Figure 3-2. An increase in energy intake results in improved nitrogen balance at both levels of protein intake, but at the lower protein intake, increments in energy intake are not effective beyond point B. *(From Munro HN: In Munro HN, Allison J (eds): Mammalian Protein Metabolism, Volume 1, New York, Academic Press, 1964, p 420)*

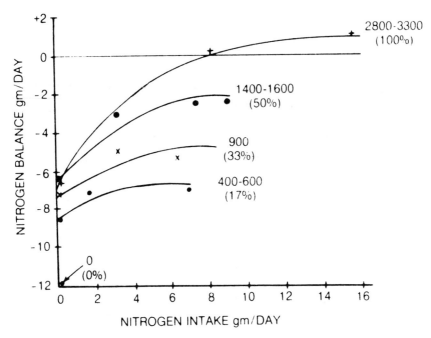

Figure 3-3. At any level of nitrogen intake, increasing caloric intake improves nitrogen balance, and at any level of caloric intake, increasing nitrogen intake improves balance. The range of caloric intake is listed to the right of each isobar. The number in parentheses below each calorie intake expresses total caloric intake as a percentage of total daily metabolic expenditure. *(From Wilmore DW: In Greene HL, et al (eds): Clinical Nutrition Update: Amino Acids. Chicago, American Medical Association, 1977, p 49. Based on data collected by Calloway and Spector[14])*

etary protein is administered. In contrast, nitrogen balance curves in nutritionally depleted patients are similar to those seen in growing children, in whom the curve increases linearly above the zero balance line and plateaus only at levels of protein consumption exceeding normal requirements (Fig. 3-4).[15] These observations suggest that the requirements for nutritional repletion of the adult are similar to those of the normal growing child.[6,15]

Protein economy decreases during most serious illnesses.[7] Nitrogen losses increase, and therefore dietary protein requirements rise (Fig. 3-5). Moreover, diseases associated with increased metabolic activity alter the usual relationship between nonprotein calories and dietary nitrogen. When nonprotein caloric intake meets 100 percent of energy demands, nitrogen balance becomes progressively negative at any fixed nitrogen dose as metabolic rate increases. Nitrogen equilibrium or retention can usually be achieved, however, by approximately doubling the quantity of nitrogen required by normal man at any given level of caloric intake. A calorie:nitrogen ratio of 150:1 is thought optimal in seriously ill patients by most investigators, although the ratio may range between 100:1 and 200:1.[7-9,15]

Amino Acid Composition of Dietary Protein

Essential amino acids.   Some required amino acids cannot be synthesized by mammals and are therefore "essential" in the sense that they must be provided in the diet. For man, the essential amino acids are isoleucine, leucine, lysine, methionine, phenylalanine, threonine, tryptophan, and valine. Histidine cannot be synthesized by humans, and since it is required by infants, it is an essential amino acid for infants. Recent studies suggest that some dietary histidine may also be required by adults.[5,20]

The pattern of essential amino acids in foods is one of the important factors influencing the total amount of protein required by man. Requirements for the individual amino acids have been estimated from studies in which single amino acids were added or deleted from the diet (Table 3-6).[12]

The "quality" or "biologic value" of a protein source is a measure of the efficiency with which the absorbed nitrogen is utilized, and the latter depends primarily on the essential amino acid composition of the protein. The quality

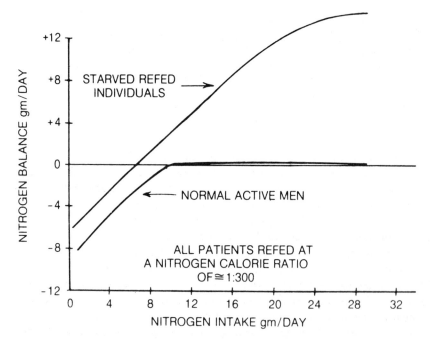

Figure 3-4. Comparison of the response to increased quantities of dietary nitrogen in normal active man and starved refed adults. *(From Wilmore DW: In Greene HL, et al (eds): Clinical Nutrition Update: Amino Acids. Chicago, American Medical Association, 1977, p 48)*

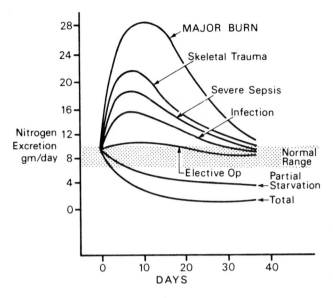

Figure 3-5. Catabolic response to serious illness. The increased nitrogen excretion depends on the magnitude of the insult. *(From Long CL: Contemp Surg 16:29–42, 1980. Reprinted with permission of Contemporary Surgery)*

of a protein can be scored by comparing its essential amino acid content with that of a reference protein the amino acid pattern of which is similar to that required by an infant.[5]

Protein requirements are greater when protein is supplied by the average American mixed diet as compared to requirements based on feeding higher quality protein, such as milk or eggs (Table 3-6).

The total protein requirement per unit body weight for the normal person falls with increasing age, and since the requirement for the essential amino acids fall even more sharply, the proportion of total amino acids that must be supplied as essential amino acids (E/T ratio) also falls with age (Table 3-6).[1] In contrast, it appears that the requirements for essential amino acids for malnourished or hospitalized patients approximate those for a normally growing 10- to 12-year-old child.[6,21]

Nonessential amino acids. The "nonessential" amino acids are those which occur in human proteins but which can be synthesized within the body from nitrogen-containing precursors. These nonessential amino acids include alanine, arginine, asparagine, aspartic acid, cystine, glycine, glutamic acid, glutamine, proline, serine, and tyrosine. Tyrosine and cystine are nonessential only because they are formed when adequate amounts of phenylalanine and methionine are present. Tyrosine can substitute for 70 to 75 percent of the phenyl-

TABLE 3-6
Protein and Amino Acid Requirements for Normal Persons

Amino Acids	Adults		Child 10–12 yr		Infants	
	MG/KG	%TPR*	MG/KG	%TPR	MG/KG	%TPR
Histidine	0	0	0	0	28	1.4
Isoleucine	10	1.8	30	3.7	70	3.5
Leucine	14	2.5	45	5.6	161	8.0
Lysine	12	2.2	60	7.5	103	5.2
Methionine + cysteine	13	2.4	27	3.4	58	2.9
Phenylalanine + tyrosine	14	2.5	27	3.4	125	6.3
Threonine	7	1.3	35	4.4	87	4.4
Tryptophan	3.5	0.65	4	0.46	17	0.85
Valine	10	1.8	33	4.1	93	4.7
Total EAA†	83.5	15.2	261	32.6	742	37.3
Protein requirement (high quality protein—gm/kg)‡	0.55		0.8		2.0	
Protein requirement (US mixed diet—gm/kg)‡	0.8		1.2		—	

*Proportion of total protein requirement (high quality protein) supplied as given amino acid.
†Essential amino acids.
‡Amount estimated to meet the needs of nearly all (97.5 percent) normal persons.
Adapted from Energy and Protein Requirements: Report of a Joint FAO/WHO Ad Hoc Expert Committee. World Health Organization Technical Report Series, 1973, No. 522, pp 55–57.

alanine requirement and cystine for about 30 percent of the methionine requirement (the fractions of these amino acids which appear to be converted to tyrosine and cystine).[12]

Although amino acids may be categorized as "essential" or "nonessential," all of the amino acids present in human proteins must be available in suitable amounts in the cell for protein synthesis to take place.

When isonitrogenous diets are compared, nitrogen balance is improved when diets consisting exclusively of essential amino acids are supplemented with nonamino acid nitrogen and is further improved when nonessential nitrogen is provided as a single nonessential amino acid. However, optimal nitrogen balance is achieved when the essential amino acids are supplemented by a combination of several but not necessarily all of the nonessential amino acids.[12,22–24] Apparently supplying nonessential amino acids spares the cellular energy requirement for the conversion of other nitrogenous compounds into the required nonessential amino acids.[12]

Taking into account the various factors influencing nitrogen requirements, a Joint FAO/WHO Ad Hoc Expert Committee on Energy and Protein Requirements estimated daily allowances of high quality protein (egg and milk) necessary to meet the requirements of nearly all (97.5 percent) healthy persons.[1] The recommendations for adults, children, and infants are 0.55 gm/kg, 0.8 gm/kg, and 2.0 gm/kg, respectively (Table 3-6). After correcting for the reduced efficiency of utilization of the protein in a mixed diet compared to the higher quality reference protein, the allowance for the mixed proteins of the American diet becomes 0.8 gm/kg for adults and about 1.2 gm/kg for the child 10 to 12 years of age.[1,5]

ROUTE OF NUTRIENT ADMINISTRATION

Because of the role of the intestine and the liver in the processing of orally consumed nutrients, it is likely that metabolic events differ to some extent when nutrients are provided enterally or intravenously.[15,25] While some authors have suggested that oral or enteral feedings are superior nutritionally,[26,27] this view has not been proven.

Blackburn and Bistrian found that mildly to moderately catabolic surgical patients required about 15 percent more calories to achieve positive nitrogen balance when nutrients were given intravenously rather than orally.[26] Thus the caloric requirement for the parenterally fed patients was equal to 1.76 times the resting metabolic expenditure (RME), whereas the orally fed patients had a caloric requirement of 1.54 × RME. In contrast, Fitzpatrick and associates found that the protein-sparing effect of glucose was optimal when the glucose was given intravenously.[19]

Munro recently reviewed data indicating that the nitrogen balance achieved with intravenously infused amino acids is comparable to that achieved with a continuous intragastric drip of the nutrient solution, but that the intravenous route is superior to intermittent, bolus enteral feedings.[25,28]

Anderson and associates found that a well balanced solution of amino acids infused intravenously was utilized as efficiently and produced the same degree of nitrogen retention as an equivalent amount of high quality protein fed orally.[21] However, differences in blood amino acid levels were observed between the orally and intravenously fed groups.

These observations suggest that while the total protein and essential amino acid requirements are probably similar for both routes of administration, the amino acid pattern best utilized parenterally may well differ from the oral pattern.[25]

TEMPORAL RELATIONSHIP OF NUTRIENT ADMINISTRATION

Carbohydrate and protein fed simultaneously interact to cause an improvement in nitrogen balance over their separate feeding.[29,30] This interaction is not observed when fat and protein are fed simultaneously.[15,30] This specific effect of carbohydrates is apparently due in part to the provision of carbon skeletons for synthetic reactions and for use in the citric acid cycle. This effect is also due in part to the stimulation of insulin secretion and hence increased uptake of amino acids by skeletal muscle.[19,30]

MACRONUTRIENTS

Minerals required in amounts exceeding 200 mg/day include sodium, chloride, potassium, calcium, magnesium, and phosphate. These mineral nutrients are essential for the maintenance of water balance, cardiac function, mineralization of the skeleton, function of nerve, muscle, and enzyme systems, and energy transformation.[5,7]

In addition, protein utilization is affected by the availability of sodium, potassium, and phosphorus in the diet. Thus nitrogen utilization is impaired when any of these mineral nutrients is withdrawn from the diet. Evidently, nutritional repletion involves the formation of tissue units containing protoplasm and extracellular fluid in fixed proportion and with fixed elemental composition. The retention of 1 gm of nitrogen is characteristically associated with the retention of 0.08 gm phosphorus, 3.1 mEq potassium, 3.5 mEq sodium, and 2.7 mEq chloride. If either a protoplasmic element (potassium, phosphorus) or an extracellular element (sodium, chloride) is not supplied, the unit of protoplasm and associated extracellular fluid apparently cannot be formed.[31]

Sodium, potassium, and chloride. The amount of sodium, potassium, and chloride in the diets of normal persons may vary widely, and balance is maintained by homeostatic mechanisms. The healthy adult with free access to salt in the diet usually consumes 100 to 300 mEq of sodium and chloride daily, and the usual adult intake of potassium is between 50 and 150 mEq/day.[5] The recommended daily allowances for healthy persons is 45 to 145 mEq each for sodium, chloride, and potassium.[5] The amounts of these elements provided during illness depend on the cardiovascular, renal, and endocrine status of the patient as well as an assessment of gastrointestinal and other losses.

During nutritional repletion, potassium, the major intracellular ion, will be deposited in the newly synthesized cells, and serum levels may fall abruptly if potassium is not supplied in sufficient amounts.

Data from patients receiving parenteral nutrition indicate a minimum daily potassium requirement of 5 to 6 mEq/gm of administered nitrogen. This recommendation of Lee and Hartley[32] is similar to the 120 to 160 mEq/day suggested by Sheldon and Kudsk.[33]

Phosphorus. Phosphorus is a critical constituent of all tissues, and its presence is essential to muscle, nervous system, and erythrocyte function and to the intermediary metabolism of carbohydrate, protein, and fat.[34] In addition, inorganic phosphorus is necessary for the synthesis of high energy organic bonds.[7] The recommended daily allowance of this mineral for healthy adults is 800 mg (25.8 mM).[5] The movement of phosphorus into newly synthesized tissue in patients receiving nutritional support is related to the magnitude of nitrogen retention, which in turn is related to caloric intake. On the basis of data from patients receiving intravenous feedings, Sheldon and Kudsk[33] and Sheldon and Grzyb[35] recommended that 15 to 25 mEq (8 to 14 mM) of phosphate be provided for each 1000 nonprotein calories administered.

Calcium. About 99 percent of the total body calcium is present in the skeleton. Nevertheless, the small amount of calcium outside of bone has a vital role, since calcium is necessary for blood coagulation, neuromuscular and myocardial function, and the integrity of intracellular cement substances and various membranes.[5,36] The recommended daily allowance of oral calcium for healthy persons is 800 mg (40 mEq). This recommendation is based on the usual 70 to 80 percent rate of absorption of calcium from the gut, as well as an adequate intake of vitamin D. According to data collected by Wittine and Freeman,[36] normal persons receiving parenteral nutrition require a minimum daily dose of 5 mg (0.25 mEq)/kg to achieve calcium equilibrium. Positive calcium balance, presumably indicating repletion of bone mineral, is not dependent on nitrogen retention, but the simultaneous administration of phosphorus, sodium, and calcium is necessary for calcium retention since bone contains these three elements in a fixed ratio.[31]

Magnesium.   Magnesium is selectively concentrated in cells and is also stored in bone. About half of the magnesium in the body is not freely exchangeable. Magnesium is one of the major intracellular ions, and it is an essential part of many enzyme systems.[5] It plays an important role in protein synthesis and in neuromuscular transmission and activity. In addition, magnesium is essential for the normal metabolism of potassium and calcium and is necessary for the mobilization of the latter from bone.[37]

The recommended daily allowance for healthy men is 350 mg (29 mEq), and for healthy women, 300 mg (25 mEq).[5] On the basis of studies in patients receiving parenteral nutrition, Lee and Hartley recommended a daily magnesium dosage of 2 mEq/gm of administered nitrogen.[32]

ESSENTIAL FATTY ACIDS

The essential fatty acids are those polyunsaturated fatty acids which cannot be synthesized in the body but which are necessary for normal growth and maintenance and the proper functioning of many physiologic processes.

The essential fatty acids play a role in the regulation of cholesterol metabolism, are important for maintaining the function and integrity of cellular and subcellular membranes, and are the precursors of the prostaglandins.[5]

Many fatty acids have essential fatty acid activity, but the two most important for man are linoleic and arachidonic.[40] Although arachidonic acid alleviates all recognized symptoms of essential fatty acid deficiency, it is not an essential dietary nutrient, since linoleic acid can be converted to arachidonic acid in the body. Linolenic acid cannot be made by mammals, and it has essential fatty acid properties in some animals. However, its essentiality for man is not clear.[5,41,42]

Thus the primary dietary essential fatty acid for man is linoleic acid, which is found widely in varying amounts in foods of both plant and animal origin and in the commercially available intravenous fat emulsions.

The amount of linoleic acid necessary to prevent the chemical and clinical evidence of deficiency has been estimated to range between 2.5 and 20 gm/day.[6,43,44] Shils recommended providing at least 4 percent of required calories as linoleic acid.[45]

Essential fatty acid deficiency is discussed in Chapter 8.

TRACE ELEMENTS

An element is considered "essential" if a clinical deficiency state develops when the substance is withdrawn from the diet and if this state is reversed when the element is again provided. Micronutrients presently recognized as

TABLE 3-7
Recommended Daily Allowances
of Trace Elements

	Oral	*Intravenous*
Zinc	10–15 mg	2.5–4.0 mg
Copper	1.2–3 mg	0.5–1.5 mg
Chromium	50–290 μg	10–15 μg
Manganese	0.7–5 mg	0.15–0.8 mg
Iodine	150 μg	1–2 μg/kg

Based on recommendations of National Research Council,[5] the AMA Expert Panel,[46] and Shils.[47]

essential for man are iron, iodine, cobalt, zinc, and copper. Fragmentary evidence supports the essentiality of chromium and manganese. On the basis of studies in experimental animals or a knowledge of their presence in human enzyme systems, selenium, vanadium, molybdenum, nickel, tin, silicon, and arsenic may also be essential for man. At present, supplements of iodine, zinc, copper, chromium, and manganese are recommended for patients receiving enteral or parenteral nutrition (Table 3-7).[46] Cobalt is supplied through vitamin B12.

Iron. Iron is a constituent of hemoglobin, myoglobin, and a number of enzymes and therefore is an essential nutrient for man. The recommended daily allowance for adult men and postmenopausal women is 10 mg, and that for menstruating women is 18 mg/day.[5]

The advisability of iron supplements in hospitalized patients is problematic, since critically ill or nutritionally depleted patients often demonstrate lack of bone marrow response, and an increased susceptibility and severity of infection has been associated with high circulating iron levels in malnourished patients.[7,38,39]

Iodine. Iodine is an integral part of the thyroid hormones and is thus an essential micronutrient. The recommended oral allowance is 150 mg/day; 1 to 2 mg/kg are recommended when iodine is to be given intravenously.[5,47]

Zinc. Zinc is an essential component of more than 70 metalloenzymes involved in the metabolism of lipids, carbohydrate, proteins, and nucleic acids, and there is a definite relationship between this element and bone growth. Thus zinc is crucial to growth, development, and normal function.[48,49] Catabolic states are associated with rapid mobilization of zinc from its intracellular stores and excretion.[7] The recommended daily oral supplement of zinc for normal persons is 10 to 15 mg. The suggested daily intravenous intake is 2.5

to 4.0 mg, and an additional 2 mg are recommended for acutely catabolic patients.[5,46] Additional supplements are recommended in the presence of significant intestinal fluid losses: 12.2 mg zinc per liter of small bowel fluid and 17.1 mg/kg of stool or ileostomy output.[46]

On the other hand, chronic ingestion of zinc in amounts exceeding 15 mg/day orally may aggravate marginal copper deficiency by depressing copper absorption.[5,50] In addition, dosage of intravenous zinc must be modified in the presence of renal dysfunction, since excessive zinc is excreted in the urine when the regulatory absorptive mechanism of the intestinal mucosa is bypassed.[46]

Copper.   Copper is a component of numerous metalloenzymes and is necessary for the proper utilization of iron in hemoglobin synthesis. In addition, this element is necessary for bone and elastic tissue development and the normal function of the central nervous system.[5,49,51] Recommendations for oral intake range between 1.2 and 3 mg/day; 0.5 to 1.5 mg/day is recommended intravenously for patients receiving parenteral nutrition. Copper is excreted primarily in the bile; therefore, intake should be decreased or omitted in patients with hepatobiliary disease.[5,46]

Chromium.   Trivalent chromium, probably acting as a cofactor for insulin, is required for maintaining normal glucose tolerance in experimental animals.[5] It apparently plays a similar role in humans.[52,53] The recommended oral allowance is 50 to 290 μg/day; 10 to 15 μg/day should be provided intravenously. When renal dysfunction is present, dosage must be adjusted, since chromium is eliminated predominantly in the urine.[5,46]

Manganese.   Manganese is an essential part of several enzyme systems involved in protein and energy metabolism and in the formation of mucopolysaccharides.[5] Recommended allowance is 0.7 to 5 mg/day orally and 0.15 to 0.8 mg/day intravenously.[5,46] Manganese is excreted primarily via the biliary tract, and dosage should therefore be modified in the presence of biliary tract obstruction.[46]

Clinical syndromes associated with trace element deficiencies are discussed in Chapter 8.

VITAMINS

Vitamins are organic compounds which are required in minute amounts for normal growth, maintenance, and reproduction. They differ from other organic foodstuffs in that they do not enter into the tissue structure and do not undergo degradation for purposes of providing energy. Vitamins cannot be synthesized in sufficient amounts by man and therefore must be provided in the diet or be synthesized by bacteria existing symbiotically in the gastrointestinal tract. The absence of a given vitamin produces a specific deficiency disease, the clinical and biochemical manifestations of which define the role of the respective vitamin.[54,55] At the present time, the vitamins recognized as essential for man are the 4 fat-soluble vitamins (A, D, E, and K) and 9 water-soluble vitamins (ascorbic acid, thiamine, riboflavin, niacin, pyridoxine, pantothenic acid, folic acid, B12, and biotin) (Table 3-8).

Allowances for normal persons are well standardized, but the requirements for persons receiving parenteral nutrition are tentative, and the altered needs associated with specific disease states remain ill-defined. The increased vitamin requirements associated with moderate or severe injury have been estimated by the National Academy of Sciences.[56] Recently, the Nutrition Advi-

TABLE 3-8
Recommended Daily Maintenance Dosage of Vitamins

Vitamin	Oral Dosage			Intravenous Dosage‡
	NORMAL*	MODERATE INJURY†	SEVERE INJURY†	
A, as retinol (IU)§	3300.0	5000.0	5000.0	3300.0
D (IU)″	400.0	400.0	400.0	200.0
E, α-tocopherol (IU)	10.0	—	—	10.0
K (mg)¶	—	2.0	20.0	—
Thiamine, B1 (mg)	1.5	2.0	10.0	3.0
Riboflavin, B2 (mg)	1.7	2.0	10.0	3.6
Niacin, B3 (mg)	19.0	20.0	100.0	40.0
Pantothenic acid, B5 (mg)	7.0	18.0	40.0	15.0
Pyridoxine, B6 (mg)	2.2	2.0	40.0	4.0
B12 (μg)	3.0	2.0	4.0	5.0
Ascorbic acid, C (mg)	60	75.0	300.0	100.0
Folic acid (μg)	400.0	1500.0	2500.0	400.0
Biotin (mg)	200.0	—	—	60.0

*Adapted from Recommended Daily Allowances.[5] Highest recommended dosage for age range 11 years to over 51 years is listed.
†Recommendations of the National Academy of Sciences.[56]
‡Recommendations of the AMA Nutrition Advisory Group for persons 11 years and over.[57]
§One IU is equivalent to 0.3 μg of retinol.
″ One IU is equivalent to 0.025 μg of vitamin D (cholecalciferol).
¶No specific recommendation for normal persons because of the synthesis of vitamin K by intestinal bacteria. Vitamin K (phylloquinone), 2 to 4 mg once weekly, is recommended in parenteral form for patients receiving intravenous nutrition and who do not require anticoagulants.[57]

sory Group of the American Medical Association set forth guidelines for vitamin allowances for patients receiving parenteral nutrition.[57] The recommendations are designed to meet the needs of the majority of patients with clinical conditions for which parenteral feeding is employed (Table 3-8).

REFERENCES

1. Energy and Protein Requirements: Report of a Joint FAO/WHO Ad Hoc Expert Committee. World Health Organization Technical Report Series, 1973, No. 522.
2. Talbot FB: Basal metabolism standards for children. Am J Dis Child 55:455–459, 1938.
3. Kinney JM: Energy requirements of the surgical patient, in Ballinger WF, Collins JA, Drucker WR, et al (eds): Manual of Surgical Nutrition. Philadelphia, WB Saunders Co, 1975, pp 223–235.
4. Cantarow A, Trumper M: Clinical Biochemistry. Philadelphia, WB Saunders Co, 1955.
5. Recommended Daily Allowances, ed 9. Food and Nutrition Board of the National Research Council, National Academy of Sciences, 1980.
6. Jeejeebhoy KN: Total parenteral nutrition. Ann R Coll Phys Surg Can 9:287–300, 1976.
7. Wilmore DW: The Metabolic Management of the Critically Ill. New York, Plenum Medical Book Co, 1977.
8. Long CL: Energy and protein needs in the critically ill patient. Contemp Surg 16:29–42, 1980.
9. Long CL, Schaffel N, Geiger JW, et al: Metabolic response to injury and illness: Estimation of energy and protein needs from indirect calorimetry and nitrogen balance. JPEN 3:452–456, 1979.
10. Duke JH, Jorgensen SB, Broell JR, et al: Contribution of protein to caloric expenditure following injury. Surgery 668:168–174, 1970.
11. Harris JA, Benedict FG: Biometric Studies of Basal Metabolism in Man, publication no. 279. Carnegie Institution of Washington, 1919.
12. Coon WW, Kowalczyk RS: Protein metabolism, in Ballinger WF, Collins JA, Drucker WR, et al (eds): Manual of Surgical Nutrition. Philadelphia, WB Saunders Co, 1975, pp 50–72.
13. Cahill GF: Starvation in man. N Engl J Med 282:668–675, 1970.
14. Calloway DH, Spector H: Nitrogen balance as related to caloric and protein intake in active young men. Am J Clin Nutr 2:405–412, 1954.
15. Wilmore DW: Energy requirements for maximum nitrogen retention, in Greene HL, Holliday MA, Munro HN (eds): Clinical Nutrition Update: Amino Acids. Chicago, American Medical Association, 1977, pp 47–57.
16. Munro HN, Crim MC: The proteins and amino acids, in Goodhart RS, Shils ME (eds): Modern Nutrition in Health and Disease, ed 6. Philadelphia, Lea and Febiger, 1980, pp 51–98.
17. Brennan MF, Fitzpatrick GF, Cohen KH, Moore FD: Glycerol: Major contribu-

tor to the short-term protein-sparing effect of fat emulsions in normal man. Ann Surg 182:386–394, 1975.

18. Wolfe BM, Culebras JM, Sim AJW, et al: Substrate interaction in intravenous feeding: Comparative effects of carbohydrate and fat on amino acid utilization in fasting man. Ann Surg 186:518–540, 1977.

19. Fitzpatrick GF, Meguid MM, O'Connell RC, et al: Nitrogen sparing by carbohydrate in man: Intermittent or continuous enteral compared with continuous parenteral. Surgery 78:105–113, 1975.

20. Kopple JD, Swendseid ME: Evidence that histidine is an essential amino acid in normal and chronically uremic man. J Clin Invest 55:881–891, 1975.

21. Anderson GH, Patel DG, Jeejeebhoy KN: Design and evaluation by nitrogen balance and blood aminograms of an amino acid mixture for total parenteral nutrition of adults with gastrointestinal disease. J Clin Invest 53:904–912, 1974.

22. Dolif D, Jurgens P: Requirement and utilization of amino-acids, in Ahnefeld FW, Burri C, Dick W, Halmagi M (eds): Parenteral Nutrition. New York, Springer–Verlag, 1976, pp 54–65.

23. Meng HC: Parenteral nutrition: Principles, nutrient requirements, and techniques. Geriatrics 30:97–107, 1975.

24. Watts JA, Bradley L, Mann AN: Total N, urea and ammonia excretions of human male subjects fed several nonessential amino acids singly as the chief source of nonspecific N. Metabolism 14:504–515, 1965.

25. Munro HN: Basic concepts in the use of amino acids and protein hydrolysates for parenteral nutrition. Proceedings of the AMA Symposium on Total Parenteral Nutrition, Nashville, Tenn, January 17–19, 1972, pp 7–35.

26. Blackburn GL, Bistrian BR: Nutritional care of the injured and/or septic patient. Surg Clin North Am 56:1195–1224, 1976.

27. Fischer JE: Hyperalimentation. Med Clin North Am 63:973–983, 1979.

28. Munro HN: Carbohydrate versus fat versus protein calories (panel discussion), in Greep JM, Soeters PB, Wesdorp RIC, et al (eds): Current Concepts in Parenteral Nutrition. The Hague, Martinus Nijoff Medical Division, 1977, p 357.

29. Elman R: Time factors in the utilization of a mixture of amino acids (protein hydrolysate) and dextrose given intravenously. Am J Clin Nutr 1:287–294, 1953.

30. Shenkin A, Wretlind A: Complete intravenous nutrition including amino acids, glucose and lipids, in Richards JR, Kinney JM (eds): Nutritional Aspects of Care in the Critically Ill. Edinburgh, Churchill Livingstone, 1977, pp 345–365.

31. Rudman D, Millikan WJ, Richardson TJ, et al: Elemental balances during intravenous hyperalimentation of underweight subjects. J Clin Invest 55:94–104, 1975.

32. Lee HA, Hartley TF: A method of determining daily nitrogen requirements. Postgrad Med J 51:441–445, 1975.

33. Sheldon GF, Kudsk KA: Electrolyte requirements in total parenteral nutrition, in Deitel M (ed): Nutrition in Clinical Surgery. Baltimore, Williams and Wilkins, 1980, pp 103–111.

34. Kreisberg RA: Phosphorus deficiency and hypophosphatemia. Hosp Pract, March 1977, pp 121–128.

35. Sheldon GF, Grzyb S: Phosphate depletion and repletion: Relation to parenteral nutrition and oxygen transport. Ann Surg 182:683–689, 1975.

36. Wittine MF, Freeman JB: Calcium requirements during total parenteral nutrition in well-nourished individuals. JPEN 1:152–155, 1977.
37. Shils ME: Major minerals: Magnesium, in Goodhart RS, Shils ME (eds): Modern Nutrition in Health and Disease. Philadelphia, Lea and Febiger, 1980, pp 310–323.
38. Alexander JW: Nutrition and surgical infection, in Ballinger WF, Collins JA, Drucker WR, et al (eds): Manual of Surgical Nutrition. Philadelphia, WB Saunders Co, 1975, pp 386–395.
39. Bothe A, Benotti P, Bistrian BR, Blackburn GL: Use of iron with total parenteral nutrition. N Engl J Med 93:1153, 1975.
40. Alfin-Slater PB, Aftergood L: Lipids, in Goodhart RS, Shils ME (eds): Modern Nutrition in Health and Disease. Philadelphia, Lea and Febiger, 1980, 113–141.
41. Holman RT: Function and biologic activities of essential fatty acids in man, in Meng HC, Wilmore DW (eds): Fat Emulsions in Parenteral Nutrition. Chicago, American Medical Association, 1976, pp 5–14.
42. Sanders TAB, Naismith DJ: Conflicting roles of polyunsaturated fatty acids. Lancet 1:654–655, 1980.
43. Collins FD, Sinclair AJ, Royle JP, et al: Plasma lipids in human linoleic acid deficiency. Nutr Metab 13:150–167, 1971.
44. Jeejeebhoy KN, Zohrab WJ, Langer B, et al: Total parenteral nutrition at home for 23 months without complication and with good rehabilitation. Gastroenterology 65:811–820, 1973.
45. Shils ME: Parenteral nutrition, in Goodhart RS, Shils ME (eds): Modern Nutrition in Health and Disease. Philadelphia, Lea and Febiger, 1980, pp 1125–1152.
46. Guidelines for essential trace element preparations for parenteral use: A statement by an expert panel, AMA Department of Foods and Nutrition. JAMA 241:2051–2054, 1979.
47. Shils ME: Minerals in total parenteral nutrition. Proceedings of the AMA Symposium on Total Parenteral Nutrition, Nashville, Tenn, January 17–19, 1972, pp 92–114.
48. Allinson R: Plasma trace elements during total parenteral nutrition. JPEN 2:35–40, 1978.
49. Ulmer DD: Trace elements. N Engl J Med 297:318–321, 1977.
50. Prasad AS, Brewer GJ, Schoomaker EB, Rabbani P: Hypocupremia induced by zinc therapy in adults. JAMA 240:2166–2168, 1978.
51. Li TK, Vallee BL: The biochemical and nutritional roles of other trace elements, in Goodhart RS, Shils ME (eds): Modern Nutrition in Health and Disease. Philadelphia, Lea and Febiger, 1980, pp 408–441.
52. Freund H, Atamian S, Fischer JE: Chromium deficiency during total parenteral nutrition. JAMA 241:496–498, 1979.
53. Jeejeebhoy KN, Chu RC, Marliss EB, et al: Chromium deficiency, glucose intolerance, and neuropathy reversed by chromium supplementation in a patient receiving long-term parenteral nutrition. Am J Clin Nutr 30:531–538, 1977.
54. Cantarow A, Schepartz B: Biochemistry, ed. 3. Philadelphia, WB Saunders Co, 1962.
55. Gann DS, Robinson HB. Salt, water, and vitamins, in Ballinger WF, Collins JA,

Drucker WR, et al (eds): Manual of Surgical Nutrition. Philadelphia, WB Saunders Co, 1975, pp 73–90.

56. Pollack H, Halpern, SL: Therapeutic Nutrition with Special Reference to Military Situations. Washington, D.C., National Academy of Sciences, National Research Council, 1951.

57. Multivitamin preparations for parenteral use: A statement by the Nutrition Advisory Group, American Medical Association Department of Foods and Nutrition, 1975. JPEN 3:258–262, 1979.

4

Enteral Nutrition

Patients unable to consume necessary nutrients orally require an alternative form of nutritional support. While some may need intravenous feeding, many such patients are capable of absorbing and utilizing nutrients delivered in a suitable form through feeding tubes introduced at various points into the alimentary tract.

HISTORICAL BACKGROUND

Enteral (tube) feeding techniques have been popularized, refined, and subjected to scientific scrutiny only in the last 30 years. However, the potential benefits of such methods were perceived as early as the Graeco-Roman era, and in the 1500s Aquapendente advocated forced feeding using a feeding tube introduced through the nose.[1] Nevertheless, starving of patients with fever was the accepted practice for centuries. In 1884, Graves advanced a revolutionary concept when he suggested that the deleterious effects of starvation compounded the consequences of disease.[2] He recommended a diet for patients with hypermetabolism secondary to infection and thyrotoxicosis consisting of sugar water, meat broths, toast crumbs, and jellies.[2,3] Later, a milk diet was proposed for patients with typhoid fever, but it was not until the classic studies of Coleman and DuBois were carried out in the early 1900s that nutritional management of the infected patient was placed on a firm scientific foundation.[3,4] Subsequently, Cuthbertson demonstrated that the catabolic response to severe trauma could be offset by high-caloric, high-nitrogen feedings.[5] Further advances in nutritional support, both parenteral and enteral, awaited the development of nutrient products and of techniques of nutrient delivery.

The advent of the electric food blender was a boon to the concept of enteral nutrition, since this appliance could be used to liquify solid foodstuffs for delivery through feeding tubes. Prior to this time, nutrients for tube feeding were virtually limited to naturally occurring liquids or semisolids.[6]

Thus the work establishing the value of nutritional support, on the one hand, and the notion of nutritionally complete liquid diets, on the other, set the stage for the development of the wide variety of enteral feeding products and feeding tubes presently available for the management of patients with various nutritional and medical requirements.

INDICATIONS FOR AND CONTRAINDICATIONS TO ENTERAL NUTRITION

The feasibility of enteral nutrition is dependent on the presence of sufficient functioning small bowel to allow the absorption of provided nutrients. Among patients meeting this criterion, suitable candidates include those in whom oral consumption is inadequate or contraindicated. Anorexia, weakness, lethargy, nausea, or oral inflammation are examples of factors contributing to poor oral intake. In addition, patients with diseases associated with markedly increased nutritional requirements, such as major burns, trauma, and sepsis, may be unable to eat enough to meet demands but often can be successfully nourished with the continuous administration of high-calorie, high-protein tube feedings. Patients in whom oral intake is contraindicated but who nevertheless may be candidates for enteral feeding include those who have certain neurologic disorders, including some patients following a cerebrovascular accident, and those who are comatose, stuporous, or extremely lethargic. Patients unable to eat because of oral, pharyngeal, or esophageal conditions, such as wired jaws, obstructing lesions, dysphagia, or recent surgery, also may be candidates for tube feeding.

In addition, enteral nutrition may be indicated for patients with certain gastrointestinal disorders that may benefit from an elemental diet since the latter is often unpalatable when taken orally. For example, nutrition can often be maintained despite mild or moderate malabsorption or pancreatic insufficiency with a slow, continuous infusion of an elemental liquid diet.[7] This regimen may also be effective in the management of inflammatory bowel disease, since the low-residue property of such elemental diets may allow bowel rest and decrease diarrhea.[8] Elemental diets also have been advocated in the management of some intestinal fistulas. With gastroduodenal and upper jejunal fistulas, the tube feedings are delivered distal to the lesion.[8,9]

In contrast, enteral feedings are contraindicated in patients with peritonitis, intestinal obstruction, paralytic ileus, gastrointestinal hemorrhage, or intractable vomiting or diarrhea.[10] In addition, enteral feedings are likely to produce a salutary effect in the management of only the most proximal and distal intestinal fistulas. Consequently, in the remaining cases, parenteral nutrition is preferred, since enteral feedings usually increase fistulous output with concomitant fluid and electrolyte disturbances and skin breakdown. In addition, enteral feedings are not recommended in the presence of severe malabsorptive states or in the early stages of short bowel syndrome, since the adequate absorption of nutrients is unlikely in these circumstances.[8,9] Finally, enteral nutrition is contraindicated when a properly managed trial of such therapy fails to meet the nutritional goals, aggravates the underlying condition, or is associated with pulmonary aspiration or unmanageable diarrhea.

NUTRIENT FORMULATIONS

A wide variety of liquid feeding preparations are presently available which differ in their content and source of protein, carbohydrate, and fat as well as in their osmolality, caloric density, sodium content, and residue. Amino acids may be derived from intact protein in the form of pureed meat, eggs, or milk; from intact protein provided as semipurified isolates from milk, soybean, or eggs; or from hydrolyzed protein with supplementary amino acids; or they may be provided as purified free amino acids.[11]

Early formulations utilizing glucose or sucrose as the carbohydrate source were high in osmolality. The current use of starches, dextrins, and glucose oligosaccharides reduces the number of active chemical components and hence the osmolality, since the latter is a colligative property. The content of fat varies considerably among liquid feeding preparations; most contain long-chain fats, such as corn oil, soy oil, and safflower oil. However, some products contain medium-chain triglycerides (MCT), which are not dependent on pancreatic lipase or bile salts for digestion; they pass through the intestinal epithelium directly into the portal system as free fatty acids.[7,11]

Commercially available products supply all the essential minerals, including trace elements and vitamins (except vitamin K), necessary to meet the requirements of *normal* persons when sufficient volume is provided to meet calorie and protein requirements. Products contain vitamin K in variable amounts (0 to 1.6 mg/liter). The highest amounts are provided in Ensure (1 mg/liter), Ensure-Plus (1.6 mg/liter), and Osmolite (1 mg/liter). The presence of vitamin K must be considered in patients who are receiving oral anticoagulants. Supplements of minerals and vitamins may be required by patients with malabsorption, marked gastrointestinal losses, increased demands associated with critical illness, or a pre-existing deficiency state.

Nutritionally complete enteral feeding preparations can be classified according to their composition, as follows:[11]

1. Formulations with intact protein containing milk (high lactose).
2. Formulations with intact protein and/or protein isolates with no lactose.
3. Formulations with hydrolyzed protein and/or amino acids with no lactose ("peptide" and "elemental" diets).

Preparations providing intact protein require normal digestive and absorptive processes for utilization and are therefore suitable only for patients with normally functioning gastrointestinal tracts (Tables 4-1, 4-2). Such patients may include those with anorexia, head and neck lesions, swallowing disorders, or dysphagia. A blenderized regular hospital diet would be nutritionally satisfactory, but the viscosity of such preparations may require an irritating, large-bore feeding tube. In contrast, formulations providing utilizable nitrogen in the form of free amino acids or di- and tripeptides plus amino acids ("elemental diets") may be suitable for patients with a variety of disorders of the small intestine, pancreas, or biliary tract, since these preparations demand no digestive effort on the part of the handicapped alimentary tract and require only a minimal absorptive surface for absorption (Table 4-3).

Formulations low in lactose are frequently indicated because of a high incidence of lactase deficiency (Tables 4-2, 4-3). Some 16 to 55 percent of North American adults are affected; a 70 percent incidence of lactase deficiency has been observed among black Americans, and a 90 percent incidence has been observed among Japanese, Thais, Formosans, and Filipinos.[12] In addition, bowel disease, fasting, starvation, protein depletion, and total parenteral nutrition have been associated with the development of lactase deficiency.[13] Lactose consumption by affected patients may result in osmotic diarrhea, bloating, gas, and abdominal cramps.[14]

The majority of commercially available formula diets have a caloric density, including both nonprotein and protein calories, of approximately 1 kcal/ml at full strength. However, enriched formulations are available which provide up to 2.0 kcal/ml. Such products with higher caloric density may be of especial value for patients who are fluid-restricted or for hypermetabolic patients with very high caloric requirements.

Defined-formula Diets (Elemental Diets)

"Defined-formula" or "elemental" diets generally include those nutritionally complete formulations in which the protein moiety is predigested and is provided as synthetic amino acids or as hydrolyzed protein supplemented with amino acids (Table 4-3). Fats, provided in variable amounts, are usually pres-

TABLE 4-1
Enteral Feeding Formulations with Intact Protein Containing Milk
(High Lactose)*—Contents per Liter at Standard Dilution (Full Strength)

	C.I.B.†,‡,§ (Carnation)	Compleat B¶ (Doyle)	Formula 2¶ (Cutter)	Meritene Liquid‡ (Doyle)
Caloric density (kcal/ml)	1.1	1.0	1.0	0.96
Protein (gm)	63	40	38	58
Protein source	Nonfat milk Soy protein Na caseinate	Beef Nonfat milk	Beef Nonfat milk	Concentrated skim milk Na caseinate
Fat (gm)	31	40	40	32
Fat source	Milk fat	Corn oil	Corn oil Egg yolks	Corn oil Mono- and diglycerides
Carbohydrate (gm)	141	120	123	111
Carbohydrate source	Sucrose Corn syrup solids Lactose	Maltodextrin Sucrose Vegetables Fruits Orange juice	Sucrose Vegetables Orange juice Wheat flour	Corn syrup solids Sucrose
Lactose (gm)	96	24	37	55
Calcium (mg)	1372	625	720	1202
Phosphorus (mg)	1105	1250	560	1202
Magnesium (mg)	459	250	100	320
Iron (mg)	18	11	13	14
Iodine (μg)	147	94	75	120
Copper (mg)	2.3	1.3	1.0	1.6
Manganese (mg)	—	2.5	0.2	3.2
Zinc (mg)	15.6	9.4	7.5	12.0
Sodium (mEq)	42	52	26	38
Potassium (mEq)	72	34	45	41
Chloride (mEq)	—	23	54	45
mOsm/kg	—	390	435–510	550–610
Vol. to meet vitamin requirements (ml), except vitamin K	1373	1600	2000	1200

*Low residue except Compleat B and Formula 2.
†C.I.B. = Carnation Instant Breakfast.
‡Data for vanilla flavor.
§Whole milk added.
¶Blenderized diet.

Meritene+ Milk‡,§ (Doyle)	Nutri-1000‡ (Cutter)	Sustacal+ Milk‡,§ (Mead–Johnson)	Sustagen+ Water‡ (Mead–Johnson)
1.1	1.0	1.3	1.7
69	39	80	100
Nonfat milk	Skim milk	Nonfat milk	Nonfat milk
Whole milk		Whole milk	Whole milk
			Ca caseinate
35	54	33	14
Milk fat	Corn oil	Milk fat	Milk fat
119	100	179	286
Corn syrup	Corn syrup	Corn syrup	Corn syrup
solids	solids	solids	solids
	Sucrose	Sucrose	Glucose
104	52	114	96
2307	1198	2148	3047
1922	938	1778	2286
384	208	500	381
17	9	22	17
145	78	185	143
1.9	1.0	2.5	1.8
3.8	1.4	3.7	4.8
14.4	7.8	18.5	14.3
42	23	54	50
76	37	86	86
62	32	50	—
690	500	756	1334
1040	1920	—	1050

Recalculated and adapted in part from Bloch AS, Shils ME: In Goodhart RS, Shils ME (eds): *Modern Nutrition in Health and Disease*, ed. 6 Philadelphia, Lea and Febiger, 1980, pp 1314–1315.

TABLE 4-2

Enteral Feeding Formulations with Intact Protein and/or Protein Isolates with No Lactose*—Contents per Liter at Standard Dilution (Full Strength)

	Ensure† (Ross)	Ensure Plus† (Ross)	Isocal (Mead-Johnson)	Isocal HCN (Mead-Johnson)
Caloric density (kcal/ml)	1.0	1.5	1.0	2.0
Protein (gm)	36	55	34	75
Protein source	Na + Ca caseinate	Na + Ca caseinate	Na caseinate	Na + Ca caseinate
	Soy protein	Soy protein	Soy protein	
Fat (gm)	36	53	44	91
Fat source	Corn oil	Corn oil	Soy oil	Soy oil
			MCT oil	MCT oil
Carbohydrate (gm)	142	200	130	225
Carbohydrate source	Corn syrup solids	Corn syrup solids	Glucose oligosaccharides	Corn syrup solids
	Sucrose	Sucrose		
Lactose (gm)	0	0	0	0
Calcium (mg)	520	630	625	667
Phosphorus (mg)	520	630	520	667
Magnesium (mg)	206	317	208	267
Iron (mg)	9	14	9	12
Iodine (μg)	78	106	78	100
Copper (mg)	1.0	1.6	1.0	2.0
Manganese (mg)	2.1	2.1	2.6	3.3
Zinc (mg)	16	24	10	20
Sodium (mEq)	32	46	23	34.8
Potassium (mEq)	37	49	33	35.9
Chloride (mEq)	29	45	29	33.8
mOsm/kg	450	600	300	650
Vol. to meet vitamin requirements (ml), except vitamin K	1887	2000	1920	1500

*Low residue, except Vitaneed.
†Data for vanilla flavor.
‡Blenderized diet with moderate residue.

Magnacal (Organon)	Nutri-1000-LF† (Cutter)	Osmolite (Ross)	Precision-HN (Doyle)	Precision Isotonic (Doyle)
2.0	1.1	1.1	1.1	1.0
70 Ca + Na caseinate	40 Ca + Na caseinate Soy protein isolate	37 Ca + Na caseinate Soy protein isolate	44 Egg white solids	29 Egg white solids
80 Soy oil Mono- and diglycerides	55 Corn oil	38 MCT oil Corn oil Soy oil	1.3 MCT oil Soy oil Mono- and diglycerides	30 Soy oil Mono- and diglycerides
250 Corn syrup solids Maltodextrin Sucrose	101 Corn syrup solids Sugar	145 Corn syrup solids	217 Maltodextrin Sugar	144 Glucose oligo-saccharides Sugar
0	0	0	0	0
1000	529	530	350	641
1000	529	530	350	641
400	211	210	140	257
18	10	10	6	12
150	79	79	53	96
2.0	1.9	1.1	0.7	1.3
—	1.4	2.1	1.4	2.6
15	8	16	5.3	9.6
43	31	25	43	33
32	38	23	23	25
27	28	24	34	29
520	380	300	557	300
1000	1920	1887	2850	1560

Recalculated and adapted in part from Bloch AS, Shils ME: In Goodhart RS, Shils ME (eds): Modern Nutrition in Health and Disease, ed 6. Philadelphia, Lea and Febiger, 1980, pp 1316–1317.

(Cont.)

TABLE 4-2 (Cont.)
Enteral Feeding Formulations with Intact Protein and/or Protein Isolates with No Lactose*—Contents per Liter at Standard Dilution (Full Strength)

	Precision-LR (Doyle)	Portagen (Mead–Johnson)	Renu (Organon)
Caloric density (kcal/ml)	1.1	1.0	1.0
Protein (gm)	26	35	33
Protein source	Egg white solids	Na caseinate	Ca + Na caseinate Soy protein isolate
Fat (gm)	1.6	48	40
Fat source	MCT oil Soy oil Mono- and diglycerides	MCT oil Corn oil Lecithin	Soy oil Mono- and diglycerides
Carbohydrate (gm)	248	115	130
Carbohydrate source	Maltodextrin Sugar	Maltodextrin Sucrose	Maltodextrin Corn syrup solids Corn and malt syrup
Lactose (gm)	0	<0.3	0
Calcium (mg)	585	938	500
Phosphorus (mg)	585	604	500
Magnesium (mg)	234	208	200
Iron (mg)	11	19	10
Iodine (μg)	88	73	75
Copper (mg)	1.2	1.6	2.0
Manganese (mg)	2.3	3.1	—
Zinc (mg)	8.8	9.4	10.0
Sodium (mEq)	31	20	22
Potassium (mEq)	22	32	32
Chloride (mEq)	31	24	18
mOsm/kg	505–549	357	330
Vol. to meet vitamin requirements (ml), except vitamin K	1710	960	2000

Sustacal Liquid (Mead–Johnson)	Sustacal HC (Mead–Johnson)	Travasorb Liquid (Travenol)	Travasorb-MCT (Travenol)	Vitaneed‡ (Organon)
1.0	1.5	1.1	1.6	1.0
60 Ca + Na caseinate Soy protein	60 Na + Ca caseinate	33 Soy bean Casein	78 Lactalbumin Casein	35 Pureed beef Ca caseinate
23 Soy oil	56.7 Soy oil	35 Corn oil	53 MCT Sunflower oil	40 Soy oil
138 Sucrose Corn syrup solids	187.5 Corn syrup solids Sucrose	136 Corn syrup solids	196 Corn syrup solids	130 Corn syrup solids Maltodextrin Beans, peaches, carrots
0	0	0	0	0
1000	833	500	800	575
917	833	500	800	525
375	333	200	320	250
17	15	9	14	12
139	125	75	120	150
1.9	1.7	1.0	1.6	1.5
2.8	2.5	2.0	3.2	—
13.9	12.5	15	24	10
40	36.3	30	24	24
53	37.5	31	71	32
44	35.4	28	56	21
625	650	488	470	400
1080	1200	2000	1250	1470

TABLE 4-3

Formulations with Hydrolyzed Protein and/or Amino Acids with No Lactose (Peptide and Elemental Diets)—Contents per Liter at Standard Dilution (Full Strength)

	Criticare HN (Mead–Johnson)	Flexical* (Mead–Johnson)	Travasorb HN (Travenol)	Travasorb STD* (Travenol)
Caloric density (kcal/ml)	1.0	1.0	1.0	1.0
Protein (gm)	37.5	22	45	30
Protein source	Casein hy-drolysate	Hydrolyzed casein Amino acids	Lactalbumin peptides Amino acids	Lactalbumin peptides Amino acids
Fat (gm)	3.3	34	13	13
Fat source	Safflower oil	Soy oil MCT oil	MCT Sunflower oil	MCT Sunflower oil
Carbohydrate (gm)	219	154	175	190
Carbohydrate source	Maltodextrins	Corn syrup solids Modified tapioca starch	Glucose oligo-saccharides	Glucose oligo-saccharides
Lactose (gm)	0	0	0	0
Calcium (mg)	521	600	500	500
Phosphorus (mg)	521	500	500	500
Magnesium (mg)	208	200	200	200
Iron (mg)	9.4	9	9	9
Iodine (μg)	79.2	75	75	75
Copper (mg)	1.0	1.0	1	1
Manganese (mg)	2.6	2.5	1.3	1.3
Zinc (mg)	10.4	10.0	7.5	7.5
Sodium (mEq)	27.1	15	40	40
Potassium (mEq)	33.1	32	30	30
Chloride (mEq)	29.2	35	39	43
mOsm/kg	650	550	560	560
Vol. to meet vitamin requirements (ml), except vitamin K	1892	2000	2000	2000

*Data are for unflavored preparation.

Vipep (Cutter)	Vital (Ross)	Standard Vivonex* (Eaton)	High Nitrogen Vivonex* (Eaton)
1.0	1.0	1.0	1.0
25 Hydrolyzed fish protein Amino acids	42 Whey, soy, and meat protein hydrolysate Amino acids	20 Crystalline amino acids	42 Crystalline amino acids
25 MCT oil Corn oil	10 Sunflower oil	1.4 Safflower oil	0.9 Safflower oil
176 Corn syrup solids Sucrose Corn starch K-gluconate Tapioca flour	185 Glucose oligo- and polysaccharides Sucrose Corn starch	230 Glucose oligo- saccharides	210 Glucose oligo- saccharides
0	0	0	0
600	667	556	333
600	667	556	333
200	267	222	133
9	12	10	6.0
75	100	83	50
0.9	1.3	1.1	0.7
1.3	1.3	1.6	0.9
7.5	10.0	8.3	5.0
33	17	20	23
22	30	30	30
48	19	20	23
520	450	550	810
2000	1500	1800	3000

Recalculated and adapted in part from Bloch AS, Shils ME: In Goodhart RS, Shils ME (eds): *Modern Nutrition in Health and Disease*, ed. 6. Philadelphia, Lea and Febiger, 1980, pp 1318–1319, 1322.

TABLE 4-3 (Cont.)

Formulations with Hydrolyzed Protein and/or Amino Acids with No Lactose (Peptide and Elemental Diets)—Contents per Liter at Standard Dilution (Full Strength)

	Amin-Aid† (McGaw)	Hepatic-Aid† (McGaw)	Travasorb Hepatic† (Travenol)	Travasorb Renal† (Travenol)
Caloric density (kcal/ml)	2.0	1.6	1.1	1.4
Protein (gm)	19	42	29.2	23.1
Protein source	Essential amino acids plus histidine	Amino acids (High in BCAA‡ low in AAA‡)	Amino acids (High in BCAA‡ low in AAA‡)	Essential amino acids plus some non-essential amino acids
Fat (gm)	70	36	14.6	17.9
Fat source	Partially hydrogenated soy oil	Partially hydrogenated soy oil Lecithin Mono- and diglycerides	MCT Sunflower oil	MCT Sunfower oil Lecithin
Carbohydrate (gm)	324	287	213	273.7
Carbohydrate source	Maltodextrins	Maltodextrins Sucrose	Glucose oligo-saccharides Sucrose	Glucose oligo-saccharides Sucrose
Lactose (gm)	0	0	0	0
Calcium (mg)	< 120	Negligible	388	0
Phosphorus (mg)	Negligible	Negligible	481	0
Magnesium (mg)	< 72	Negligible	189.5	0
Iron (mg)	Negligible	Negligible	8.7	0
Iodine (µg)	Negligible	Negligible	72.9	0
Copper (mg)	Negligible	Negligible	1.0	0
Manganese (mg)	Negligible	Negligible	1.2	0
Zinc (mg)	Negligible	Negligible	7.3	0
Sodium (mEq)	< 6.0	Negligible	19.4	0
Potassium (mEq)	< 6.0	Negligible	29.2	0
Chloride (mEq)	Negligible	Negligible	19.5	0
mOsm/kg	1125	900	690	590
Vol. to meet vitamin requirements (ml), except vitamin K	—	—	2000	—

†Incomplete nutrient formulations that may be of value in renal failure (Amin-Aid, Travasorb Renal) and hepatic insufficiency (Hepatic-Aid, Travasorb Hepatic).
‡BCAA, branched-chain amino acids; AAA, aromatic amino acids.

ent in a finely emulsified form, often with a proportion as medium-chain tri-glycerides.[15] Some preparations contain only enough fat to meet essential fatty acid requirements and to provide a vehicle for fat-soluble vitamins.[8]

Extensive studies in the 1950s demonstrated the ability of such diets to support normal longevity, reproduction, growth, and lactation in rats. In the 1960s, long-term studies of humans receiving chemically formulated, bulk-free, virtually fat-free, elemental diets were conducted under the sponsorship of the National Aeronautics and Space Administration (NASA) in order to explore the applicability of these diets to in-flight space feeding. Sixteen male volunteers received 2100 to 3700 kcal/day of the elemental diet as their sole nutritional source for 19 weeks. They remained physically active and healthy and had normal blood and urine values; their body weights remained stable after a slight loss during the initial period of adaption. Fecal elimination in all individuals was strikingly reduced; the subjects had smaller than normal bow-el movements at regular intervals of 5 to 6 days.[16-18]

In 1969, Thompson and associates demonstrated that an elemental diet can be successfully used for the nutritional management of patients with markedly reduced intestinal absorptive surface and rapid transit times.[19] Nu-trition can usually be maintained with such a diet when 100 cm or more of functioning small bowel remain, but with adaption, as little as 65 cm of jeju-num may prove adequate.[20] Subsequent studies have suggested the utility of elemental diets in a variety of clinical situations, including:

1. Diarrheal states.
2. Enteritis of radiotherapy or chemotherapy.[21,22]
3. Selected gastrointestinal fistulas.[23-25]
4. Inflammatory bowel disease.[8,26]
5. Malabsorption syndrome.[7]
6. Pancreatitis.[27]
7. Pancreatic insufficiency.[7]
8. Short bowel syndrome.[15,19]
9. To decrease fecal output ("medical colostomy").
10. To prevent stress-induced gastric ulceration.[28,29]
11. To protect enteric mucosa from toxicity of chemotherapy.[21]
12. To provide a nonallergic food source.[8,17]

However, the value of an elemental diet has not been established conclusively in all of these conditions. The nutritional management of specific conditions is discussed in Chapter 10.

When elemental diets were first formulated, it was generally believed that dietary protein required complete hydrolysis to free amino acids before absorption occurred. Consequently, solutions of free amino acids were thought to be ideal nitrogen sources. More recent evidence, however, suggests that there are specific systems which mediate the transport of intact small peptides through the enteric mucosa and that these transport systems are separate and independent from those for free amino acids.[30,31] Thus the major route of absorption of di- and tripeptides involves active transport of the intact peptide across the brush border membrane, bypassing the brush border peptidases, with subsequent hydrolysis to free amino acids by intracellular cytoplasmic enzymes.[31,32] However, these peptides may also be absorbed by intraluminal hydrolysis by brush border peptidases, followed by uptake of free amino acids. The relative importance of these two absorptive processes apparently varies from one peptide to another. In addition, hydrolysis followed by amino acid uptake is also a more prominent component of peptide absorption in the ileum than in the jejunum.[32]

A potentially clinically relevant aspect of peptide absorption is the fact that absorption of amino acid residues from a solution of di- and tripeptides is frequently more rapid than absorption from an equimolar solution of free amino acids.[32] For example, the rate of absorption of glycine and leucine is greater when the dipeptide glycylleucine is presented to the intestinal mucosa than when an equimolar mixture of free glycine and free leucine is presented.[33] This difference in absorption kinetics has been observed with the majority of di- and tripeptides studied, but it is not necessarily demonstrable at all concentrations. Thus, at some concentrations, absorption of amino acids from a peptide may occur at about the same rate as that of the equivalent free amino acids. Although available data indicate that the absorptive capacity of the small bowel is usually considerably greater for oligopeptide–amino acid mixtures than for mixtures of free amino acids,[32] the kinetic advantage varies among the different peptide-containing protein hydrolysates. Silk and associates observed that total α-amino nitrogen absorption was greater from casein or lactalbumin hydrolysates than from the respective equivalent free amino acid mixtures.[30] However, when a fish protein hydrolysate was studied, several individual amino acid residues were absorbed to a greater extent from the hydrolysate than from the corresponding free amino acid mixture, but there was no significant difference in the proportions of total α-amino nitrogen absorbed from the two test solutions.

Prolonged starvation and various intestinal disorders generally have a more severe effect on the transport of free amino acids than on peptide transport, thus suggesting a therapeutic role for nutrient preparations providing di- and tripeptides. For example, no appreciable increase in plasma amino acid levels is observed after feeding free amino acids to patients with hereditary deficiencies of free amino acid carrier systems involving either neutral amino acids (Hartnup disease) or basic amino acids (cystinuria). However, when these patients receive the same amino acids in dipeptide form, their plasma amino acid levels increase.[34] In patients with celiac sprue, free amino acid absorption is markedly reduced, but dipeptide absorption is less severely affected. Similarly, free amino acid absorption is reduced in tropical sprue and short bowel syndrome.[32] In the protein–calorie malabsorption that follows jejunoileostomy for obesity, jejunal absorption of the free amino acid leucine is reduced, but absorption of the dipeptide glycylleucine is unaffected.[31,35] In contrast, *short-term* dietary restriction may *increase* the absorption of the free amino acids without altering peptide absorption.[32]

Finally, experiments in rats with pancreatic insufficiency disclose that oligopeptide diets are better utilized than diets consisting exclusively of free amino acids.[36]

In summary, amino acids generally are more rapidly absorbed from di- and tripeptides than from free amino acid solutions, but this kinetic advantage varies with the specific peptide, the peptide concentration, and the nature of the protein hydrolysate. Laboratory data suggest a therapeutic role for peptide diets, but it has not been established in clinical practice that such formulations are superior to solutions of free amino acids.

Supplementary and Special-purpose Formulations

Some supplements available for special nutritional needs, including protein, carbohydrate, and fat sources, are listed in Table 4-4, and formulas for the treatment of renal failure (Amin-Aid) and severe hepatic insufficiency (Hepatic-Aid) are listed in Table 4-3. The nutritional management of the latter two conditions is considered in Chapter 10.

NONNUTRITIONAL EFFECTS OF ENTERAL FEEDING

Effects on the Stomach

Bury and Jambunathan studied the effect of two elemental diets, Vivonex and Flexical, on gastric emptying in humans.[37] Intragastric bolus feedings of either 300 or 600 ml of the elemental diets produced a significant delay in gastric emptying compared to equal volumes of a blenderized diet or water. However, continuous intragastric feedings at rates of 100 to 150 ml/hr were associated with a constant rate of gastric emptying of all tested diets.[8]

Bury and Jambunathan also observed a significant inhibition of gastric acid secretion in response to intragastric feedings of elemental diets.[37] These findings are consistent with those of Rivilis and associates, who observed an eight-fold reduction in hydrogen ion output in dogs receiving an orally ingested casein hydrolysate as compared to the output in dogs receiving normal dog chow.[38]

Voitk and associates studied the protective effect of a casein hydrolysate

TABLE 4-4
Some Supplementary Formulations (Contents per 1000 kcal)

	Cal-Power (General Mills)	Casec (Mead–Johnson	Citrotein (Doyle)	Controlyte (Doyle)
Protein (gm)	0.6	237.6	60.5	Trace
Fat (gm)	0	5.4	2.6	48.0
Carbohydrate (gm)	272.0	0	184.2	143.0
Sodium (mEq)	2.4	6.0	45.8	0.9
Potassium (mEq)	0.7	2.1	26.8	0.2
Amount needed to give 1000 kcal	550.0 gm liquid	270.0 gm dry weight	263.4 gm dry weight	198.0 gm dry weight
Type of supplement	Carbohydrate source	Protein source	Protein, vitamin, mineral supplement	Low protein, low electrolyte calorie source

From Block AS, Shils ME: In Goodhart, RS, Shils ME (eds): Modern Nutrition in Health and Disease, ed 6, Philadelphia, Lea and Febiger, 1980, pp 1320–1321.

diet in pigs subjected to the stress of hemorrhagic shock.[29] A substantially reduced incidence (20 percent) of gastric stress ulcers was observed in the experimental group receiving the elemental diet as compared to that observed in the control group receiving a regular diet (90 percent). Choctaw and associates studied the effects of an elemental diet, Vivonex-HN, on the incidence of gastrointestinal bleeding in patients who had sustained burn injuries involving 20 to 80 percent of body surface area.[28] A significantly reduced incidence of all upper gastrointestinal bleeding as well as major bleeding (that is, bleeding requiring transfusion) was observed in the group of patients fed the elemental diet as compared to the group receiving a regular hospital diet (Fig. 4-1). Patients in the former group received the elemental diet as a continuous tube infusion around the clock if the burn involved 40 percent or more of the body surface area.

Effects on the Small Intestine

Both starvation and protein deprivation have adverse effects on the morphology and function of the small bowel (see Chapter 1). Since similar though less marked changes are observed when all necessary nutrients are provided intravenously (see Chapter 8), it is apparent that other factors besides malnutrition play a major etiologic role.[13,39] Evidently, nutrients in the lumen of the small bowel are important not only for the maintenance of normal intestinal mass but are also essential for normal adaptive responses to major small bowel resections.[39] Thus Levine and associates found significant changes in the small

EMF Liquid (Control Drugs)	Gevral (Lederle)	Hy-cal (Beecham–Massengill)	Lipomul-Oral (Upjohn)	Liprotein (Upjohn)
243.0	170.9	0.1	0.1	82.7
0	5.7	0.1	111.1	64.3
6.97	66.8	244.1	1.1	22.1
51.0	18.6	2.4	2.90	8.0
4.91	3.65	0.07	0.09	42.5
481.2 ml liquid	284.8 gm dry weight	407 ml liquid	166.7 ml liquid	183.7 gm dry weight
Protein source	Protein–calorie supplement	Carbohydrate source	Fat source	Calorie source

(Cont.)

bowel of rats fed intravenously compared to rats receiving the same solution orally.[13] Lower gut weight (22 percent lower), mucosal weight (28 percent lower), mucosal protein (35 percent lower), mucosal DNA (25 percent lower), and mucosal height were observed in the parenterally fed animals, which also had lower intestinal disaccharidase activity.

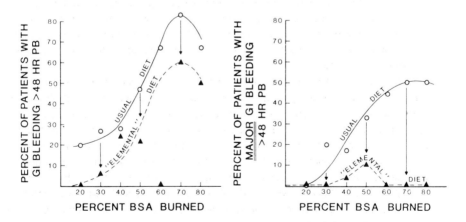

Figure 4-1. Effect of diet on gastrointestinal hemorrhage occurring after 48 hours postburn (PB) in patients with various size burns. Elemental diet is most effective in preventing major upper gastrointestinal (GI) bleeding in severely burned patients. BSA = body surface area. *(From Choctaw WT, et al: Arch Surg 115: 1073–1076, 1980. Copyright 1980, American Medical Association)*

TABLE 4-4 (Cont.)
Some Supplementary Formulations (Contents per 1000 kcal)

	Lonalac (Mead–Johnson)	Lytren (Mead–Johnson)	MCT Oil (Mead–Johnson)	Microlipid (Organon)
Protein (gm)	53.0	0	0	0
Fat (gm)	54.7	0	120.5	111.1
Carbohydrate (gm)	74.2	253.0	0	0
Sodium (mEq)	1.7	100.0	0	0
Potassium (mEq)	48.1	83.3	0	0
Amount needed to give 1000 kcal	1500 ml standard dilution or 196 gm dry weight	268 gm dry weight or 3333 ml standard dilution	120.5 gm liquid	222 ml liquid
Type of supplement	Low sodium–high protein source	Calorie and electrolyte source	Medium–chain triglycerides	Fat source

Experiments by Dworkin and associates [40] and Adams and associates[41] indicated that even the integrity of bypassed segments of bowel can be protected by ingested nutrients. However, the former investigators found that the in-continuity small intestine was heavier per centimeter than the bypassed segments of the same animal.

Apparently, ingested diets exert their trophic effect by two mechanisms: a direct effect related to contact of the intraluminal nutrients with the intestinal epithelial cells with direct utilization of the nutrients by the absorptive cells, and an indirect, systemic effect related to the release of trophic hormones.[39]

The relative effectiveness of various forms of ingested nutrients in maintaining small bowel integrity has not been studied thoroughly. Available data from animal studies indicate that solid diets are more effective than liquid formula diets. Similarly, in the short bowel syndrome, regular diets are more effective than elemental diets in stimulating compensatory hyperplasia.[39] Young and associates compared orally chow-fed rats with rats receiving continuous intragastric infusions of isocaloric amounts of Vivonex, Vivonex-HN, Flexical, or Ensure.[42] Mucosal weight, DNA, or protein concentration per segment were decreased significantly in most bowel segments of the animals receiving the liquid formula diets.

Effects on the Pancreas

The effect of liquid formula diets on exocrine pancreatic function has been analyzed by many investigators, but the data are confusing because they have

Polycose (Ross)	Pro Mix (Beatrice Scientific)	Sumacal (Organon)	Sumacal Plus (Organon)
0	227.0	0	0
0	0	0	0
250.0	22.7	250.0	312.5
12.0	18.52	4.34	4.6
2.5	116.51	2.94	4.2
263.0 gm dry weight	284.0 gm dry weight	1000 ml liquid	400 ml liquid
Oligo-saccharides	Protein source	Carbohydrate source	Concentrated carbohydrate source

been derived from studies employing varying experimental methods. Thus pancreatic function has been assessed in man, dogs, and rats receiving a variety of liquid formulas fed orally or infused into the stomach, duodenum, or jejunum. Moreover, the results have been compared with those of different control groups, including subjects who were fasted, received saline, were fed regular diets, or were treated with parenteral nutrition.

Effects of oral or intragastric feedings. McArdle and associates compared pancreatic exocrine output in orally fed dogs receiving either the elemental diet, Flexical, or regular dog food.[43] The concentration of the enzymes, amylase, lipase, and trypsinogen, did not change significantly with the elemental diet. However, a 60 percent reduction in the total volume of pancreatic juice was observed, resulting in an overall reduction in the total amount of enzyme secreted.

Neviackas and Kerstein found that when dogs were fed Vivonex orally in amounts that maintained or were associated with only slight decreases in body weight, pancreatic enzyme production fell compared to enzyme production following consumption of regular dog chow.[44] However, when the dosage of the elemental diet was increased to a level that produced weight gain, enzyme production increased and was not significantly different from that occurring with regular food.

Young and associates studied rats receiving oral chow, Vivonex, Vivonex-HN, Flexical, or Ensure.[42] Amylase activity per gram of pancreas was significantly reduced in the animals fed Vivonex, Flexical, and Ensure. Serum amylase levels were also lowered with these diets.

When dogs receiving oral Vivonex were compared with saline-fed controls, Kelly and Nahrwold found that the elemental diet stimulated a significant increase in the total volume and in the total protein and bicarbonate output from the pancreas.[45] Ragins and associates also found marked stimulation of volume, protein, and bicarbonate when dogs receiving Vivonex intragastrically were compared to fasting controls.[46]

Effects of intraduodenal feedings.   Data are also available on the pancreatic stimulating effect of intraduodenal infusion of elemental diets. Ragins found that dogs respond only with an increase in volume,[46] whereas Wolfe and associates observed an increase in protein output as well.[47] In a similar experiment, Kelly and Nahrwold also observed increased protein output, but in contrast to the other investigators found an enhanced output of bicarbonate.[45] When the latter investigators compared the stimulating effects of oral and intraduodenal Vivonex, they observed that total protein secretion was similar with both modes of feeding, but the oral feedings stimulated greater total volume and increased concentration and total output of bicarbonate. These differences may be due to the release of gastrin, secretin, and cholecystokinin following oral or intragastric feedings, whereas only cholecystokinin is released with intraduodenal feedings at the pH of Vivonex (pH 5.4).[45]

Effects of intrajejunal feedings.   Ragins and associates[46] and Ertan and associates[48] studied the response to intrajejunal feedings in dogs and man, respectively. The latter investigators found that an isotonic mixture of amino acids (pH 6.0) was as potent a stimulus to pancreatic secretion as intravenous cholecystokinin. In contrast, Ragins and associates found that no significant stimulation occurred when Vivonex (pH 5.4) was infused.[46] The difference in results may be due to the presence of carbohydrates in Vivonex, since intrajejunal glucose is known to inhibit pancreatic secretion.[46]

Finally, Kelly and Nahrwold compared the pancreatic responses to oral Vivonex, intraduodenal Vivonex, and glucose-based parenteral nutrition.[45] Parenteral nutrition had the least effect on pancreatic exocrine function. The protein and bicarbonate output was comparable to that observed in the control dogs receiving intraduodenal saline.

Tentative conclusions can be drawn from available data. It appears that various feeding regimens stimulate pancreatic exocrine secretion in the following descending order of magnitude: oral solid diets, oral elemental diets, intraduodenal elemental diets, intrajejunal elemental diets, total parenteral nutrition, and fasting.

TECHNIQUES OF ENTERAL FEEDING

Access to the Alimentary Tract
Feeding tubes may be introduced into the alimentary tract at various points using bedside or operative techniques:

1. Bedside techniques.
   a. Nasogastric intubation.
   b. Nasoduodenal intubation.
2. Operative techniques.
   a. Cervical pharyngostomy
   b. Gastrostomy
   c. Jejunostomy

Intubation of the gastrointestinal tract using a feeding tube passed through the nose is satisfactory for most patients for whom the eventual resumption of oral feeding is anticipated. When an operation is performed for an underlying surgical condition, it may be desirable to place a feeding tube at the conclusion of the procedure, thereby eliminating the need for a nasal tube, which may be irritating and less cosmetic. An operation exclusively for the purpose of establishing access for feeding generally is indicated only for patients requiring enteral nutrition indefinitely or permanently.

Intragastric feedings, either by nasogastric feeding tube or gastrostomy, have the advantage that the osmotic load reaches the duodenum in gradual fashion, limiting the incidence of the dumping syndrome.[49] However, pulmonary aspiration is the major complication to be avoided, so that candidates for intragastric feedings must be alert with gag and cough reflexes intact, and gastric emptying should be normal. Suitable patients should have conditions which allow them to assume the semi-Fowler position (30° upright) for the duration of tube feeding therapy. Thus intragastric feedings are contraindicated in comatose, stuporous, or lethargic patients, in severely debilitated or weak patients, in those with tracheostomy tubes, and in those with persistently high gastric residual volumes. Candidates for enteral nutrition who have a condition making intragastric feeding inadvisable can often be successfully managed by introducing nutrient solutions distal to the pylorus through nasoduodenal or jejunostomy tubes.

Nasogastric and nasoduodenal intubation. Enteral nutrition has been greatly advanced by the advent of small diameter feeding tubes which are constructed of materials that are pliable and nonirritating. An array of tubes which vary in construction, diameter, and length are commercially available (Table 4-5). Plastic tubes have been replaced with those constructed of mate-

TABLE 4-5
Some Commercially Available Feeding Tubes

Feeding Tube	Manufacturer	Composition	Specifications
Argyle Quest Duo-Tube*	Argyle Div., Sherwood Medical, St. Louis, MO.	Silicone Rubber	Silicone or mercury weighted tip; Fr sizes 5, 6, 8; 42" length; ensheathed in removable plastic tube.
Entriflex	Biosearch Medical Products, Inc., Raritan, N.J.	Polyurethane	Mercury weighted bolus tip; Tip and lumen surface coated with hydrophilic substance; 8 Fr; 30" and 43" lengths; stylets available.
Hydromer-Dobbhoff	Biosearch Medical Products, Inc., Raritan, N.J.	Polyurethane	Large mercury weighted bolus tip; Tip and lumen surface coated with hydrophilic substance; 8 Fr; 43" length; stylets available.
Keofeed	Hedeco, Mountain View, CA.	Silicone Rubber	Mercury weighted bolus tip available; Fr sizes 6.0, 7.3, 9.6, 14.6, 18.0; 36" and 43" lengths; pre-lubricated with pre-inserted guide.
Vivonex	Norwich-Eaton Pharmaceuticals, Norwich, NY.	Polyurethane	Tungsten weighted bolus tip; 8 Fr; 45" length.

Formerly Pro-Med.

rials that are softer, less reactive, and more resilient such as silicone rubber and polyurethane. The viscosity of the nutrient solution to be used determines the diameter of the tube employed. Commercially prepared liquid formulas generally flow easily through small-bore tubes (8 Fr or less). However, blenderized hospital diets are viscous and require larger diameter tubes; for this reason they are used infrequently at present. Patients tolerate 8 Fr tubes well, and therefore this size tube can usually be employed for feeding any of the commercially prepared enteral formulations. The elemental diets are the least viscous preparations and can be introduced through smaller diameter tubes (e.g., 5 to 6 Fr), but these are so flaccid that placement is often more difficult and dislodgement occurs more easily. The length of tube that is chosen varies, depending on whether gastric (30 to 36 inch length) or duodenal (42 to 43 inch length) feeding is desired. Many tubes have radiopaque, weighted tips to aid introduction and to reduce the incidence of dislodgement. Finally, since these tubes are very pliable, passage may be facilitated by using a stylet provided with some tubes or by attaching the feeding tube to a stiffer plastic tube (for example, with a dissolvable gelatin capsule) which is subsequently withdrawn.

A feeding tube is placed while the patient is in the semi-Fowler or sitting position (Figs. 4-2–4-6). The appropriate length to be advanced for gastric feeding can be estimated before introduction by extending the tube from the patient's earlobe to the bridge of his nose and from there to the tip of the xiphoid process. The tip of the tube is placed in the patient's nose, and the tube is slowly advanced. If feasible, the patient is asked to swallow water through a straw during the procedure. After passage, air is insufflated through the tube, and a bubbling sound on auscultation over the stomach in the left-upper quadrant suggests that the tip of the tube is properly located. However, an abdominal x-ray should always be obtained to confirm the appropriate location of the tube before feedings are started. When the tube is in the proper location, it is taped to the cheek or forehead without any tension so that the tube does not press against the nose.

For intraduodenal feedings, the tube is passed into the stomach as above, but, in addition, a 6 to 8 inch untaped loop of tubing is left extending from the nose. One or 2 inches of the tube are advanced each hour. In addition, the patient is placed in the right-lateral decubitus position to facilitate spontaneous peristaltic advancement of the tube through the pylorus into the duodenum. Placement of the tip of the tube at the pylorus under fluoroscopy may

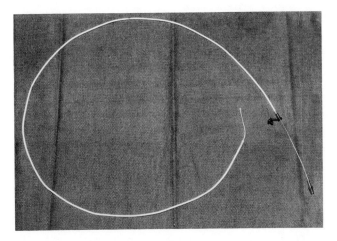

Figure 4-2. A 43 inch duodenal feeding tube (Entri-Flex), with stylet in place.

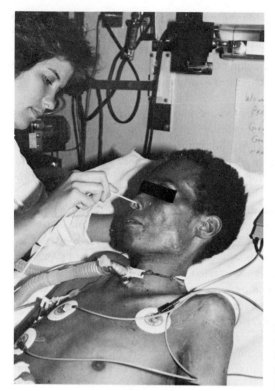

Figure 4-3. Passage of a tube for duodenal feedings. The tube is advanced into the stomach with the patient in the semi-Fowler position.

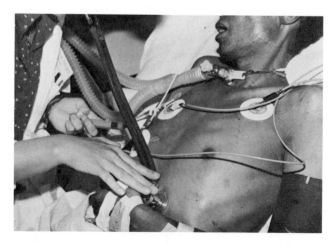

Figure 4-4. A bubbling sound over the stomach during air insufflation suggests the proper location of the tube in the stomach.

expedite passage. Again, x-ray confirmation of proper location is mandatory before feeding is begun.

When the usual methods of intubation are unsuccessful, tubes can be properly placed under direct endoscopic guidance.[50,51]

Cervical esophagastomy. Access to the alimentary tract by means of cervical esophagostomy (or pharyngostomy) is particularly applicable when performed in conjunction with extensive head and neck surgery—for example, radical mandibular resection.[52] However, this procedure also may be of value for patients requiring long-term or permanent tube feeding, since celiotomy is not required and the procedure has been performed using local anesthesia.[53] A tube esophagostomy is usually created, but a permanent stoma can be constructed, if indicated. It should be noted that this method of access does not alter the risk of pulmonary aspiration in patients otherwise subject to this complication.

Gastrostomy. Constructing a tube gastrostomy is a simple procedure associated with little additional risk when performed in conjunction with another

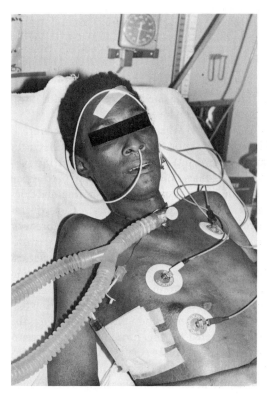

Figure 4-5. A 6 to 8 inch loop of duodenal tube extends from the nose; 1 to 2 inches of tubing are advanced each hour.

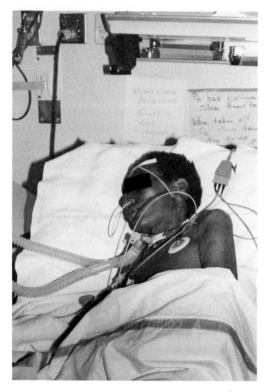

Figure 4-6. Patient is placed in the right-lateral decubitus position to facilitate passage of the tube into the duodenum.

intra-abdominal procedure. It is, therefore, indicated when the need for intra-gastric feeding is anticipated in the postoperative period.

More careful consideration is required when an operative procedure is contemplated solely for establishing access for feeding. Local anesthesia for gastrostomy (or jejunostomy) is preferred by some authors,[54–56] but the supplementary sedation and narcotic analgesia so often required may produce an obtunded patient without the benefit of the respiratory monitoring and control afforded patients receiving general endotracheal anesthesia. Consequently, general anesthesia may be preferable despite its inherent risks. Moreover, the malnourished, debilitated state of many of the patients for whom gastrostomy is indicated may increase not only the anesthetic risk but the surgical morbidity, as well. Meguid and Williams observed a 6.5 percent complication rate occurring in 46 patients receiving gastrostomies.[54] Complications included one case each of wound infection, wound dehiscence, and gastrostomy disruption. The mortality rate was 37 percent, undoubtedly reflecting the underlying condition of patients considered for this procedure. More recently, Wasiljew and associates reviewed a series of 147 patients who had undergone operation solely for the placement of a feeding gastrostomy.[55] Twenty-three patients (15.7 percent) experienced a complication, 9 of which were considered major. These latter included wound dehiscence in 4 patients, stomal leak in 3, and gastric hemorrhage in 2. Nine patients (6.1 percent) died within 30 days of operation, and 5 of the deaths were associated with pulmonary conditions such as retained secretions, lung abscess, or aspiration pneumonia.

Consequently, severely debilitated patients requiring a gastrostomy for long-term or permanent enteral nutrition may benefit from a period of preoperative nutritional repletion using nasogastric or intravenous feedings.

Jejunostomy. Nutrients infused into the jejunum generally are not subject to regurgitation, and therefore the risk of pulmonary aspiration associated with intragastric feedings is substantially reduced. Another advantage of a jejunostomy is that it provides a feeding route for patients with more proximal obstruction or disease. In addition, effective and safe nutrition has been described in the immediate postoperative period following abdominal surgery using newer techniques, including needle–catheter jejunostomy (see Chapter 10). Finally, jejunostomy feedings may produce less pancreatic stimulation than intragastric or intraduodenal diets.

In contrast, symptoms of the dumping syndrome associated with hyperosmolar nutrient solutions are more likely to occur with intrajejunal perfusion. In addition, digestion may be depressed because of inadequate mixing of the intrajejunal nutrient formulas with bile and pancreatic juice.[9] Thus predigested formulations are indicated.

The anesthetic and surgical considerations discussed in relation to gastrostomy are equally applicable here.

Initiating Therapy

An appropriate nutrient formulation is chosen on the basis of the patient's status. Considerations include caloric requirements, fluid and electrolyte balance, site of alimentary tract access, and digestive and absorptive function of the small intestine.

Following selection of a nutrient formulation, the volume of full-strength solution which will meet calorie and protein demands is determined (see Chapter 3). Initially, the enteral feeding solution is diluted to one-third strength, placed in an enteral feeding container (Table 4-6), and then delivered continuously to the patient in the semi-Fowler position (30° upright). Infusion is begun at a rate of 50 ml/hr. Thereafter, the rate of administration is increased in increments of 25 ml/hr every 12 hours, so that by 24 to 36 hours, a rate which will provide the predetermined volume generally has been attained. As therapy proceeds, the patient is observed for manifestations of intolerance, such as abdominal cramps, diarrhea, glucosuria, and, in the case of intragastric feedings, gastric retention. The presence of any of these findings early in the course of therapy is an indication to slow the rate of advancement to allow a longer period of adaption. Until sufficient volume of solution is tol-

TABLE 4-6
Some Commercially Available Enteral Feeding Containers

Container	Manufacturer	Capacity (ml)
Dobbhoff Enteric Feeding Bag	Biosearch Medical Products, Inc.	1000
Ethox/Barron Gavage-Bag Set	Ethox Corporation	1000
Flexitainer Enteral Nutrition Container	Ross Laboratories	1000
Flip Top Tube Feeding Bag	Seamless Hospital Products Co.	1500
Kangaroo Feeding Set	Chesebrough-Pond's Inc.	1000
Keofeed Enteric Feeding Bag	Hedeco	1500,500
Plastic Irrigating Container	American McGaw	500
Stomach Feeding Bag	Concord	500
Travenol Enteral Feeding Container	Travenol Laboratories	1300
Vivonex Delivery System	Norwich-Eaton	1000

Adapted from Matarese LE: Nutritional Support Services, vol 2, February 1982, pp 48–52.

erated, supplemental intravenous fluid may be required to maintain water and electrolyte balance.

After the dilute solution is administered for 24 hours at full volume with no manifestations of intolerance, the concentration of the nutrient solution is increased to two-thirds strength for 12 to 24 hours, and finally to full strength without alteration in volume.[57]

Use of hyperosmolar nutrient solutions may be associated with hypernatremic dehydration. Consequently, patients are allowed to consume clear liquids *ad libitum* if feasible. In other patients, especially those unable to communicate thirst, free water should be given[8] and can be provided with the tube feedings. Water is conveniently administered when the feeding bag is changed, usually every 8 hours. Thus, 100 to 200 ml of water can be administered over 30 minutes every 8 hours through the feeding tube. This arrangement has the advantage that the tube is flushed after each container of liquid formula is administered, thus reducing the incidence of tube occlusion.

The amounts of vitamins and minerals provided in the volume of nutrient formulation prescribed should be noted in order to determine the necessity for supplements. In addition, vitamin K may be required by some patients, depending on the feeding product being used.

Continuous, around-the-clock delivery of liquid formula diets is preferred to intermittent, bolus feedings.[10,57-59] Greater total daily volumes are tolerated with less gastric retention[37] and fewer manifestations of dumping syndrome. In addition, some data suggest that the nutrient value is enhanced when substrates are infused continuously.[60,61] Administration by gravity infusion is usually successful; however, some patients develop manifestations of intolerance which can be relieved or ameliorated by employing an infusion pump to provide a more constant rate of flow.[10] Jones and associates found that the diarrhea and abdominal distention and cramping that developed during gravity infusion could be controlled when an infusion pump was used, but the incidence of regurgitation and aspiration was unaffected.[62] When a pump is employed, a model should be chosen that develops pressures which do not exceed the bursting strength of the feeding tube being used.

MONITORING PATIENTS RECEIVING ENTERAL FEEDINGS

Patients receiving enteral feedings should be closely monitored. The feeding tube and delivery system are checked regularly, and patients are observed for signs of intolerance. Gastric residual volumes are measured in patients receiving intragastric feedings every 3 to 4 hours initially and then once a day after

TABLE 4-7
Monitoring Schedule for Patients Receiving Enteral Feedings: Required Procedures

Procedure	Before Therapy	Daily	Mondays	Tuesdays	Wednesdays	Thursdays	Fridays	Notes
Body weight	X	X						
Input/output record		X						
Fractional urine (sugar/acetone)		X						
CBC	X		X			X		Daily first 5 to 7 days
Chemistry panel*	X		X			X		Daily first 5 to 7 days
Liver panel†	X		X			X		
Prothrombin time	X					X		
Gastric residuals‡		X						Every 3 to 4 hours until full volume is tolerated

*Serum glucose, urea, creatinine, sodium, potassium, chloride, bicarbonate, calcium, phosphate, magnesium, total protein, and albumin.
†Serum bilirubin, SGOT, SGPT, and alkaline phosphatase.
‡In patients receiving intragastric feedings.

TABLE 4-8
Monitoring Schedule for Patients Receiving Enteral Feedings:
Optional Determinations

Procedure	Interval
Nutritional assessment*	Weekly
Skin tests	Every 2 to 3 weeks
Serum B-12†	Initially and p.r.n.
Serum folate†	Initially and p.r.n.
Serum iron†	Initially and p.r.n.
Transferrin	Weekly
Zinc	Weekly
Copper	Weekly
24-hour urine nitrogen‡	1 to 7 times per week

*See Chapter 1.
†Essential if anemia present.
‡Nitrogen balance studies based on urinary nitrogen invalidated by significant fecal nitrogen losses, as in diarrhea.

full volume has been reached and tolerated. During the initial period of adaption, the residual volume after 3 to 4 hours should not exceed two times the volume infused during the preceding 1 hour. After full volume has been reached, residuals should not exceed 150 to 200 ml. If high residual volumes are present, feedings should be withheld for a few hours, or a decreased infusion rate may be necessary. Persistent delay in gastric emptying contraindicates intragastric feedings.

Metabolic parameters are also closely monitored (Tables 4-7 and 4-8). Pretreatment studies identify metabolic abnormalities requiring correction prior to or during treatment. Periodic evaluation during the course of enteral feeding permits early diagnosis of metabolic derangements related to nutritional repletion (for example, hyperglycemia) as well as those due to the infusion of hyperosmolar solutions (for example, prerenal azotemia).

COMPLICATIONS OCCURRING DURING ENTERAL NUTRITION

Untoward effects occurring during the course of enteral nutrition can be classified as mechanical, gastrointestinal, or metabolic, as follows:[10]

1. Mechanical.
   a. Depressed cough.
   b. Dysphagia.

    c. Esophageal erosions.
    d. Esophageal reflux.
    e. Esophagitis.
    f. Increased airway secretions.
    g. Otitis media.
    h. Parotitis.
    i. Pharyngitis.
    j. Pulmonary aspiration.
    k. Rhinitis.
    l. Tube obstruction.
2. Gastrointestinal.
    a. Abdominal cramping.
    b. Abdominal distention.
    c. Aggravation of GI disease.
    d. Diarrhea.
    e. Malabsorption.
    f. Nausea and vomiting.
3. Metabolic.
    a. Essential fatty acid deficiency.
    b. Fluid and electrolyte disturbances.
    c. Hyperglycemia.
    d. Hyperosmolar dehydration.
    e. Hyperosmolar nonketotic coma.
    f. Hypoprothrombinemia.
    g. Inadvertent IV administration.
    h. Liver abnormalities.
    i. Prerenal azotemia.
    j. Vitamin deficiencies.

Regurgitation with pulmonary aspiration of stomach contents is among the most serious potential complications. Thus candidates for intragastric feedings must be carefully chosen and observed, as previously discussed. Most of the remaining mechanical problems relate to the irritating effect of nasal feeding tubes. Morbidity has been reduced substantially by the advent of the new generation of small-diameter, pliable tubes.

Gastrointestinal symptoms of the dumping syndrome—vomiting, cramping, distention, and diarrhea—are usually responses to the infusion of hyperosmolar feeding mixtures. However, diarrhea may also be due to prolonged antibiotic administration, malabsorption, lactose intolerance, and microbial contamination of the nutrient formula. The last factor is avoided by freshly preparing nutrient solutions and refrigerating them until used. Enteral feedings, usually administered from a 1 liter bottle or bag, can be safely infused at room temperature over an 8 to 12 hour period.[63] Diarrhea due to the dumping syndrome may be controlled by pump-assisted administration, by switching to another nutrient preparation, or by adding antidiarrheal agents—such as codeine, paregoric, or diaphenoxylate with atropine (Lomotil)—to the nutrient solution.[57] In addition, Frank and Green reported marked reduction in the incidence of diarrhea when they added the bulk laxative Metamucil, 7 gm/liter, to the liquid formula.

If underlying gastrointestinal conditions, such as enterocutaneous fistulas or Crohn's disease, are aggravated by tube feedings, then these feedings should be discontinued in favor of parenteral nutrition.

Potential metabolic derangements associated with enteral feedings are similar to those reported in patients receiving intravenous feedings (see Chapter 8). Blood sugar should be carefully monitored. Hyperglycemia is managed by the administration of insulin. However, when insulin is given, uninterrupted flow of the nutrient solution is critical to avoid hypoglycemia. Prerenal azotemia and hypernatremia may occur in patients receiving hyperosmolar feedings, especially in those unable to communicate thirst and those with impaired renal concentrating ability.[65,66] These conditions also may be associated with or aggravated by the fluid losses accompanying glycosuria, diarrhea, or enterocutaneous fistulas. Prerenal azotemia is averted by the routine administration of free water, as well as by careful replacement of obligatory losses. Patients with cardiac and renal diseases are subject to fluid overload; feeding with a higher caloric density preparation may be advisable in these patients.

Patients receiving elemental diets which contain minimal amounts of fat may develop a deficiency of fat-soluble vitamins and essential fatty acids after prolonged periods of treatment.[67-70] These problems can be averted by administering vitamin supplements and linoleic acid supplements. The latter can be provided in the form of margarine or eggs added to feedings or by the intravenous infusion of a fat emulsion.

Young and associates studied liver histology in rats who had received 2 weeks of intragastric feedings with regular chow, Vivonex, Vivonex-HN, Flexical, or Ensure.[71] Total liver lipid accumulation was significantly increased in rats fed Vivonex, and the percent of liver lipid was significantly greater in rats fed either Vivonex or Flexical. The etiology of these changes is uncertain, but a kwashiorkor-like mechanism or inadequate fat supplementation have been suggested.[72]

SUMMARY

Enteral feeding is an effective method of therapy for many patients unable to consume sufficient nutrients orally. The utility of this technique has been enhanced by the availability of a wide range of nutrient formulations, allowing the therapeutic program to be tailored to the requirements of a given patient. In fact, many patients referred for parenteral nutrition may be managed successfully using the enteral route.[73]

The safety and effectiveness of enteral nutrition can be improved by the use of small-bore, pliable feeding tubes, by continuous rather than intermittent infusion of the liquid diet, and by diligent metabolic monitoring.

REFERENCES

1. Mettler CC: History of Medicine. Philadelphia; Blakiston Co, 1947, p 870.
2. Graves RJ: Lectures on the Practice of Medicine. Dublin, New Sydenham Society, 1884.
3. Wilmore DW, McDougal WS, Peterson JP: Newer products and formulas for alimentation. Am J Clin Nutr 30:1498–1505, 1977.
4. Coleman W, DuBois EF: Clinical calorimetry, VII: Calorimetric observations on the metabolism of typhoid patients with and without food. Ann Intern Med 15:887–892, 1915.
5. Cuthbertson DP: Observations on disturbance of metabolism produced by injury to the limbs. Q J Med 1:233–246, 1932.
6. Robinson CH: Liquid diets. J Clin Nutr 1:476–477, 1953.
7. Shils ME: Enteral nutrition by tube. Cancer Res 37:2432–2439, 1977.
8. Bury KD: Elemental diets, in Fischer JE (ed): Total Parenteral Nutrition. Boston, Little, Brown and Co, 1976, pp 395–411.
9. Shils ME, Randall HT: Diet and nutrition in the care of the surgical patient, in Goodhart RS, Shils ME (eds): Modern Nutrition in Health and Disease, ed 6. Philadelphia, Lea and Febiger, 1980, pp 1082–1124.
10. Heymsfield SB, Bethel RA, Ansley JD, et al: Enteral hyperalimentation: An alternative to central venous hyperalimentation. Ann Intern Med 90:63–71, 1979.
11. Bloch AS, Shils ME: Appendix, in Goodhart RS, Shils ME (eds): Modern Nutrition in Health and Disease, ed 6. Philadelphia, Lea and Febiger, 1980, pp 1244–1330.
12. Broitman SA, Zamcheck N: Nutrition in diseases of the intestines, in Goodhart RS, Shils ME (eds): Modern Nutrition in Health and Disease, ed 6. Philadelphia, Lea and Febiger, 1980, pp 912–952.
13. Levine GM, Deren JJ, Steiger E, Zinno R: Role of oral intake in maintenance of gut mass and disaccharide activity. Gastroenterology 67:975–982, 1974.
14. Stephenson LS, Latham MC: Lactose intolerance and milk consumption: The relation of tolerance to symptoms. Am J Clin Nutr 27:296–303, 1974.
15. Voitk AJ, Echave V, Brown RA, Gurd FN: Use of elemental diet during the adaptive stage of short gut syndrome. Gastroenterology 65:419–426, 1973.
16. Shapiro R: Historical development and limitations of "elemental" diets, in Shils ME (ed): Defined-formula Diets for Medical Purposes. Chicago, American Medical Association, 1977, pp 1–5.
17. Stephens RV, Randall T: Use of a concentrated, balanced liquid elemental diet for nutritional management of catabolic states. Ann Surg 170:642–667, 1969.

18. Winitz M, Graff J, Gallagher N, et al: Evaluation of chemical diets as nutrition for man-in-space. Nature 205:741–743, 1965.
19. Thompson WR, Stephens RV, Randall HT, Bowen JR: Use of the "space diet" in the management of a patient with short bowel syndrome. Am J Surg 117:449–459, 1969.
20. Randall HT: Enteric feeding, in Ballinger WF, Collins JA, Drucker WR, et al (eds): Manual of Surgical Nutrition. Philadelphia, WB Saunders Co, 1975, pp 267–284.
21. Bounous G, Hugon J, Gentile JM: Elemental diet in the management of the intestinal lesion produced by 5-fluorouracil in the rat. Can J Surg 14:298–311, 1971.
22. Hugon JS, Bounous G: Elemental diet in the management of the intestinal lesions produced by radiation in the mouse. Can J Surg 15:18–26, 1972.
23. Bury KD, Stephens RV, Randall HT: Use of a chemically defined, liquid, elemental diet for nutritional management of fistulas of the alimentary tract. Am J Surg 121:174–183, 1971.
24. Rocchio MA, Cha CM, Haas KF, Randall HT: Use of chemically defined diets in the management of patients with high output gastrointestinal cutaneous fistulas. Am J Surg 127:148–156, 1974.
25. Voitk AJ, Echave V, Brown RA, et al: Elemental diet in the treatment of fistulas of the alimentary tract. Surg Gynecol Obstet 137:68–72, 1973.
26. Voitk AJ, Echave V, Feller JH, et al: Experience with elemental diet in the treatment of inflammatory bowel disease. Arch Surg 107:329–333, 1973.
27. Voitk AJ, Brown RA, Echave V, et al: Use of an elemental diet in the treatment of complicated pancreatitis. Am J Surg 125:223–227, 1973.
28. Choctaw WT, Fujita C, Zawacki BE: Prevention of gastrointestinal bleeding in burn patients: A role for "elemental" diet. Arch Surg 115:1073–1076, 1980.
29. Voitk AJ, Chiu C, Gurd FN: The prophylactic effect of an elemental diet on porcine stress ulcers. Surg Forum 22:328–329, 1971.
30. Silk DBA, Fairclough PD, Clark ML, et al: Use of a peptide rather than free amino acid nitrogen source in chemically defined "elemental" diets. JPEN 4:548–553, 1980.
31. Sleisenger MH, Kim YS: Protein digestion and absorption. N Engl J Med 300:659–663, 1979.
32. Mathews DM, Adibi SA: Peptide absorption. Gastroenterology 71:151–161, 1976.
33. Adibi SA: Intestinal transport of dipeptides in man: Relative importance of hydrolysis and intact absorption. J Clin Invest 50:2266–2275, 1971.
34. Adibi SA: Oligopeptides as carriers of amino acids for chemically defined diet, in Shils ME (ed): Defined-formula Diets for Medical Purposes. Chicago, American Medical Association, 1977, pp 15–20.
35. Fogel, MR, Ravitch MM, Adibi SA: Absorptive and digestive function of the jejunum after jejunoileal bypass for treatment of human obesity. Gastroenterology 71:729–733, 1976.
36. Imondi AR, Stradley RP: Utilization of enzymatically hydrolyzed soybean protein and crystalline amino acid diets by rats with exocrine pancreatic insufficiency. J Nutr 104:793–801, 1974.
37. Bury KD, Jambunathan G: Effects of elemental diets on gastric emptying and

gastric secretion in man. Am J Surg 127:59–64, 1974.

38. Rivilis J, McArdle AH, Wlodek GK, Gurd FN: Effect of an elemental diet on gastric secretion. Ann Surg 179:226–229, 1974.

39. Tilson MD: Pathophysiology and treatment of the short bowel syndrome. Surg Clin North Am 60:1273–1284, 1980.

40. Dworkin LD, Levine GM, Farber NJ, Spector MH: Small intestinal mass of the rat is partially determined by indirect effects of intraluminal nutrition. Gastroenterology 71:626–630, 1976.

41. Adams PR, Copeland EM, Dudrick SJ, et al: Maintenance of gut mass in bypassed bowel of orally vs. parenterally nourished rats. J Surg Res 24:421–427, 1978.

42. Young EA, Cioletti LA, Winborn WB, et al: Comparative study of nutritional adaption to defined formula diets. Am J Clin Nutr 33:2106–2118, 1980.

43. McArdle AH, Echave W, Brown RA, Thompson AG: Effect of elemental diet on pancreatic secretion. Am J Surg 128:690–692, 1974.

44. Neviackas JA, Kerstein MD: Pancreatic enzyme response with elemental diet. Surg Gynecol Obstet 142:71–74, 1976.

45. Kelly GA, Nahrwold DL: Pancreatic secretion in response to an elemental diet and intravenous hyperalimentation. Surg Gynecol Obstet143:87–91, 1976.

46. Ragins H, Levenson SM, Signer R, et al: Intrajejunal administration of an elemental diet at neutral pH avoids pancreatic stimulation. Am J Surg 126:606–614, 1973.

47. Wolfe BM, Keltner RM, Kaminski DL: The effect of an intraduodenal elemental diet on pancreatic secretion. Surg Gynecol Obstet 140:241–245, 1975.

48. Ertan A, Brooks FP, Ostrow JD, et al: Effect of jejunal amino acid perfusion and exogenous cholecystokinin on the exocrine pancreatic and biliary secretions in man. Gastroenterology 61:686–692, 1971.

49. Barrocas A: ABC's of tube feeding. J Louisiana State Med Soc 130:83–86, 1978.

50. Tomczak D, Engel JJ: Rapid intubation of the small intestine under direct endoscopic guidance. Gastrointest Endosc 25:51–52, 1979.

51. Chung RSK, Denbesten L: Improved technique for placement of intestinal feeding tube with the fibreoptic endoscope. Gut 17:264–266, 1976.

52. Graham WP III, Royster HP: Simplified cervical esophagostomy for long term extraoral feeding. Surg Gynecol Obstet 125:127–128, 1967.

53. Farndon JR, Taylor RMR: Cervical pharyngostomy. Ann R Coll Surg Engl 59:507–510, 1977.

54. Meguid MM, Williams LF: The use of gastrostomy to correct malnutrition. Surg Gynecol Obstet 149:27–32, 1979.

55. Wasiljew BK, Ujiki GT, Beal JM: Feeding gastrostomy: Complications and mortality. Am J Surg 143:194–195, 1982.

56. Matino JJ: Feeding jejunostomy in patients with neurologic disorders. Arch Surg 116:169–171, 1981.

57. Kaminski MV: Enteral hyperalimentation. Surg Gynecol Obstet 143:12–16, 1976.

58. Meguid MM: The enteral alternative. Contemp Surg 13:41–52, 1978.

59. Hiebert JM, Brown A, Anderson RG et al: Comparison of continuous vs. intermittent tube feedings in adult burn patients. JPEN 5:73–75, 1981.

60. Fitzpatrick GF, Meguid MM, O'Connell RC et al: Nitrogen sparing by carbohydrate in man: Intermittent or continuous enteral compared with continuous parenteral glucose. Surgery 78:105–113, 1975.
61. Munro HN: Carbohydrate versus fat versus protein calories (panel discussion), in Greep JM, Soeters PB, Wesdorp RIC, et al (eds): Current Concepts in Parenteral Nutrition. The Hague, Martinus Nijoff Medical Division, 1977, p 357.
62. Jones BJM, Payne S, Silk DBA: Indications for pump assisted enteral feeding. Lancet 1:1057–1058, 1980.
63. White WT III, Acuff TE, Sykes TR, Dobbie RP: Bacterial contamination of enteral nutrient solution: A preliminary report. JPEN 3:459–461, 1979.
64. Frank HA, Green LC: Successful use of a bulk laxative to control the diarrhea of tube feeding. Scand J Plast Reconstr Surg 13:193–194, 1979.
65. Gault MH, Dixon ME, Doyle M, Cohen WM: Hypernatremia, azotemia, and dehydration due to high-protein tube feeding. Ann Intern Med 68:778–791, 1968.
66. Telfer N: The effect of tube feeding on the hydration of elderly patients. J Gerontol 20:536–543, 1965.
67. Freeman JB, Egan MC, Millis BJ: The elemental diet. Surg Gynecol Obstet 142:925–932, 1976.
68. Farthing MJG, Jarrett EB, Williams G, Crawford MA: Essential fatty acid deficiency after prolonged treatment with elemental diet. Lancet 2:1088–1089, 1980.
69. Dodge JA, Salter DG, Yassa JG: Essential fatty acid deficiency due to artificial diet in cystic fibrosis. Br Med J 2:192–193, 1975.
70. Dodge JA, Yassa JG: Essential fatty acid deficiency after prolonged treatment with elemental diet. Lancet 2:1256–1257, 1980.
71. Young EA, Cioletti LA, Winborn WB, Weser E: The effect of defined formula diets on fat accumulation in rat liver. Gastroenterology 74:1115, 1978.
72. Young EA, Cioletti LA, Traylor JB, Balderas V: Gastrointestinal response to nutrient variation of defined formula diets. JPEN 5:478–484, 1981.
73. Bethel RA, Jansen RD, Heymsfield SB, et al: Nasogastric hyperalimentation through a polyethylene catheter: An alternative to central venous hyperalimentation. Am J Clin Nutr 32:1112–1120, 1979.

5

Parenteral Nutrition: General Principles

Parenteral nutrition, total parenteral nutrition (TPN), hyperalimentation, intravenous hyperalimentation (IVH), and *intravenous feedings* are terms used synonymously to denote methods of providing all required nutrients intravenously. The solutions administered are designed to meet not only basal and maintenance requirements, but also the additional demands of growth and development, nutritional repletion, and stress states, including critical illness and injury.

HISTORICAL BACKGROUND

Effective nutrition by vein independent of alimentary tract function is a relatively recent achievement. In a remarkable series of investigations, Dudrick, Rhoads, Wilmore, and their associates, working at the University of Pennsylvania in the 1960s, demonstrated for the first time that their system of "intravenous hyperalimentation" could support normal growth and development in children and not only maintain nutrition in adults, but replete malnourished, starving, and seriously ill individuals as well.[1-3]

The scientific foundation upon which the Pennsylvania group built in bringing parenteral nutrition to clinical fruition had been laid during the preceding 100 years. The landmark developments in parenteral nutrition can be listed as follows:[4]

- 1891: Intravenous infusion of saline in man by Matas.
- 1896: Intravenous infusion of glucose in man by Biedl and Kraus.
- 1911: First use of intravenous glucose for nutritional purposes by Kausch.
- 1913: Nitrogen balance achieved in animals by Henriques and Anderson using intravenous casein hydrolysates.
- 1915: Intravenous infusion of fats in animals by Murlin and Lusk.
- 1925: Discovery of pyrogens in intravenous solutions by Siebert.
- 1939: Protein hydrolysates infused in man by Elman with positive nitrogen balance.
- 1946: Protein-sparing effect of glucose in fasting man described by Gamble.
- 1949: Central venous nutrition in dogs by Rhode, Parkins, and Vars.
- 1952: Percutaneous subclavian catherization in man by Aubaniac.
- 1955: Essential and nonessential amino acid requirements for man identified by Rose after 14 years of investigation.
- 1961: Development of a nontoxic fat emulsion, Intralipid, by Wretlind.
- 1967: Normal growth and development in animals receiving hyperalimentation, reported by Dudrick.
- 1967: Positive nitrogen balance achieved by Dudrick in patients receiving long-term total parenteral nutrition.
- 1968: Normal growth and development in an infant receiving intravenous nutrients, reported by Wilmore.

Saline was first infused intravenously for treatment of shock by Matas in 1891. In 1896, Biedl and Kraus injected glucose intravenously,[4] but it was not until 1911 that glucose was first infused specifically for nutritional purposes.[5] In the 1940s, Gamble demonstrated the protein-sparing effect of glucose in fasting man, thereby establishing the scientific basis for glucose infusion in fasting patients.[6] Although the magnitude of nitrogen catabolism was reduced, nitrogen equilibrium could not be established, and maximum protein-sparing benefit was achieved with approximately 100 gm of glucose. These pioneering studies by Gamble emphasized the necessity for providing not only calories, but also protein for patients starved for prolonged periods.

Successful efforts to provide protein intravenously in animals date to 1913, when Henriques and Anderson reported nitrogen equilibrium in animals receiving infusions of protein hydrolysates.[7] However, it was not until 1939 that such hydrolysates were successfully administered to patients. In that year, Elman and Weiner reported positive nitrogen balance in several patients receiving mixtures of glucose and amino acids, which were obtained from an acid hydrolysate of casein fortified with tryptophan and methionine or cystine.[8] Each liter of the nutrient solution contained about 20 gm of amino acids and 80 gm of glucose.

During the next 25 years, efforts to consistently achieve positive nitrogen balance and nutritional repletion in seriously ill patients were hampered by a variety of factors. Infusing glucose and amino acids in isotonic solutions in sufficient amounts to meet all energy and protein demands required excessive volumes of fluid. This problem was ameliorated to some extent by the concomitant administration of diuretics, but still only limited positive nitrogen balance was achieved.[4,9] It was hoped that the greater caloric density of an isotonic fat emulsion, Lipomul, would allow the infusion of sufficient calories in a physiologic volume. However, this preparation, derived from cottonseed oil, proved too toxic. Addition of protein hydrolysates to concentrated glucose solutions resulted in preparations that could potentially provide all required nutrients in practical volumes, but such hypertonic solutions inevitably produced thrombophlebitis of the peripheral veins. Nevertheless, the potential clinical value of such concentrated solutions was perceived by Dudrick and his associates.[2,3] These investigators designed a series of laboratory and clinical experiments in which such hypertonic solutions were infused directly into the superior vena cava, where they were rapidly diluted. They used modifications of techniques for central venous catheterization described in dogs by Rhode et al,[10] and subsequently in humans by Aubaniac.[4] These experiments culminated in the development of parenteral nutrition as we know it today.

In 1971, synthetic crystalline amino acids became clinically available, and the amino acid mixtures were patterned after Rose's recommendations for essential and nonessential amino acids.[11] Clinically safe fat emulsions derived from soybean oil and safflower oil were approved for use in the United States in 1975 and 1979, respectively.

INDICATIONS FOR AND CONTRAINDICATIONS TO PARENTERAL NUTRITION

Although the clinical benefits derived from substrates infused intravenously appear equivalent to those derived from substrates absorbed from the alimentary tract (see Chapters 3 and 9), the less invasive and less expensive alimentary route is preferable when feasible. However, many hospitalized patients have conditions in which alimentary tract nutrition is inadequate, inadvisable, or would require an operative procedure (e.g., gastrostomy or jejunostomy) to establish access (see Chapter 4). It is for these patients that parenteral feedings should be considered.

Normally nourished patients unable to eat for as long as 7 to 10 days generally do not require parenteral nutrition; the protein-sparing effect of 100 to 150 gm of glucose provided in a 5 percent solution is sufficient. Patients in this category include those undergoing gastrointestinal surgery in whom several days of ileus can be anticipated postoperatively. However, if the resumption of adequate intake is not imminent after 7 to 10 days, parenteral feedings are recommended.

In contrast, normally nourished patients should receive TPN promptly when initial evaluation discloses gastrointestinal dysfunction which is expected to persist beyond 7 to 10 days. In addition, malnourished or markedly hypercatabolic patients (e.g., those with severe burns, sepsis, or multiple trauma) with gastrointestinal dysfunction are begun on parenteral nutrition immediately.

In some patients parenteral feedings have benefits in addition to nutrition *per se.* When all nutrients are provided intravenously, a state of bowel rest can be achieved in which the mechanical and secretory activity of the alimentary tract declines to basal levels. This may be beneficial in the management of gastrointestinal fistulas and acute inflammatory disease, including pancreatitis and regional enteritis. In addition, parenteral nutrition may be useful as a "medical colostomy." The reduction or elimination of the fecal stream associated with intravenous feedings may benefit patients with inflammation or decubitus ulcers adjacent to the anus or an intestinal stoma or fistula.[12]

The nutritional management of specific diseases is discussed in Chapter 10.

Acute metabolic derangements should be treated before parenteral nutrition is begun. In addition, TPN should not be used during periods of acute hemodynamic instability or during surgical operations since the nutrient solution may be used inadvertently for fluid resuscitation.[12] Furthermore, parenteral nutrition is not indicated for patients with malnutrition due to a rapidly progressive disease which is not amenable to curative or palliative therapy. For example, parenteral feedings are not warranted in patients with disseminated malignancy when it has been determined that there is no reasonable probability of benefit from surgery, chemotherapy, or irradiation. Thus parenteral nutrition is not used to sustain the hopelessly ill.

Because nutrient solutions must be prepared precisely under sterile conditions, and since patients receiving such solutions require careful and frequent metabolic monitoring, parenteral nutrition should be used only in institutions with personnel and facilities able to meet these criteria of safe practice. Although a parenteral nutrition "team" may improve efficiency, it is not an essential feature of effective or safe therapy.

FORMULATION OF NUTRIENT SOLUTIONS

To maintain or restore nutrition parenterally requires the infusion of nonprotein calories and a protein source, usually amino acids, in sufficient amounts, in the appropriate ratio, and in a volume of fluid consistent with normal water balance.

Vitamins, electrolytes, trace metals, and insulin may be added to solutions of glucose and amino acids, but reagents must be chosen which take into account their mutual chemical, physical, and pharmacologic compatibilities. In contrast, fat emulsions, providing calories and essential fatty acids, are usually infused separately.

The requirements for the various nutrients depend on the initial nutritional status of the patient and his underlying disease process (see Chapter 3). Although the precise requirements of an individual patient can be determined by metabolic balance studies and direct or indirect calorimetry, such techniques generally are not employed in routine clinical practice. However, on the basis of data from clinical investigations applying such methods to patients with various diseases, injuries, and degrees of stress, it is possible to estimate requirements and, on the basis of these estimates, to formulate basic nutrient solutions of essentially fixed composition which can be used to meet the needs of most patients. The requirements for a given patient can usually be met by varying the volume of the basic formulation and by making simple adjustments in the electrolyte content of the solution.

The efficient use of nitrogen for protein synthesis requires the provision of sufficient nonprotein calories to meet full caloric expenditure.[13] For optimal nitrogen utilization, ill patients require in the range of 100 to 200 nonprotein calories for each gram of nitrogen infused.[14] Nutrient solutions are, therefore, prepared with such a calorie–nitrogen ratio, and the volume prescribed is determined by the caloric requirement of the patient.

In clinical practice, the caloric requirement is usually estimated from tables or from simple formulas (e.g., the Harris–Benedict equation), which are adjusted for activity and stress (see Chapter 3). Although nitrogen requirements can likewise be determined or estimated, nitrogen needs are usually met as a consequence of the fixed calorie–nitrogen ratio of the nutrient solutions. Thus, as the volume of infusate is increased to meet increased caloric demands, the additional nitrogen requirements, which generally parallel the rising caloric needs,[15] are likewise met.

Although such standard preparations of nutrient solutions can be used to satisfy the needs of most individuals, fluid-restricted patients, those with renal or hepatic failure, or severely hypermetabolic patients may require special nutrient formulations. The nutritional management of specific diseases is discussed in Chapter 10.

CALORIE SOURCES IN PARENTERAL NUTRITION

Carbohydrates

Glucose.   Glucose is the carbohydrate of choice in parenteral nutrition, since it is the normal physiologic substrate, it naturally occurs in blood, and it is abundant, inexpensive, and readily purified for parenteral administration. It can be given in high concentrations (25 percent or more) and in large amounts which are well tolerated by most patients after a period of adaption.[16-18] The rate of glucose metabolism in human subjects varies between 0.4 and 1.4 gm/kg/hr. Under normal conditions, the average adult utilizes about 0.5 gm/kg/hr.[19,20] Impaired glucose tolerance is observed in patients with diabetes mellitus, in patients with diseases associated with insulin resistance (e.g., sepsis, severe burns, or other injuries), and in patients receiving corticosteroids. Although glucose is virtually nontoxic, the hypertonic solutions generally employed may be associated with potentially serious complications usually related to alterations in blood glucose levels (see Chapter 8).

Glucose may be used as the exclusive nonprotein calorie source, or it may be administered in varying proportions with lipids. When used with lipids, at least 100 to 150 gm of glucose should be supplied in order to achieve maximum impact on nitrogen balance and to provide the energy substrate for certain key tissues, notably the central nervous system, peripheral nerves, red blood cells, white blood cells, active fibroblasts, and certain phagocytes, which normally require glucose as the sole or major energy source.[21-23] When lesser amounts of glucose are infused, the required substrate is provided via gluconeogenesis.

Glucose should be infused together with the nitrogen source, since simultaneous feeding of these substances is associated with an improvement in nitrogen balance as compared to their consecutive or separate administration.[23-25]

Glucose for parenteral infusion is commercially available in concentrations from 5 to 70 percent and is provided as glucose monohydrate with a caloric density of 3.4 kcal/gm (Table 5-1).

Fructose. Fructose has been considered a potential substitute for glucose, with the hope that it would provide an insulin-independent carbohydrate of

TABLE 5-1
Glucose Preparations

Glucose Concentration (%)	Caloric Content (kcal/liter)	Osmolarity (mOsm/liter)
5	170	252
10	340	505
20	680	1010
40	1360	2020
50	1700	2525
60	2040	3030
70	2380	3535

TABLE 5-2
Metabolic Properties of Carbohydrates for Parenteral Nutrition

	Glucose	Fructose	Sorbitol	Xylitol
Normal metabolite	+	±		
Metabolized by cells in all tissues	+			
Increases nitrogen utilization	+	+	+	+
Antiketogenic	+	+	+	+
Partial insulin independency		+	+	+
Increased lactic acid		+	+	+
Incrased uric acid		+	+	+
Depletion of liver ATP		+	+	+
Depletion of liver inorganic phosphate		+	+	+
Urinary loss			+	+
Oxalate crystal deposition				+

From Shenkin A, Wretlind A: In Richards JR, Kinney JM (eds): Nutritional Aspects of Care in the Critically Ill. Edinburgh, Churchill Livingstone, 1977, p 347.

value—for example, in diabetics or during stress states associated with glucose intolerance.[26] However, fructose metabolism is insulin-independent only for the initial stage of transit and initial phosphorylation. Since the majority of adult tissues do not readily utilize the fructose directly but can utilize it only after conversion to glucose, mainly in the liver, fructose appears to offer no advantage over glucose. Moreover, rapid infusion of fructose has been reported to induce lactic acidosis, hypophosphatemia, depletion of hepatic adenine nucleotides, and elevation of bilirubin and uric acid (Table 5-2).[18,23,26-29]

Sorbitol and xylitol. The sugar alcohols, sorbitol and xylitol, have also been evaluated as glucose substitutes because of their partial insulin independence. However, both sorbitol, which is dehydrogenated to fructose, and xylitol are insulin-independent again only in the initial steps of their metabolism, and neither substance can be directly used by peripheral tissues prior to conversion to glucose in the liver.[29] In addition, each has been associated with serious metabolic derangements (Table 5-2).

In contrast to these findings, Ahnefeld and associates presented data from Germany indicating that the complications associated with fructose and xylitol are dose-related.[30] Using a combination of fructose, glucose, and xylitol in a ratio of 2:1:1 with a total dose of 0.5 gm/kg/hr, these investigators reported improved glucose tolerance without exogenous insulin and no side-effects.

Maltose. Maltose, a disaccharide consisting of two linked glucose units, would be an attractive calorie source, since a maltose solution contains twice as many calories as an isosmotic solution of glucose. Available data are limited. Young and Weser demonstrated that a bolus infusion of 25 gm of maltose was as efficiently utilized as a similar amount of glucose.[31] However, when Forster and Hoos continuously infused maltose at a rate of 0.25 gm/kg/hr, urinary loss exceeded 25 percent of the administered load, making this substance unsuitable for parenteral nutrition, at least at present.[32]

Lipids

Lipids are a major component of oral diets, generally providing about 40 percent of total caloric intake. In addition to reflecting the composition of the normal oral diet, use of lipid emulsions in intravenous regimens is attractive because the high caloric density (9 kcal/gm) and isotonicity of these preparations allow high caloric infusions in relatively small volumes via peripheral veins.

Early experience with lipids using the cottonseed oil emulsion Lipomul was unsatisfactory because of the toxicity of this preparation, which was evidently due to the large size of the emulsified particles and to the emulsifying agents, soybean phospholipid and pluronic F68.[33] More recently, however, emulsions of soybean oil (Intralipid) and safflower oil (Liposyn) have been prepared which are safe for clinical use. These newer preparations are purified plant oils emulsified in water. Egg phospholipids are added to regulate the size of the fat particles, stabilize the emulsion, and prevent fusion of the oil drops. Glycerol is added to make the emulsion isosmotic, since oil-in-water emulsions have no osmolal effect.[34] The resulting fat droplets have characteristics which are similar to those of naturally occurring chylomicrons found in the circulation after absorption of dietary lipid from the small intestine.[33-35] Thus the particle size and the plasma elimination characteristics of these fat emulsions appear comparable to those of chylomicrons.

Studies of the elimination kinetics of soybean emulsion triglycerides indicate that at very low concentrations, the rate of removal from the plasma is dependent on the triglyceride concentration. Above a certain critical concentration representing saturation of binding sites of lipoprotein lipase enzymes, a maximum elimination capacity is reached which is independent of concentration. This maximum elimination capacity is influenced by the clinical state of the patient. It is increased during periods of starvation, after trauma, and in severely catabolic states. Hallberg found that the rate of clearance after a 15 hour fast varied from 1.9 to 5.7 gm of triglyceride/kg/day, and this increased to 4.43 to 8.23 gm of triglyceride/kg/day after a 39 hour fast. If the 39 hour fast was associated with a surgical procedure, then the clearance of lipid rose to between 5.06 and 30.39 gm triglyceride/kg/day.[33-37]

That intravenously infused fats are used for energy is demonstrated by an increase in heat production, an increase in oxygen consumption, a decrease in respiratory quotient, and the appearance of carbon-14 (C-14) in the expired air of patients receiving C-14-labeled fat.[36]

Soybean emulsion (Intralipid). Intralipid is available as a 10 or 20 percent emulsion derived from soybean triglycerides and is comprised of 10 or 20 percent soybean oil, 1.2 percent egg yolk phospholipids, 2.25 percent glycerin, and pyrogen-free water. These preparations are mixtures of neutral triglycerides of predominantly unsaturated fatty acids. The major component fatty are linoleic (50 percent), oleic (26 percent), palmitic (10 percent), and linolenic (9 percent). The osmolarity of the 10 and 20 percent emulsions is approximately 280 and 330 mOsm/liter, respectively. Both preparations contain fat particles of approximately 0.5 μ size. The total caloric value of the 10 percent emulsion, including triglyceride, phospholipid, and glycerol, is 1.1 kcal/ml, of which about 0.1 kcal/ml is derived from added glycerol. The corresponding value for the 20 percent emulsion is 2 kcal/ml, of which 0.1 kcal/ml is provided by the added glycerol (Table 5-3).

Intralipid has been used clinically for nearly 20 years in Europe and for about 7 years in the United States. This lengthy experience forms the basis for most of the current knowledge concerning the clinical utility, metabolism, safety, and toxicity of intravenous fat emulsions.

Toxicity associated with intravenous infusion has been minimal. The most frequent acute adverse reactions are fever, sensations of warmth, chills, shivering, chest or back pain, anorexia, and vomiting. Hallberg and associates observed fever in 2.7 percent of 2781 infusions, chills in 1 percent, and sensation of warmth in 8 percent.[36]

Greene and associates reported that 6 of 20 patients had decreases in pulmonary membrane diffusion lasting several hours following Intralipid infusion.[38] There were no significant changes in Po_2 values, nor were there any clinical signs of ischemia. The changes in pulmonary diffusion reverted to basal levels when serum lipids were cleared. The transient elevation of serum lipids seen with fat infusion was prevented by the administration of heparin (60 IU/kg), which as a consequence prevented the changes in pulmonary function. In contrast, Wilmore and associates found no changes in pulmonary function in a series of burn patients receiving single or multiple units of the fat emulsion.[39] Blood gas tensions and pulmonary diffusion capacity, determined by xenon-133 perfusion–diffusion and carbon monoxide rebreathing techniques, were normal.

Adverse reactions associated with chronic infusions of Intralipid are quite uncommon. Clinically significant alterations in liver function are unusual, but transient mild elevations of transaminase and alkaline phosphatase levels have been observed. Histologic and ultrastructural changes associated with chronic infusions included focal proliferation and enlargement of the Kupffer cells, accumulation of fat pigment within the cytoplasm, and the occurence of a brown, lipofuscin-like pigment in the reticuloendothelial cells ("intravenous fat pigment").[33,36,40,41]

Anemia has been reported following prolonged administration of soybean emulsion,[33] but Hansen and associates found no significant alterations in

TABLE 5-3
Intravenous Fat Emulsions

	10% Safflower Oil	20% Safflower Oil	10% Soybean Oil	20% Soybean Oil
Proprietary name	Liposyn 10%	Liposyn 20%	Intralipid 10%	Intralipid 20%
Triglyceride source (wt./vol.)	Safflower oil 10%	Safflower oil 20%	Soybean oil 10%	Soybean oil 20%
Emulsifier (wt./vol)	Egg phospholipids 1.2%	Egg phospholipids 1.2%	Egg phospholipids 1.2%	Egg phospholipids 1.2%
Tonicity adjuster (wt./vol.)	Glycerol 2.5%	Glycerol 2.5%	Glycerol 2.25%	Glycerol 2.25%
Osmolarity	300 mOsm/liter	340 mOsm/liter	280 mOsm/liter	330 mOsm/liter
Fat droplet size	0.4 μ	0.4 μ	0.5 μ	0.5 μ
Total caloric value	1.1 kcal/ml	2.0 kcal/ml	1.1 kcal/ml	2.0 kcal/ml
Calories from fat	1.0 kcal/ml	1.9 kcal/ml	1.0 kcal/ml	1.9 kcal/ml
Calories from added glycerol	0.1 kcal/ml	0.1 kcal/ml	0.1 kcal/ml	0.1 kcal/ml
Major component fatty acids				
Linoleic	77%	77%	50%	50%
Oleic	13%	13%	26%	26%
Palmitic	7%	7%	10%	10%
Linolenic	0.5%	0.5%	9%	9%
Stearic	2.5%	2.5%	2.5%	2.5%

hemoglobin or hematocrit in their study of 292 patients.[42] Studies of blood co-agulation in association with fat infusions have been variable. Hypercoagula-bility and decreased platelet adhesiveness have been noted by some investigators but remained unconfirmed by others.[33,41]

The most serious adverse effects have been observed in infants or chil-dren. The "fat overload syndrome" associated with the cottonseed emulsion Lipomul has rarely been observed with Intralipid infusion. However, Belin and associates reported the occurrence of this syndrome in a 5-month-old in-fant receiving Intralipid, 4 gm/kg/day.[43] After 114 days, the child developed marked hyperlipidemia, gastrointestinal disturbances, hepatosplenomegaly with impaired hepatic function, anemia, thrombocytopenia, prolonged clot-ting time, elevated prothrombin time, and spontaneous bleeding. The syn-drome resolved completely within 6 weeks.

Of 159 pediatric patients reviewed by Hansen and associates, 4 had se-vere reactions.[42] One child had an allergic reaction with wheezing, erythema, wheals, and urticaria occurring after 11 days of the fat emulsion. The remain-ing 3 children evidently received excessive doses of fat emulsion. One of these children developed tachycardia, tachypnea, hepatomegaly, elevated SGOT and LDH, and thrombocytopenia. The second child had hepatosplenomegaly leukopenia, and thrombocytopenia, and the third had hepatosplenomegaly and jaundice.

Safflower oil (Liposyn).   This recently available fat emulsion contains 10 or 20 percent safflower oil, 1.2 percent egg phospholipids, and 2.5 percent glyc-erin and is a mixture of neutral triglycerides of predominantly unsaturated fatty acids. The fatty acids forming the major components of the emulsion are linoleic, 77 percent; oleic, 13 percent; palmitic, 7 percent; and stearic, 2.5 per-cent. Linolenic acid content is 0.5 percent. Liposyn 10 percent has an osmo-larity of about 300 mOsm/liter and a total caloric value, including fat, phospholipid, and glycerol, of 1.1 kcal/ml. The corresponding values for the 20 percent emulsion are 340 mOsm/liters and 2.0 kcal/ml. Both preparations contain emulsified fat particles of approximately 0.4 μ in diameter (Table 5-3). The experience with Liposyn is less extensive than that with Intralipid, but it is assumed to be comparable to the soybean emulsion both in its mode of metabolism and in its very low incidence of clinical toxicity.[44-46]

The use of fat emulsions in parenteral nutrition is discussed in Chapters 7, 9, and 10.

Alcohol
Ethanol provides 7.1 kcal/gm and is therefore a potential high-energy source for use in parenteral nutrition. Infusion of up to 1.5 gm/kg/day with corre-sponding blood levels below 50 mg percent appears well tolerated, at least in younger patients.[17,47,48] Although occasionally used to supplement caloric in-take, there is little enthusiasm for the use of ethanol as a primary or major

caloric source because of its dose-related adverse pharmacologic effects.[18,20,49,50] It is toxic to muscle, brain, and liver, and the effect on the latter occurs despite adequate nutrition.[50,51]

Through its inhibitory effect on gluconeogenesis, ethanol can induce hypoglycemia, a response which is more pronounced in starved patients.[47] In addition, ethanol impairs leukocyte migration and phagocytosis, and its degradation product, acetaldehyde, is exhaled and is irritating to the pulmonary alveoli. The sedative and inebriating effects of ethanol are generally undesirable, and tolerance is reduced even with dilute infusions in older, debilitated patients. Its use in those with pulmonary disease, pancreatitis, or cirrhosis is especially undesirable.[18,48,50]

Solutions of 5 or 10 percent ethanol in 5 percent dextrose are commercially available.

PROTEIN SOURCES IN PARENTERAL NUTRITION

Achieving nutritional homeostasis or repletion is dependent not only on sufficient calories but also on the quantity and quality of dietary protein whether provided orally or intravenously. Optimal impact on nitrogen balance requires a sufficient quantity of both the essential and nonessential amino acids, the relative requirements for which vary with age and clinical state (see Chapter 3). Whereas nitrogen equilibrium can be achieved in normal adults when about 15 percent of the amino acid intake is in the form of essential amino acids, nutritional repletion in adult patients requires a spectrum of amino acids comparable to that required by a 10- to 12-year-old child. Thus the proportion of essential amino acids required increases to about 33 percent. (See Table 3-6). In addition, all of the amino acids present in human protein must also be available in suitable amounts for protein synthesis. Although the carbon skeletons of the nonessential amino acids can be synthesized from available precursors, improved nitrogen balance occurs when a combination of several, but not necessarily all, of the nonessential amino acids is supplied in addition to the essential amino acids.[48,52]

Thus nutrient solutions for use in adult patients should have a pattern of amino acids reflecting these general requirements. Currently available preparations which provide a biologically utilizable nitrogen source material for protein synthesis include the protein hydrolysates and solutions of pure crystalline L-amino acids (Tables 5-4, 5-5, and 5-6).

Hydrolysates of casein or fibrin were the protein sources originally used during the development of parenteral nutrition. Protein hydrolysates are mixtures of free amino acids and low molecular weight peptides derived from the acid hydrolysis of fibrin or the enzymatic digestion of casein by pancreatic proteolytic enzymes. That these preparations can supply the nitrogenous sub-

TABLE 5-4
Commercially Available Protein Sources for Parenteral Nutrition

Generic Name	Proprietary Name	Manufacturer
5% Casein Hydrolysate	Amigen (Travamin), 5%	Travenol Laboratories
5% Casein Hydrolysate with 5% dextrose	Amigen (Travamin), 5% with dextrose, 5%	Travenol Laboratories
10% Casein Hydrolysate	Amigen (Travamin), 10%	Travenol Laboratories
10% Crystalline amino acids	Aminosyn, 10%	Abbott Laboratories
10% Crystalline amino acids	Travasol, 10%	Travenol Laboratories
8.5% Crystalline amino acids	Aminosyn, 8.5%	Abbott Laboratories
8.5% Crystalline amino acids	FreAmine III, 8.5%	McGaw Laboratories
8.5% Crystalline amino acids	Travasol, 8.5%	Travenol Laboratories
8.5% Crystalline amino acids with electrolytes	Aminosyn, 8.5% with electrolytes	Abbott Laboratories
8.5% Crystalline amino acids with electrolytes	Travasol, 8.5% with electrolytes	Travenol Laboratories
8% Crystalline amino acids	Veinamine	Cutter Laboratories
7% Crystalline amino acids	Aminosyn 7%	Abbott Laboratories
7% Crystalline amino acids with electrolytes	Aminosyn, 7% with electrolytes	Abbott Laboratories
5.5% Crystalline amino acids	Travasol, 5.5%	Travenol Laboratories
5.5% Crystalline amino acids with electrolytes	Travasol, 5.5% with electrolytes	Travenol Laboratories
5% Crystalline amino acids	Aminosyn, 5%	Abbott Laboratories
3.5% Crystalline amino acids with electrolytes*	Aminosyn, 3.5% M	Abbott Laboratories
3.5% Crystalline amino acids with electrolytes*	Travasol, 3.5% M	Travenol Laboratories
3% Crystalline amino acids with electrolytes*	Freamine III, 3%	McGaw Laboratories
5.4% Essential amino acids†	Nephramine, 5.4%	McGaw Laboratories
5.2% Essential amino acids†,‡	Aminosyn-RF	Abbott Laboratories

*Designed for "protein-sparing" therapy (see Chapter 10).
†Designed for use in renal failure (see Chapter 10).
‡Supplemented with arginine.

TABLE 5-5
Proportion of Essential Amino Acids in Protein Sources, Compared to Requirements for Normal Individuals*

	Requirements (%) ADULTS	Requirements (%) CHILDREN 10-12 YR	Travenol Casein Hydrolysates (%)	Abbott Amino Acids (%)†	Cutter Amino Acids (%)	McGaw Amino Acids (%)†	Travenol Amino Acids (%)
Isoleucine	1.8	3.7	5.3	7.5	6.2	6.9	4.8
Leucine	2.5	5.6	8.4	9.7	4.3	9.1	6.3
Lysine	2.2	7.5	6.4	5.3‡	6.7‡	7.3‡	4.7‡
Methionine + cysteine	2.4	3.4	2.7	4.1	5.3	5.5	5.9
Phenylalanine + tyrosine	2.5	3.4	5.3	5.0	5.0	5.6	6.7
Threonine	1.3	4.4	3.9	5.4	2.0	4.0	4.2
Tryptophan	0.65	0.46	0.7	1.7	1.0	1.5	1.8
Valine	1.8	4.1	6.4	8.3	3.2	6.6	4.6
Total essential amino acids§	15.2	32.6	39	47	34	47	39

*Calculated as a percentage of total amino acids.
†Not applicable to products for renal failure.
‡Calculated as lysine as a free base.
§Does not include histidine.

strates necessary to support normal growth and development and positive nitrogen balance has been demonstrated conclusively.

Despite demonstrated clinical effectiveness, however, protein hydrolysates have several drawbacks. The composition of the hydrolysates reflects the composition of the parent protein rather than the requirements of the patient. About 40 percent of the nitrogen provided is present as peptides, a variable proportion of which (36 to 53 percent) is believed to be metabolically unavailable and excreted in the urine.[18,53] Consequently, the evaluation of the essential amino acid pattern of hydrolysates is somewhat imprecise.[54] The protein hydrolysates contain a variable amount of ammonia, which may produce adverse clinical effects. Hyperammonemia is of special significance in infants, as it can result in mental retardation. In addition, protein hydrolysates occasionally produce allergic reactions.

At present, solutions of crystalline amino acids are used in nearly all centers as the nitrogen source in TPN regimens. These newer preparations provide all of the nitrogen in the form of free L-amino acids, and no ammonia or peptide products are present. The composition of these solutions has been tailored to include the essential and nonessential amino acids in amounts and proportions thought necessary to meet the demands of most hospitalized patients. Special solutions of amino acids for specific diseases (for example, renal failure) are also available.

In comparing the two nitrogen sources, Anderson and associates found that 0.8 gm/kg of casein hydrolysate was required to achieve nitrogen equilibrium in malnourished adults, whereas only 0.4 gm/kg of amino acids was required when a solution of crystalline amino acids was used which had a composition approximating the needs of a normally growing child.[55]

Commercially available parenteral protein sources include 5 and 10 percent casein hydrolysates and solutions of crystalline L-amino acids in various concentrations (Table 5-4). The composition of the amino acid solutions varies somewhat, depending on the manufacturer, but for each manufacturer the proportions of individual and total essential and nonessential amino acids are constant regardless of the total amino acid concentration (Tables 5-5 and 5-6). Thus the percent composition of 3.5, 5.5, 8.5, and 10 percent Travasol are identical. Varying protein concentrations allow the same amounts and proportions of amino acids to be provided in more or less total fluid volume.

SOURCES OF ESSENTIAL FATTY ACIDS

Linoleic acid is the primary and perhaps the only essential fatty acid for man. This substance is effective in preventing and alleviating the recognized clinical abnormalities attributed to fatty acid deficiency (see Chapter 8). The role of linolenic acid in human nutrition is unclear (see Chapter 3).[56] Intravenous

TABLE 5-6
Composition of Parenteral Protein Sources

	Amigen, 10%	Amigen, 5%	Aminosyn, 10%	Travasol, 10%	Aminosyn, 8.5%	Aminosyn, 8.5% with Electrolytes	Freamine III, 8.5%	Travasol, 8.5%	Travasol, 8.5% with Electrolytes	Veinamine	Aminosyn, 7%	Aminosyn, 7% with Electrolytes	Travasol, 5.5%	Travasol, 5.5% with Electrolytes	Aminosyn, 5%	Aminosyn, 3.5% M	Travasol, 3.5% M	Freamine III, 3%	Nephramine, 5.4%	Aminosyn-RF
Protein concentration (%)	10	5	10	10	8.5	8.5	8.5	8.5	8.5	8	7	7	5.5	5.5	5	3.5	3.5	3	5.4	5.2
Nitrogen (gm/100 ml)	1.3	0.65	1.57	1.68	1.33	1.33	1.30	1.42	1.42	1.33	1.10	1.10	0.924	0.924	0.786	0.55	0.59	0.46	0.64	0.79
Essential amino acids (mg/100 ml)																				
L-Isoleucine	520	260	720	480	620	620	590	406	406	493	510	510	263	263	360	252	168	210	560	462
L-Leucine	820	410	940	620	810	810	770	526	526	347	660	660	340	340	470	329	217	270	880	726
L-Lysine (salt)	620	310	720	580	624	624	870	492	492	667	510	510	318	318	360	252	203	310	900	—
L-Lysine (free base)*	?	?	513	464	445	445	620	394	394	534	363	363	255	255	257	179	163	219	640	535
L-Methionine	260	130	400	580	340	340	450	492	492	427	280	280	318	318	200	140	203	160	880	726
L-Phenylalanine	400	200	440	620	380	380	480	526	526	400	310	310	340	340	220	153	217	170	880	726
L-Threonine	380	190	520	420	460	460	340	356	356	160	370	370	230	230	260	182	147	120	400	330
L-Tryptophan	70	35	160	180	150	150	130	152	152	80	120	120	99	99	80	56	63	46	200	165
L-Valine	620	310	800	460	680	680	560	390	390	253	560	560	252	252	400	280	161	200	640	528

Nonessential amino acids (mg/100 ml)																				
L-Alanine	300	150	1280	2080	1100	1100	600	1760	1760	0	900	900	1140	1140	640	448	728	210	0	0
L-Arginine	360	180	980	1040	850	850	810	880	880	749	690	690	570	570	490	343	364	290	0	600
Aspartic acid	700	350	0	0	0	0	0	0	0	400	0	0	0	0	0	0	0	0	0	0
L-Cysteine	0	0	0	0	0	0	20	0	0	0	0	0	0	0	0	0	0	7	20	0
L-Histidine	260	130	300	440	260	260	240	372	372	237	210	210	241	241	150	105	154	85	250	429
Glutamic acid	2600	1300	0	0	0	0	0	0	0	426	0	0	0	0	0	0	0	0	0	0
Glycine	220	110	1280	2080	1100	1100	1190	1760	1760	3387	900	900	1140	1140	640	448	728	420	0	0
L-Proline	900	450	860	420	750	750	950	356	356	107	610	610	230	230	430	300	147	340	0	0
L-Serine	600	300	420	0	370	370	500	0	0	0	300	300	0	0	210	147	0	180	0	0
L-Tyrosine	120	60	44	40	44	44	0	34	34	0	44	44	22	22	44	31	14	0	0	0
Electrolytes																				
Calcium (mEq/liter)	10	5	0	0	0	0	0	0	0	0	0	0	0	0	0	0	0	0	0	0
Magnesium (mEq/liter)	4	2	0	0	0	0	0	0	10	6	0	10	0	10	0	3	5	5	0	0
Potassium (mEq/liter)	31	19	5.4	0	66	5.4	0	0	60	30	5.4	66	0	60	5.4	13	15	24.5	0	5.4
Sodium (mEq/liter)	60	35	0	0	70	70	10	52	70	40	88	70	35	70	60	47	25	35	6	0
Acetate (mEq/liter)	?	?	148	87	90	142	0	34	135	50	0	124	22	100	60	68	54	44	44	105
Chloride (mEq/liter)	44	20	0	40	35	98	0	0	70	50	0	96	0	70	0	40	25	40	0	0
Phosphate (mM/liter)	30	15	0	0	15	15	10	0	30	0	0	15	0	30	0	0	7.5	3.5	0	0
Osmolarity (mOsm/liter)	860	430	1000	1060	850	1160	810	860	1160	950	700	1013	520	850	500	460	450	405	440	475

*Calculated from salt forms and actually present in solution.

131

sources of linoleic acid include safflower oil (Liposyn) and soybean emulsion (Intralipid). Only the latter supplies significant amounts of linolenic acid (Table 5-3). Linoleic acid may also be provided by the topical application of safflower seed oil.[57,58] The requirement for linoleic acid for adults has been estimated to range between 2.5 and 20 gm/day.[35,59,60] Shils recommends providing at least 4 percent of calories as linoleic acid.[61]

TRACE ELEMENT SOLUTIONS

Many trace elements have been identified in human tissues, but the essentiality of the various individual elements has not been conclusively determined. At present, it is suggested that parenteral nutrition solutions include supplements of iodine, zinc, copper, chromium, and manganese. Cobalt is provided as vitamin B12. Guidelines for the administration of these micronutrients have been established (see Table 3-7),[62] but the determination of dosage is imprecise owing to the variable concentration of these substances occurring as contaminants in the commercially available nutrient solutions.[63] In addition, human requirements undoubtedly fluctuate, depending on the clinical status of the patient.

Until recently, patients received periodic transfusions of blood or plasma to supply trace elements, a method often providing inadequate amounts. Alternatively, trace elements were omitted entirely, sometimes resulting in clinical deficiency states which have only recently been recognized. At present, trace elements may be provided in multiple trace element solutions which are prepared in the hospital pharmacy. Aliquots of such a preparation are then added to the parenteral nutrition solution. An example of such a multiple trace element solution appears in Table 5-7.

TABLE 5-7
USC Trace Element Solution*

Compound	Amount Dissolved in a 150 ml Solution†,‡	Ionic Concentration
$ZnCl_2$ (48.3% zinc)	620 mg	2.0 mg/ml
$CuSO_4 \cdot 5H_2O$ (25.5% copper)	300 mg	0.5 mg/ml
$MnSO_4 \cdot H_2O$ (32.5% manganese)	200 mg	0.4 mg/ml
NaI (84.75% iodine)	10 mg	56 μg/ml
$CrCl_3 \cdot 6H_2O$ (19.5% chromium)	4.6 mg	6 μg/ml
Distilled Water	q.s. ad 150 ml	—

*Dosage: 2 ml/day for stable adults. See Chapter 3 for discussion of requirements. Modified after Shils [18].
†Solution transferred to sterile vials through a 0.22 millipore filter and then autoclaved.
‡pH adjusted to 2.0 with HCl.

TABLE 5-8
Individual Trace Metal Additives for Parenteral Nutrition*

Compound	Ionic Concentration	Recommended Daily Dosage†
Zinc chloride	Zinc, 1 mg/ml	4–6 ml
Chromic chloride	Chromium, 4 μg/ml	3 ml
Manganese chloride	Manganese, 0.1 mg/ml	4 ml
Cupric chloride	Copper, 0.4 mg/ml	3 ml

*Available from Abbott Laboratories, North Chicago, ILL., and USV Laboratories, Tuckahoe, N.Y.
†See Chapter 3 for intravenous requirements.

Multielement solutions have the advantage that they can be prepared in large volumes, and the trace elements can all be provided by a single addition to the nutrient solution. On the other hand, such mixtures of fixed composition have the drawback that dosage cannot be individualized, and overdosage is possible when the need for one element is appreciably higher than that for the other trace elements present in the formulation.[62]

Individual solutions providing zinc, manganese, copper, and chromium are now commercially available (Table 5-8).

Since zinc and chromium are excreted in the urine, these substances should be reduced or omitted from the nutrient solutions when renal function is impaired. Similarly, when biliary tract obstruction is present, intake of copper and manganese should be reduced or omitted, because these elements are excreted primarily in the bile.[62]

Although some recommend iron supplements, others withhold iron from critically ill or nutritionally depleted patients because of the frequent lack of bone marrow response in the critically ill and the increased susceptibility and severity of infection associated with high circulating iron levels in malnourished patients.[26,64,65] Bothe and associates recommend blood transfusions when iron deficiency anemia occurs.[65] In contrast, iron supplements may be given to stable patients after nutritional repletion. Under the latter circumstances, iron deficiency can be treated with iron dextran infused through a separate intravenous line. Following a test dose, the entire calculated corrective dose can be given in normal saline over 4 to 6 hours.[66,67]

VITAMINS

Vitamin regimens have varied from center to center because of the uncertainty of intravenous requirements and the altered needs associated with malnutrition and various disease states. Early protocols recommended the

TABLE 5-9
Parenteral Vitamin Preparations (Vitamins/ml)

Vitamins	Berocca C	Bejex	Folbesyn	MVI Concentrate	MVI-12
A (IU)	—	—	—	2000	330
D (IU)	—	—	—	200	20
Thiamine, B1 (mg)	5	2	5	10	0.3
Riboflavin, B2 (mg)	5	2	5	2	0.36
Niacin, B3 (mg)	40	50	37.5	20	4
Pantothenic acid, B5 (mg)	10	10	5	5	1.5
Pyridoxine, B6 (mg)	10	1	7.5	3	0.4
B12 (μg)	—	5	7.5	—	0.5
Ascorbic acid, C (mg)	50	100	150	100	10
E (IU)	—	—	—	1	1
Folic acid (μg)	—	—	500	—	40
Biotin (mg)	0.1	—	—	—	6

administration of combinations of commercially available vitamin preparations (Table 5-9) in an attempt to meet requirements for both the water-soluble and the fat-soluble vitamins.[7,26,61,68] However, in 1975, guidelines for parenteral vitamin administration were proposed by the Nutrition Advisory Group of the Department of Foods and Nutrition of the American Medical Association (see Table 3-8),[69] and on the basis of these guidelines, a new intravenous multivitamin preparation, MVI-12 (USV Pharmaceutical Corporation), has been formulated (Table 5-9). Ten ml/day of this preparation meet the AMA recommendations.

Patients with multiple vitamin deficiencies or with markedly increased requirements may be given multiples of the AMA recommended daily dosage for 2 or more days, as indicated by clinical status. Supplementation of the daily multivitamin dosage with one or more specific vitamins may be necessary in cases of specific vitamin deficiencies. Separate intramuscular administration of vitamin K is recommended for patients not receiving anticoagulants.[69]

To prevent excessive excretion of water-soluble vitamins, the daily dosage should be infused over a number of hours.[68] Vitamins are generally added to the first liter of the nutrient solution each day.

FLUID AND ELECTROLYTE BALANCE

Nutrients must be provided in a volume consistent with maintaining or restoring water balance. Thus fluid requirements are based on pre-existing excess or deficiency states, ongoing losses, and cardiac and renal function. Patients with normal fluid balance and normal cardiorenal function can receive up to 4000 ml or more per day of nutrient solution, depending on their calorie and nitrogen requirements. Sodium requirements are influenced by the same factors that affect fluid requirements (see Chapter 3).

In contrast, requirements for the major intracellular ions—potassium, magnesium, and phosphate—bear a significant relationship to caloric and nitrogen intake and the nutritional state of the patient. As the anabolic state is achieved with nutritional therapy, these ions are deposited or incorporated in the newly synthesized cells, and deficiencies of these elements in the extracellular fluid routinely develop when insufficient amounts are provided in the nutrient solutions.

Jeejeebhoy found that balance was maintained in patients on long-term parenteral nutrition when these average amounts were provided daily: potassium, 86 mEq; magnesium, 29 mEq; and phosphorus, 46 mEq.[35] In their study of phosphate balance in parenteral nutrition patients, Sheldon and Grzyb found that normal serum levels of inorganic phosphate could be maintained when 15 to 25 mEq (8 to 14 mM) of phosphate as potassium dihydrogen phosphate were administered with each 1000 nonprotein kcal.[70] Calcium equilibrium can be achieved in most patients when approximately 5 mg (0.25 mEq)/kg is provided.[71,72]

These recommendations, detailed in Chapter 3, are average figures derived from studies of series of patients receiving parenteral nutrition. The requirements for any given individual patient vary, depending on the pre-existing nutritional status and the underlying disease process. Thus conscientious metabolic monitoring is required and provides the basis for making adjustments in the composition of the nutrient solution to meet the demands of the individual patient. In this way, metabolic complications can be avoided. Monitoring protocols for the various TPN systems are discussed in Chapters 6 and 7.

INSULIN

Many patients receiving concentrated glucose solutions require insulin to maintain normal blood glucose levels and to achieve maximum utilization of this energy substrate. Acute hyperglycemic episodes are managed by intravenous or subcutaneous administration of crystalline insulin. Maintenance insulin, however, is best provided by the addition of an appropriate amount to the nutrient solution by the pharmacist at the time of solution preparation. Although some insulin loss may occur when insulin is added to parenteral nutrition solutions,[73,74] such loss can be overcome by increasing the dose. On the other hand, this method has the advantage that alterations in the rate of glucose infusion, for whatever reason, are automatically accompanied by concomitant and appropriate alteration in the rate of insulin administration.

ALBUMIN

Although parenterally administered albumin gradually undergoes degradation, yielding nitrogen-containing residues capable of supporting the anabolic state, the essential amino acid content of albumin is poor, and its half-life, 18 days, is too long for it to be an immediate or efficient source of utilizable protein. Therefore, albumin is not used for nutritional purposes, but it is administered to increase or maintain colloid osmotic pressure so that concomitantly administered amino acids, rather than being diverted to albumin synthesis, will be readily available for tissue protein synthesis.[26,75]

SYSTEMS OF TOTAL PARENTERAL NUTRITION

At present, 2 systems of total parenteral nutrition are used clinically. The "glucose system" provides all calories as glucose and requires central venous administration. In the "lipid system," lipid is the major, though not exclusive, caloric source. Solutions in this system can be infused through peripheral veins. The indications, the methods of preparation and administration, and the relative advantages and disadvantages of these 2 systems are described in Chapters 6, 7, and 9.

REFERENCES

1. Dudrick SJ, Rhoads JE: New horizons for intravenous feeding. JAMA 215:939–949, 1971.
2. Dudrick SJ, Wilmore DW, Vars HM: Long-term total parenteral nutrition with growth in puppies and positive nitrogen balance in patients. Surg Forum 18:356–357, 1967.
3. Dudrick SJ, Wilmore DW, Vars HM, Rhoads JE: Long-term total parenteral nutrition with growth, development, and positive nitrogen balance. Surgery 64:134–142, 1968.
4. Rhoads JE: The history of nutrition, in Ballinger WF, Collins JA, Drucker WR, et al (eds): Manual of Surgical Nutrition. Philadelphia, WB Saunders, 1975, pp 1–9.
5. Abbott WM: Parenteral nutrition, in Hardy JD (ed): Textbook of Surgery: Principles and Practice. Philadelphia, Lippincott, 1977, pp 168–176.
6. Gamble JL: Physiologic information gained from studies on the life raft ration. Harvey Lect 42:247–273, 1946–47.
7. Fleming CR, McGill DB, Hoffman HN II, Nelson RA: Total parenteral nutrition. Mayo Clin Proc 51:187–199, 1976.

8. Elman R, Weiner DO: Intravenous alimentation with special reference to protein (amino acid) metabolism. JAMA 112:796–802, 1939.

9. Rhoads JE: Diuretics as an adjuvant in disposing of extra water employed as a vehicle in parenteral hyperalimentation. Fed Proc 21:389, 1962.

10. Rhode CM, Parkins WM, Vars HM: Nitrogen balances of dogs continuously infused with 50 percent glucose and protein preparations. Am J Physiol 159:415–425, 1949.

11. Rose WC, Wixom RL, Lockhard HB, Lambert GF: The amino acid requirement of man, XV: The valine requirement: summary and final observations. J Biol Chem 217:987–995, 1955.

12. Dudrick SJ, Ruberg RL, Long JM, et al: Uses, nonuses, and abuses of intravenous hyperalimentation, in Cowan GSM, Scheetz WL (eds): Intravenous Philadelphia, Lea and Febiger, 1972, pp 111–121.

13. Heird WC, Winters RW: Total parenteral nutrition: The state of the art. J Pediatr 86:2–16, 1975.

14. Kinney JM: Hyperalimentation. Acta Anaesthesiol Scand [Suppl] 55:127–130, 1974.

15. Long CL, Schaffel N, Geiger JW, et al: Metabolic response to injury and illness: Estimation of energy and protein needs from indirect calorimetry and nitrogen balance. JPEN 3:452–457, 1979.

16. Geyer RP: Parenteral nutrition. Physiol Rev 40:150–186, 1960.

17. Lee HA: Intravenous nutrition. Br J Hosp Med 2:719–728, 1974.

18. Shils ME: Guidelines for total parenteral nutrition. JAMA 220:1721–1729, 1972.

19. Dudrick SJ, MacFadyen BV Jr, VanBuren CT, et al: Parenteral Hyperalimentation: Metabolic problems and solutions. Ann Surg 176:259–264, 1972.

20. Ryan JA Jr: Complications of total parenteral nutrition, in Fischer JE (ed): Total Parenteral Nutrition. Boston, Little, Brown and Co, 1976, pp 55–100.

21. Azar GJ, Bloom WL: Similarities of carbohydrate deficiency and fasting. Arch Intern Med 112:338–343, 1963.

22. Levenson SM, Crowley LV, Seifter E: Starvation, in Ballinger WF, Collins JA, Drucker WR, et al (eds): Manual of Surgical Nutrition. Philadelphia, WB Co, 1975, pp 236–264.

23. Shenkin A, Wretlind A: Complete intravenous nutrition including amino acids, glucose and lipids, in Richards JR, Kinney JM (eds): Nutritional Aspects of Care in the Critically Ill. Edinburgh, Churchill Livingstone, 1977, pp 245–365.

24. Elman R: Time factors in the utilization of a mixture of amino acids (protein hydrolysate) and dextrose given intravenously. Am J Clin Nutr 1:287–294, 1953.

25. Nube M, Bos LP, Winkelman A: Simultaneous and consecutive administration of nutrients in parenteral nutrition. Am J Clin Nutr 32:1505–1510, 1979.

26. Wilmore DW: The Metabolic Management of the Critically Ill. New York, Plenum Medical Book Co, 1977.

27. Bergstrom J, Hultman E, Roch-Norlund AE: Lactic acid accumulation in connection with fructose infusion. Acta Med Scand 184:359–364, 1968.

28. Krebs HA: Some general considerations concerning the uses of carbohydrates in parenteral nutrition, in Johnston IDA (ed): Advances in Parenteral Nutrition. Baltimore, University Park Press, 1978, pp 23–44.

29. Lee HA, Wretlind A: Non-protein energy sources in parenteral nutrition. Acta Chir Scand [Suppl] 466:6–7, 1976.
30. Ahnefeld FW, Bassler KH, Bauer BL, et al: Suitability of non-glucose carbohydrates for parenteral nutrition. Eur J Intensive Care Med 1:105–13, 1975.
31. Young EA, Weser E: The metabolism of maltose after intravenous injection in normal and diabetic subjects. J Clin Endocrinol 38:181–188, 1974.
32. Forster H, Hoos I: The suitability of maltose for parenteral nutrition. Eur J Intensive Care Med 1:141–144, 1975.
33. McNiff BL: Clinical use of 10% soybean oil emulsion. Am J Hosp Pharm 34:1080–1086, 1977.
34. Hallberg D: Therapy with fat emulsion. Acta Anaesthesiol Scand [Suppl] 55:131–136, 1974.
35. Jeejeebhoy KN: Total parenteral nutrition. Ann R Coll Phys Surg Can 9:287–300, 1976.
36. Hallberg D, Holm I, Obel AL, et al: Fat emulsions for complete intravenous nutrition. Postgrad Med J 43:307–316, 1967.
37. Hallberg D: Studies on the elimination of exogenous lipids from the blood stream: The effect of fasting and surgical trauma in man on the elimination rate of a fat emulsion injection intravenously. Acta Physiol Scand 65:153–163, 1965.
38. Greene HL, Hazlett D, Demaree R: Relationship between Intralipid-induced hyperlipemia and pulmonary function. Am J Clin Nutr 29:127–135, 1976.
39. Wilmore DW, Moylan JA, Helmkamp GM, Pruitt BA Jr: Clinical evaluation of a 10% intravenous fat emulsion for parenteral nutrition in thermally injured patients. Ann Surg 178:503–513, 1973.
40. Jacobson S, Ericsson JLK, Obel AL: Histopathological and ultrastructural changes in the human liver during complete intravenous nutrition for 7 months. Acta Chir Scand 137:335–349, 1971.
41. Wretlind A: Current status of Intralipid and other fat emulsions, in Meng HC, Wilmore DW (eds): Fat Emulsions in Parenteral Nutrition. Chicago, American Medical Association, 1976, pp 109–122.
42. Hansen LM, Hardie WR, Hidalgo J: Fat emulsion for intravenous administration: Clinical experience with Intralipid 10%. Ann Surg 184:80–88, 1976.
43. Belin RP, Bivins BA, Jona JZ, Young VL: Fat overload with a 10% soybean oil emulsion. Arch Surg 111:1391–1393, 1976.
44. Barlow AL: Liposyn Research Conference Proceedings. North Chicago, Abbott Laboratories, 1979.
45. Bivins BA, Rapp RP, Record K, et al: Parenteral safflower oil emulsion (Liposyn 10%): Safety and effectiveness in treating or preventing essential fatty acid deficiency in surgical patients. Ann Surg 191:307–315, 1980.
46. Connors RH, Coran AG, Wesley JR: Pediatric TPN: Efficacy and toxicity of a new fat emulsion. JPEN 4:384–386, 1980.
47. Heuckenkamp PU, Sprandel U, Liebhardt EW: Studies concerning ethanol as a nutrient for intravenous alimentation in man. Nutr Metab 21 (Suppl 1): 121–124, 1977.
48. Meng HC: Parenteral nutrition: Principles, nutrient requirements, and techniques. Geriatrics 30:97–107, 1975.

49. Vanamee P: Parenteral nutrition, in Nutrition Reviews' Present Knowledge in Nutrition. New York, Nutrition Foundation, 1976, pp 415–436.
50. Wretlind A, Schmer W: Carbohydrates and fats colloquium, in White PL, Nagy ME (eds): Total Parenteral Nutrition. Acton, Mass, Publishing Sciences Group, Inc., 1974, pp 186–238.
51. Rubin E, Lieber CS: Fatty liver, alcoholic hepatitis and cirrhosis produced by alcohol in primates. N Engl J Med 290:128–135, 1974.
52. Coon WW, Kowalczyk RS: Protein metabolism, in Ballinger WF, Collins JA, WR, et al (eds): Manual of Surgical Nutrition. Philadelphia, WB Saunders Co, 1975, pp 50–72.
53. Christensen HN, Lynch EL, Powers JH: The conjugated, non-protein amino acids of plasma, III: Peptidemia and hyperpeptiduria as a result of the intravenous administration of partially hydrolyzed casein (Amigen). J Biol Chem 166:649–652, 1946.
54. Munro HN: Basic concepts in the use of amino acids and protein hydrolysates for parenteral nutrition. Proceedings of the AMA Symposium on Total Parenteral Nutrition, Nashville, Tennessee, January 17–19, 1972, pp 7–35.
55. Anderson GH, Patel DG, Jeejeebhoy KN: Design and evaluation by nitrogen balance and blood aminograms of an amino acid mixture for total parenteral nutrition of adults with gastrointestinal disease. J Clin Invest 53:904–912, 1974.
56. Recommended Dietary Allowances, ed 9. Washington, DC, National Academy of Sciences, 1980.
57. Press M, Hartop PJ, Prottey C: Correction of essential fatty-acid deficiency in man by the cutaneous application of sunflower-seed oil. Lancet 1:597–598, 1974.
58. Skolnik P, Eaglstein WH, Ziboh VA: Human essential fatty acid deficiency: Treatment by topical application of linoleic acid. Arch Dermatol 113:939–941, 1977.
59. Collins FD, Sinclair AJ, Royle JP, et al: Plasma lipids in human linoleic acid deficiency. Nutr Metab 13:150–167, 1971.
60. Jeejeebhoy KN, Zohrab WJ, Langer B, et al: Total parenteral nutrition at home for 23 months without complications and with good rehabilitation. Gastroenterology 65:811–820, 1973.
61. Shils ME: Parenteral nutrition, in Goodhart RS, Shils ME (eds): Modern Nutrition in Health and Disease. Philadelphia, Lea and Febiger, 1980, pp 1125–1152.
62. Guidelines for essential trace element preparations for parenteral use. JAMA 241:2051–2054, 1979.
63. Hauer EC, Kaminski MV Jr: Trace metal profile of parenteral nutrition solutions. Am J Clin Nutr 31:264–268, 1978.
64. Alexander JW: Nutrition and surgical infection, in Ballinger WF, Collins JA, Drucker WR, et al (eds): Manual of Surgical Nutrition. Philadelphia, WB Saunders Co, 1975, pp 386–395.
65. Bothe A Jr, Benotti P, Bistrian BR, Blackburn GL: Use of iron with total parenteral nutrition. N Engl J Med 93:1153, 1975.
66. Byrne WJ, Ament ME, Burke M, Fonkalsrud E: Home parenteral nutrition. Surg Gynecol Obstet 149:593–599, 1979.
67. Mays T, Mays T: Intravenous iron-dextran therapy in the treatment of anemia

occurring in surgical, gynecologic and obstetric patients. Surg Gynecol Obstet 143:381–384, 1976.

68. Lowry SF, Goodgame JT, Maher MM, Brennan MF: Parenteral vitamin requirements during intravenous feeding. Am J Clin Nutr 31:2149–2158, 1978.

69. Multivitamin preparations for parenteral use: A statement by the Nutrition Advisory Group. JPEN 3:258–262, 1979.

70. Sheldon GF, Grzyb S: Phosphate depletion and repletion: Relation to parenteral nutrition and oxygen transport. Ann Surg 82:683–689, 1975.

71. Jeejeebhoy KN, Anderson GH, Sanderson I, Bryan M: Total parenteral nutrition: Nutrient needs and technical tips, Part 1. Mod Med Can 29:832–841, 1974.

72. Wittine MF, Freeman JB: Calcium requirements during total parenteral nutrition in well-nourished individuals. JPEN 1:152–155, 1977.

73. Oh TE, Dyer H, Wall BP, et al: Insulin loss in parenteral nutrition systems. Intensive Care 4:342–346, 1976.

74. Weber SS, Wood WA, Jackson EA: Availability of insulin from parenteral nutrient solutions. Am J Hosp Pharm 34:353–357, 1977.

75. Duke JH, Dudrick SJ: Parenteral feeding, in Ballinger WF, Collins JA, Drucker WR, et al (eds): Manual of Surgical Nutrition. Philadelphia, WB Saunders Co, 1975, pp 285–317.

6

Parenteral Nutrition: The Glucose System

In the glucose system of parenteral nutrition, glucose is used exclusively as the caloric source, and synthetic amino acids are generally used as the protein source.

PREPARATION OF NUTRIENT SOLUTIONS

The nutrient solution contains equal volumes of 40 to 50 percent glucose and 8.5 percent crystalline amino acids, appropriate electrolytes, vitamins, and trace elements. Methods of preparation include the bulk method, the single unit method, and the kit method.

In the bulk method, large volumes of solutions are prepared in vats in a manufacturing pharmacy. Bulk chemicals are used and large-volume filtering, sterilizing, and bottling devices are employed.[1,2] Such a method may be useful in large institutions where many patients receive TPN daily. In contrast, commercially available kits are useful in smaller institutions with minimal facilities and low demand for TPN.* Such kits consist of a 500 ml container with amino acids with or without added electrolytes and a partially filled 1 liter bottle containing 40 to 50 percent glucose. This liter container

---

*Available from McGaw Laboratories, Travenol Laboratories, and Abbott Laboratories.

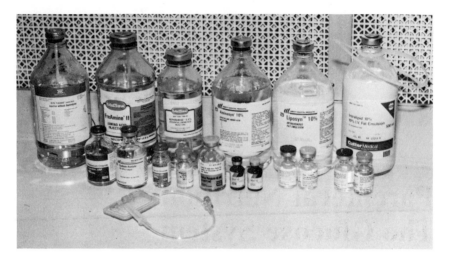

Figure 6-1. Materials for preparation of the glucose system assembled in the pharmacy under a laminar flow hood.

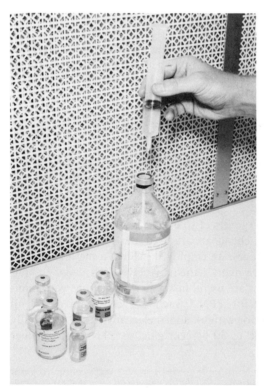

Figure 6-2. Electrolytes added to amino acid solution aseptically.

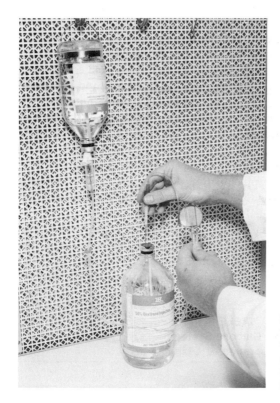

Figure 6-3. Amino acid–electrolyte solution being transferred to a bottle containing 50 percent glucose; the solution is passed through a 0.22 μ bacterial filter during transfer.

has a partial vacuum to allow easy transfer of the amino acids with transfer sets provided with the kit.

The most common method of preparation is the single unit method. Here individual components—including glucose, amino acids, electrolytes, trace elements, vitamins, and insulin, if needed—are mixed in an evacuated liter container. Preparing the solutions, determining the compatibility of the various components, and monitoring quality control are under the supervision of the parenteral nutrition pharmacists.[3] Solutions are prepared aseptically in the pharmacy under a laminar flow filtered air hood and are sterilized by passage through a 0.22 μ membrane filter which screens all bacteria (Figs. 6-1–6-3). The compatibilities of the various components are determined in part by their concentration, the pH of the additives as well as that of the receiving solution, and the order of admixture.* One of the most common considerations is the compatibility of calcium and phosphate supplements. A

*An extensive discussion of compatibility with parenteral nutrition solutions is presented in King JC: Guide to Parenteral Admixtures, St. Louis, Cutter Laboratories, 1978.

precipitate will form if calcium and phosphate ions are combined in too small a volume or in too high a concentration. One way to avoid precipitation is to add the calcium supplement to the glucose solution and the phosphate to the amino acid solution prior to mixing the glucose and amino acid components together. Using such a method, supplements of both calcium and phosphate sufficient for maintenance can usually be added safely to the nutrient solution. However, the greater amount of phosphate required for phosphate-depleted patients may require a phosphate infusion through a separate intravenous line.

Following mixture of the various components, the nutrient solution is visually inspected for evidence of precipitation or particulate matter. Bacteriologic monitoring is an essential feature of quality control. At the Massachusetts General Hospital, 10 percent of all TPN units are randomly sampled and cultured.[3] After preparation, the nutrient solution is refrigerated until used, generally within 24 hours. Darkening of the solution due to the interaction of organonitrogenous agents and glucose (Maillard's reaction) may occur with prolonged storage at room temperature, or more rapidly if

TABLE 6-1
The Glucose System:
Preparation of 1 Liter

8.5 percent Amino Acids*	500 ml
50 percent Glucose	500 ml
Additives to each liter:	
Sodium (as acetate)	45 mEq
Potassium† (as chloride)	35 mEq
Potassium† (as acid phosphate)	8.8 mEq
Phosphate (as potassium acid phosphate)	6 mM
Magnesium (as sulfate)	8 mEq
Calcium (as chloride)	5 mEq
Additives to 1 liter per day:	
MVI-12‡	10 ml
USC Trace Element Solution§	2 ml

*As FreAmine III, 8.5 percent. Contains 10 mEq/ℓ of sodium and 20 mEq (10 mM)/ℓ of phosphate. Equivalent amino acid solutions (Aminosyn, 8.5 percent; Travasol, 8.5 percent) have different electrolyte contents (see Table 5-6).
†Provided as potassium phosphate, Abbott Laboratories. One ml contains 4.4 mEq potassium and 3 mM phosphate (equivalent to approximately 5.4 mEq assuming average valence of 1.8). See Turco and Burke.[4]
‡Manufactured by USV Pharmaceutical Corporation.
§See Table 5-7.
Note: Essential fatty acids and vitamin K are supplied separately (see text).

TABLE 6-2
The Glucose System:
Nutrients Provided in Each Liter

Nutrient	Amount
Non-protein calories	850 kcal
Caloric density	0.85 kcal/ml
Glucose	250 gm
Nitrogen	6.5 gm
Protein equivalent	40.6 gm
Calorie*/nitrogen ratio	131:1
Sodium	50 mEq
Potassium	43.8 mEq
Magnesium	8 mEq
Calcium	5 mEq
Chloride	40 mEq
Acetate	45 mEq
Phosphate	11 mM
Sulfate	8 mEq

*Non-protein kcal.

the solution is steam autoclaved. Prolonged storage may also be associated with loss of potency of additives, especially vitamins, and an increased risk of significant microbial contamination.

The protocol employed for the preparation of the glucose system at the Los Angeles County–University of Southern California Medical Center is presented in Table 6-1. The nutrients provided in each liter of the glucose system are outlined in Table 6-2. Essential fatty acids are provided by infusing 500 ml of a 10 percent fat emulsion twice weekly through a separate intravenous line. Both safflower oil and soybean oil emulsions provide linoleic acid, but only the latter contain linolenic acid, the necessity for which in humans is uncertain. Intramuscular injections of vitamin K are given as needed in accordance with periodic measurements of prothrombin time.

The composition of the nutrient solution presented here is appropriate for the vast majority of patients. The variable caloric and nitrogen requirements of individual patients can usually be met by altering the volume infused. Biochemical monitoring, discussed below, determines the necessity for adjustments in the mineral supplements and the need for insulin. Some patients, however, have medical conditions which require significant modification of this standard protocol. These patients include those requiring fluid and sodium restriction and patients with renal and hepatic failure. The nutritional management of these specific conditions is discussed in Chapter 10.

VASCULAR ACCESS

Because of the osmolar contribution of not only the glucose but also the amino acids and electrolytes, the nutrient solution has a final concentration exceeding 2000 mOsm/liter. Such a solution can never be safely infused through peripheral veins. Consequently, these solutions must be delivered into a central vein, where the infusate is rapidly diluted. The incidence of morbidity associated with establishing and maintaining central venous access is influenced by the site and technique of insertion of the venous cannula, the length and composition of the cannula, and the diligence with which the infusion apparatus is managed during the course of nutrition therapy.

The location of the infusion apparatus is important, since motion of the body part to which the apparatus is attached may disrupt the connection between the infusion tubing and the venous cannula or may disturb the overlying occlusive dressing. Ideally, the apparatus should be arranged so that the patient is able to move about freely. Since the inception of total parenteral nutrition, the standard route of administration in hospitalized patients has been through a percutaneously placed subclavian venous catheter. Other routes are used occasionally with variable success.

Subclavian Catheterization

Percutaneous subclavian catheterization is a blind procedure, since the vessel can be neither visualized nor palpated. Successful catheterization therefore depends on a certain degree of skill and rigid discipline in following the details of technique.[5]

Many techniques of percutaneous cannulation have been described, including both supraclavicular and infraclavicular approaches. At the Los Angeles County–USC Medical Center, the use of the infraclavicular approach described in Figures 6-4–6-13 has resulted in a higher rate of successful cannulation with fewer complications than with other techniques. This approach is used in all patients requiring the glucose system except those in whom a specific contraindication exists. Thus subclavian catheterization is avoided when the tissues at or adjacent to the proposed site of catheter insertion are affected by infection, hematoma, recent or anticipated surgical procedure, radiation therapy, fistulas, drainage, extensive tumor, or burns. Deformities of the neck or spine increase the risk of pneumothorax during percutaneous subclavian catheterization, and therefore other routes of vascular access are preferable in patients with such conditions. Percutaneous catheterization is also contraindicated in patients with severe pulmonary disease, in whom a pneumothorax would produce severe morbidity or even death. Maintaining the sterility of the catheter and overlying dressings is much more difficult in patients with a tracheostomy because of the purulent secretions associated with such a stoma. Consequently, a tracheostomy is a relative contraindication to percutaneous subclavian catheterization.

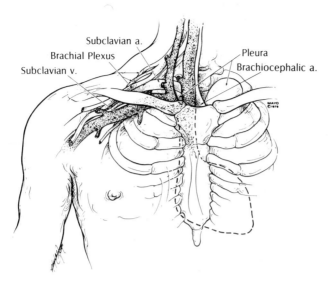

Subclavian a.

Brachial Plexus

Subclavian v.

Pleura

Brachiocephalic a.

Insertion of Subclavian Catheter Figures 6-4–6-13

Figure 6-4. This diagram illustrates the anatomic relationship between the subclavian vein and the medial one-third of the clavicle. The junction of the medial and middle thirds of the clavicle under which the subclavian vein passes is a key reference point in subclavian catheterization. *(From Linos DA, Mucha P Jr, Van Heerden JA: Mayo Clin Proc 55:315–321, 1980)*

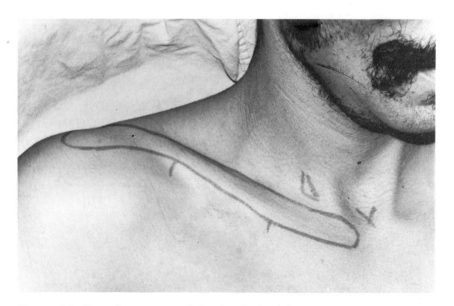

Figure 6-5. The relevant anatomic landmarks have been outlined on this patient. They include the clavicle, divided into thirds, the suprasternal notch (marked X), and the easily palpable triangle between the sternal and clavicular heads of the sternocleidomastoid muscle (marked △). This last landmark is the second key reference point in subclavian catheterization.

147

When an attempt at cannulation is unsuccessful, the contralateral sub-clavian vein may be cannulated, but only after a chest x-ray demonstrates the absence of a pneumothorax or other complication resulting from the original attempt.

The side to be cannulated is generally a matter of personal preference, except when one side is contraindicated by conditions already discussed or when a thoracostomy tube is in place. In the latter circumstance, the catheter is introduced on the ipsilateral side, since the chest tube protects against po-tential pneumothorax.

Catheter management.   After successful insertion, careful attention is paid to the subclavian catheter and its dressings, since cutaneous bacteria are impor-tant in the genesis of catheter-related sepsis. Theoretically, such organisms may gain access to the tip of the catheter by migrating along the moist film between the catheter and the subcutaneous tissue. This view is supported by studies demonstrating that organisms colonizing the skin and those coloniz-ing the catheter tip are often identical.[6,7] When meticulous technique is em-ployed in the maintenance of venous catheters, the incidence of catheter-related sepsis may fall to nearly zero.[7] At the Los Angeles County–

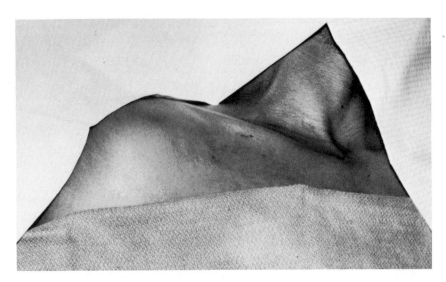

Figure 6-6. The procedure is done at the bedside using sterile gloves. The side to be cannulated is scrubbed with povidone–iodine soap (Betadine) for ten minutes. The area prepared includes the neck and the upper anterior chest from the shoul-der to the contralateral midclavicular line. Sterile towels are draped about the oper-ative field as illustrated.

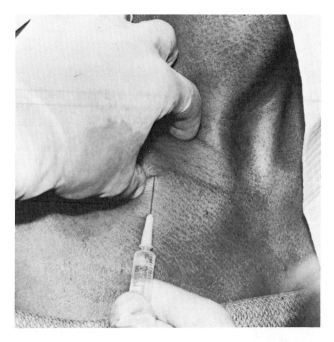

Figure 6-7. After draping, the patient is placed in the deep Trendelenburg position (head down, feet up). This is a critical aspect of the technique, since the increase in venous pressure associated with this position results in (1) a distended subclavian vein, making this target more easily punctured, and (2) a reduced risk of aspirating air into the vein and air embolism. In the Trendelenburg position, the two key reference points are again identified and are marked by the placement of the thumb and index finger at the junction of the medial and middle thirds of the clavicle and the triangle between the two heads of the sternocleidomastoid muscle, respectively. The skin along the inferior border of the clavicle at the junction of the medial and middle thirds is infiltrated with 1 percent xylocaine, as illustrated.

USC Medical Center, the nurse assigned to the Parenteral and Enteral Nutrition Service changes the subclavian catheter dressings on Mondays, Wednesdays, and Fridays using aseptic technique. All dressings are removed and the skin surrounding the catheter insertion site is defatted with ether or acetone. The insertion site, the surrounding skin, and the junction between the cannula and the intravenous extension tubing (which is interposed between the intravenous administration set and the cannula) are scrubbed with povidone–iodine solution. Such an iodine-containing solution significantly reduces the skin flora.[8] With the patient in the Trendelenburg position, the old extension tubing is disconnected and new, sterile tubing (previously connected to the intravenous administration set and filled with the nutrient solution) is quickly

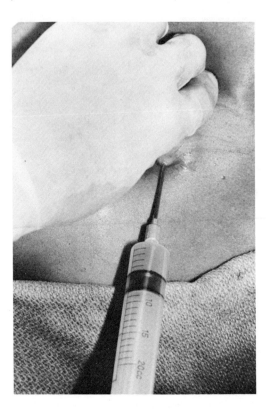

Figure 6-8. The apparatus used for cannulating the subclavian vein is the Deseret Intracath intravenous catheter placement unit with wire stylet (Deseret Company, Sandy, Utah, Catalog Number 3162). This apparatus consists of a 16 gauge (1.7 mm), 8 inch (20.3 cm) plastic catheter which is introduced through the lumen of a 14 gauge (2.1 mm) needle. The needle is attached to a 20 ml syringe and is then introduced just beneath the clavicle while gentle suction is applied to the syringe. The needle traverses a path described by a line joining the two key reference points. The syringe and needle form an angle with the anterior chest wall of 30° to 45°

connected to the venous cannula. Thereafter, an antimicrobial ointment is applied at the catheter insertion site and a 1 inch × 1 inch gauze dressing is placed over it. The surrounding area is sprayed with benzoin and, finally, an airtight, occlusive, adhesive bandage is applied. The choice of topical antimicrobial ointment is problematic. Jarrard and Freeman studied the skin flora beneath subclavian catheter dressings in patients receiving either povidone–iodine ointment (Betadine) or an ointment containing a mixture of bacitracin, neomycin, and polymyxin B (Neosporin).[8] The particular ointment did not appear to affect the results materially. Neither eradicated all organisms, but both ointments appeared superior to sterile petroleum jelly. In a subsequent study, Jarrard and associates found that when subclavian dressings were changed in the manner described above on a daily basis instead of on alternate days, all skin organisms beneath the dressings could be eliminated.[9] These investigators suggested daily dressing changes for patients who are at high risk for septic complications.

Functioning subclavian catheters may remain in place for the duration of nutrition therapy unless catheter-related sepsis or thrombophlebitis develop.

Occasionally, vascular access in extensively burned patients can be achieved only by cannulating through burned skin. In such patients, the catheter is changed every 48 to 72 hours to avoid sepsis and septic thrombosis of the great veins.[10] In some centers, subclavian catheters are changed prophylactically every 72 hours in all patients with extensive burns.[11,12]

Complications.   Although once mastered, subclavian cannulation is a simple procedure, complications nevertheless do occur. They most commonly develop during attempts by inexperienced persons. The procedure should therefore be learned under the supervision of an experienced operator. In addition, Bernard and Stahl found in their series of subclavian catheterizations that nearly half the complications occurred in the 2.5 percent of patients in whom the procedure was done as an emergency—for example, for central venous pressure monitoring or emergency fluid resuscitation.[13] Thus morbidity occurring in patients receiving subclavian catheters for parenteral nutrition is likely to be less common than morbidity reflected in series including emergency cannulations.

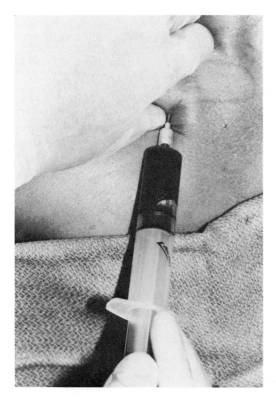

Figure 6-9. When the subclavian vein is entered, blood freely returns into the syringe. Then the syringe is detached and the thumb of the left hand occludes the orifice of the needle (to prevent aspiration of air) until the catheter is brought into position.

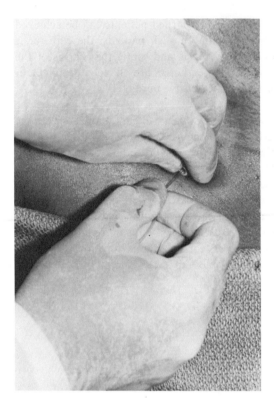

Figure 6-10. The catheter is then passed through the needle and advanced its full length. The catheter should only be advanced, never withdrawn, through the needle. Attempts to withdraw the catheter with the needle in a fixed position may result in shearing off the end of the catheter, which may then embolize. After the catheter is inserted its full length, it is engaged in the hub of the needle and the wire stylet is removed. A syringe is attached to demonstrate free flow of blood through the catheter. Thereafter, an infusion of 5 percent dextrose is begun through sterile extension tubing which had previously been attached to an adjacent non-sterile intravenous administration set by an assistant.

Cannulation is successful in 85 to 97.5 percent of attempts.[5,14] Failure may result from inability to insert the catheter into the subclavian vein or from improper advancement of the catheter tip into one of the jugular veins or the contralateral innominate vein instead of into the superior vena cava.

Complications can be classified as those occurring during insertion of the venous cannula and those involving the indwelling catheter after successful insertion, as follows:

1. Potential complications during subclavian catheter insertion.
   a. Air embolus.
   b. Arterial puncture.
   c. Arteriovenous fistula.
   d. Brachial plexus injury.
   e. Cardiac arrhythmia.
   f. Cardiac perforation with tamponade.
   g. Catheter embolus.
   h. Hemomediastinum.
   i. Hemothorax.

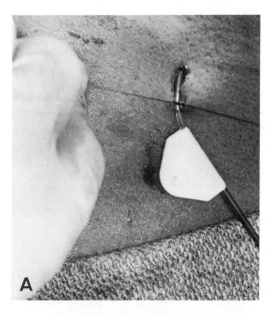

A

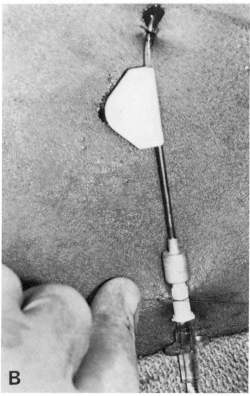

B

Figure 6-11. The needle is then withdrawn from the subclavian vein and the catheter is protected from the sharp tip of the needle by applying the needle cover. Next the patient's position is changed from the Trendelenburg position to the semi-Fowler position. The low or negative venous pressure present in this latter position minimizes any bleeding from the subclavian puncture site. Now the apparatus is secured to the anterior chest wall by two sutures. **A.** The first is placed about the catheter at its entrance beneath the clavicle. **B.** The second suture is placed around the catheter adapter.

153

      j. Hydromediastinum.

      k. Hydrothorax.

      l. Pneumothorax.

     m. Subcutaneous emphysema.

      n. Thoracic duct injury.

2. Potential complications of indwelling subclavian catheters.

      a. Air embolism.

      b. Cardiac perforation with tamponade.

      c. Catheter occlusion.

      d. Catheter leak.

      e. Catheter-related sepsis.

      f. Central vein thrombophlebitis.

      g. Endocarditis.

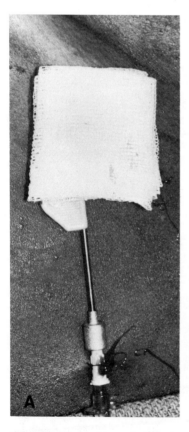 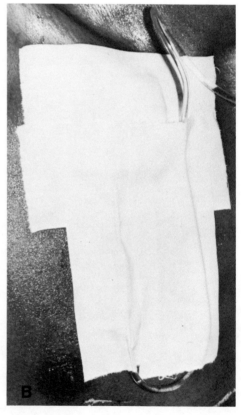

Figure 6-12. Povidone–iodine ointment is applied at the catheter insertion site and at the site of the two sutures. **A.** A small gauze dressing (1 inch × 1 inch) is placed over the skin insertion site, the surrounding skin is painted with tincture of benzoin, and then **B**, an air-tight, occlusive adhesive bandage is applied.

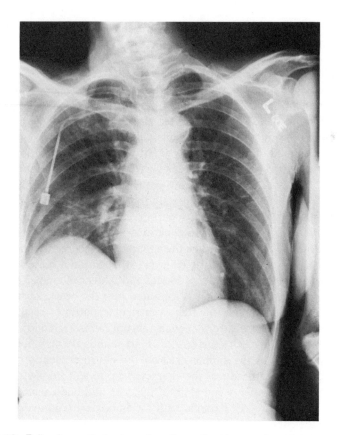

Figure 6-13. Following catheter insertion, the patient is examined for any evidence of pneumothorax. A chest x-ray is obtained shortly after the procedure. The film confirms the absence of chest complications and demonstrates the appropriate location of the tip of the catheter in the superior vena cava. Now the nutrient solution can replace the isotonic glucose infusion.

Overall complication rates have been reported to be 1.5 percent,[14] 2.74 percent,[15] 4 percent,[10] 4.5 percent,[13] and 8.5 percent[16] in various series of subclavian catheterizations.

PNEUMOTHORAX. Pneumothorax resulting from inadvertent entrance into the pleural cavity is probably the most common complication of attempted subclavian catheterization. Pneumothorax occurred in 0.47, 1, 1.7, 3, and 6 percent of attempts in five reported series.[10,13,14,16,17] Large or total pneumothoraces require treatment with tube thoracostomy, but minor pulmonary collapse often requires only close observation. Bilateral or tension pneumothoraces are uncommon but severe complications which may result in death without prompt treatment.

AIR EMBOLISM. Venous air embolism occurs when air under atmospheric pressure passes through the subclavian catheter into the lower pressure central veins and the heart. Air may enter during catheter insertion when the finger over the hub of the inserting needle is removed to allow passage of the catheter. Air embolism may also occur when the intravenous tubing or the venous cannula becomes disconnected from the rest of the infusion apparatus. Aspiration of air has also been reported through a crack in the catheter hub and through the skin tract of a previously removed subclavian catheter.[18-20]

The likelihood of air embolus is greatly increased in situations in which the patient's central venous pressure is very low, as in the upright position or in markedly dehydrated patients. Thus catheter insertion should be undertaken in the Trendelenburg position, preferably after restoration of normal fluid volume. Separation of the infusion apparatus can be avoided by taping all connections and securing the infusion apparatus on the anterior chest wall. The risk of separation is increased when the apparatus is secured to moveable parts of the body such as the shoulder (Fig. 6-14). Separation may occur in this position when ambulatory patients abduct and adduct the upper extremity.

When a large amount of air is aspirated into the heart, air bubbles produce acute obstruction of the right ventricular outflow tract causing an abrupt rise in venous pressure, an equally abrupt fall in systemic arterial pressure, and, ultimately, cardiac arrest.[21-23] Heart sounds are inaudible in the upright position, but in the supine position the churning action of the heart mixing blood and air produces the characteristic to-and-fro, swishing, "millwheel" murmur.[24] Patients complain of dyspnea and chest pain and may be disoriented or comatose.[10] Patients with air embolus are immediately placed in the Trendelenburg position with the left side down. In this position, the ventricular outflow tract is below the air, which therefore rises, hopefully relieving the air lock.[21,23,25] Aspiration of right ventricular air through the subclavian catheter may be helpful. Other reported therapeutic maneuvers include external or internal cardiac message, percutaneous aspiration of the right ventricle, and emergency cardiopulmonary bypass.[19]

In a review of 14 cases of air embolism associated with central venous catheters reported in the world literature through 1977, Peters and Armstrong found that 5 patients were resuscitated without sequelae, 3 patients recovered with transient central nervous system signs (for example, hemiplegia), and 6 patients died.[20] In animal studies, Durant and associates found that the prognosis of air embolism depends on the amount of air aspirated, the speed with which the air enters, the position of the body at the time of embolism, the efficacy of the respiratory excretory mechanism, and proper positioning following diagnosis.[21]

CENTRAL VEIN THROMBOSIS. Venous thrombosis is associated with stasis of blood flow, local trauma or inflammation of the vessel wall, or altered coagulability of blood (Virchow's triad). A lower incidence of thrombophlebi-

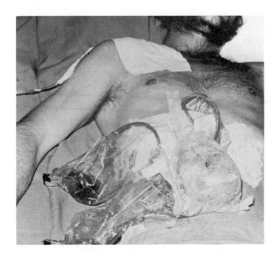

Figure 6-14. The infusion apparatus is inappropriately secured to the shoulder rather than the anterior chest wall. Air embolism is likely if separation of the tubing from the cannula occurs during arm motion, especially if the patient is upright when venous pressure at the catheter tip is negative.

tis occurs with subclavian cannulation than with cannulation of peripheral veins, presumably because of greater blood flow around the cannula in large-caliber veins and the shorter catheter required for subclavian catheterization. Nevertheless, central vein thrombosis does occur and may involve the subclavian, jugular, and innominate veins and the superior vena cava. Patients in whom this complication is most likely to occur include those with low flow states (for example, in shock and dehydration), sepsis, and extensive burns. The last group of patients is additionally subject to the complication of suppurative thrombophlebitis. Thrombophlebitis is also more likely to occur when the tip of the catheter is inappropriately placed in the smaller caliber innominate or jugular veins rather than the superior vena cava. In this case, the irritating effect of the hypertonic nutrient solution may provoke thrombosis. Although a reduced incidence of thrombophlebitis in peripheral veins has been observed when peripherally inserted central venous catheters are made of silastic, this beneficial effect has not been seen when silastic catheters replace the short plastic catheters used for percutaneous subclavian insertion.[26]

Clinical manifestations of central vein thrombosis include edema of the upper extremity and sometimes of the neck and face, as well. Pulmonary embolus has also been reported. Venograms can be obtained to confirm the diagnosis of central vein thrombosis. Evidently, many patients are asymptomatic, since autopsy series suggest a higher incidence of venous thrombosis than is recognized clinically.[27]

Treatment consists of removing the venous cannula, the tip of which is cultured; elevating the extremity; and administering anticoagulants. Intensive antibiotic therapy is required for suppurative thrombophlebitis. The incidence of this latter complication may be reduced in burn patients if the venous cannula is prophylactically changed every 48 to 72 hours.[11,12] Blackett diagnosed central vein thrombosis in 4.5 percent of 178 patients receiving parenteral nutrition through a subclavian catheter.[17] In each case the clinical manifestations resolved completely in days to weeks after removal of the catheter.

CATHETER EMBOLUS. During subclavian catheterization, the venous cannula can be inadvertently divided by the sharp tip of the inserting needle; it may then embolize into the central circulation. The mechanism by which this complication occurs is generally the inappropriate attempt to withdraw the catheter through the inserting needle; the tip of the needle engages the catheter and continued traction severs it. To avoid this accident, the needle and catheter must be withdrawn simultaneously.

Severed catheters may lodge anywhere from the subclavian vein to the pulmonary artery and cause thrombosis or cardiac arrhythmia or act as a nidus for sepsis. It is generally recommended, therefore, that catheter fragments be removed, preferably by a nonoperative approach. This approach includes transvenous snare techniques using hooked catheters, wire loops, stone baskets, and endoscopic forceps.[10,19]

CATHETER-RELATED SEPSIS (See page 169).

Internal Jugular Vein Catheterization

Internal jugular venous catheters, inserted percutaneously by a variety of techniques,[28] are commonly used for infusing crystalloid solutions and for measuring central venous pressure. Long-term use for infusing nutrient solutions is hampered by patient discomfort and difficulty maintaining a sterile, occlusive dressing because of motion of the neck and beard growth in men. As a consequence, this method of vascular access may be associated with a higher rate of catheter sepsis and local thrombosis.[29] Benotti and associates suggested that this route can be used safely for 3 to 4 weeks if the percutaneously placed catheter is drawn through a subcutaneous tunnel created between the puncture site in the neck and a point 2 to 3 cm below the clavicle.[29] In this way the catheter and the overlying dressing are placed on the anterior chest wall. This technique may be useful when subclavian catheterization has been unsuccessful.

Broviac Right Atrial Silcone Rubber Catheters

The Broviac catheter* was specifically designed for long-term use in patients receiving parenteral nutrition at home (Fig. 6-15).[30] It is particularly useful in this group of patients because of the nonreactive, minimally thrombogenic nature of silicone rubber (Silastic). In addition, the catheter is fitted with a

---

*Available from Evermed, P.O. Box 296, Medina, Washington. A similar catheter with a larger internal diameter (Hickman catheter) is also available.

Dacron cuff which lies within a subcutaneous tunnel and provokes a fibrotic reaction which presumably seals the tunnel and prevents ascending infection.[31]

The Broviac catheter is of value for limited indications in hospitalized patients. Such indications may include technical inability to insert a subclavian catheter percutaneously or one of the absolute or relative contraindications to subclavian catheterization discussed previously. The latter include deformities of the neck or spine and severe pulmonary disease. In addition, it may be advisable to use a Broviac catheter in patients who have an increased susceptibility to catheter sepsis. Such patients include those with chronic debilitating illness, those receiving immunosuppressive or cytotoxic drugs, and those with a tracheostomy. However, a reduced rate of sepsis associated with the use of a Broviac catheter in these circumstances is unproved. One potential drawback of the Broviac catheter is that because of the effort expended to introduce it, there may be reluctance or delay in removing it when unexplained fever develops.

The Broviac catheter is inserted under local anesthesia in the operating room. One end of the catheter is advanced through a vein into the right atri-

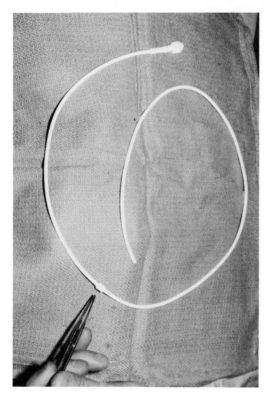

Figure 6-15. A Broviac catheter. The forceps points to a Dacron cuff which is placed in the subcutaneous tunnel to prevent ascending infection.

um, and the other end transverses a long subcutaneous tunnel and exits on the anterior chest wall.

The catheter may be introduced into the right atrium through the cephalic vein which is exposed in the deltopectoral groove, or it may be introduced through the external jugular vein. However, insertion through the internal jugular vein is often easier and faster (Figs. 6-16–6-21). The internal jugular vein is exposed through a 2 to 5 cm vertical incision placed between the two heads of the sternocleidomastoid muscle. Following exposure of the vein, a subcutaneous tunnel is created between the incision in the neck and a point on the anterior chest wall between the nipple and the lateral sternal border. The tunnel is made with a small (No. 3–4) Hegar cervical dilator. A hole drilled in the tip of the dilator allows a heavy silk suture to be drawn through the tunnel which is then tied to the tip of the catheter. The catheter is advanced through the tunnel so that the Dacron cuff lies within the tunnel 2 to 3 cm above the entrance of the catheter and within an intercostal space. The catheter, now exiting in the neck incision, is cut so that the tip will just reach the right atrium. At this point, proximal and distal control of the previously exposed internal jugular vein is obtained with vascular loops or clamps, and the tip of the catheter is introduced through a venotomy around which a 7-0 cardiovascular purse-string suture had been placed. Thereafter, the purse-string suture is secured, the catheter is sutured to the adjacent sternocleidomastoid muscle, and the neck incision is closed with a subcuticular suture. The appropriate location of the catheter is confirmed fluoroscopically or by chest x-ray before the patient leaves the operating room.

Recently a technique for percutaneous placement of the Broviac catheter has been described which utilizes apparatus designed for transvenous pacemaker insertion.[32] A subcutaneous tunnel is created in the usual fashion so that the catheter exits through a 1 cm infraclavicular incision. The subclavian

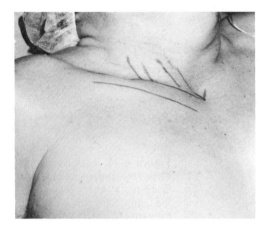

Insertion of Broviac Catheter Figures 6-16–6-21.

Figure 6-16. Pertinent landmarks (the clavicle and the sternal and clavicular heads of the sternocleidomastoid muscle) are outlined. The internal jugular vein is exposed through a vertical incision between the two muscle heads just above the clavicle.

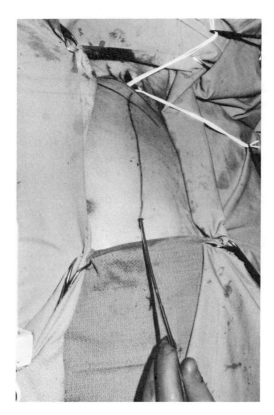

Figure 6-17. The internal jug-ular vein has been exposed and surrounded by vessel loops. A subcutaneous tunnel is made with a Hegar cervical dilator.

vein is then punctured with an 18-gauge needle through the infraclavicular incision, and a flexible J wire is introduced through the needle and advanced centrally. The needle is removed, and a 10.5 F strip-away sheath introducer and vein dilator* are passed over the J wire after which the dilator and wire are removed. Then the Broviac catheter is quickly inserted through the sheath introducer. At this point the sheath introducer is withdrawn and stripped away from the catheter. The procedure is completed by closing the infraclavicular incision.

Peripherally Inserted Central Venous Catheters
Long plastic catheters advanced into the superior vena cava through the basi-lic or cephalic vein are not satisfactory routes for parenteral nutrition because of a high incidence of phlebitis and thrombosis. Recently, however, satisfac-tory results have been reported using long catheters of silicone elastomer (Si-

---

*Available from Medtronic Inc., Minneapolis, Minnesota.

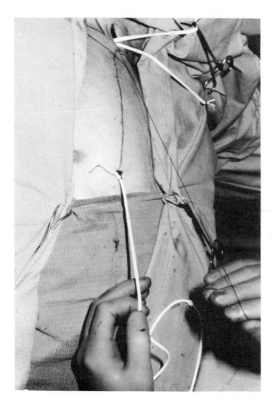

Figure 6-18. A heavy silk suture previously carried through the tunnel with the Hegar dilator is now tied to the tip of the Broviac catheter. The latter is then pulled through the tunnel.

lastic).* The properties of silicone rubber have been previously discussed and evidently contribute to the reduced morbidity and increased longevity with such peripherally inserted catheters. In a prospective study of patients receiving parenteral nutrition, MacDonald and associates found that the peripherally inserted silicone catheter was comparable to plastic or silicone subclavian catheters.[26] The average duration of use exceeded 29 days; only 1 of 20 such peripherally inserted catheters had to be removed because of phlebitis, and there were no instances of thrombosis or catheter-related sepsis. However, other authors using the same apparatus reported a somewhat higher complication rate. Bottino and associates reported 20 instances of phlebitis in 87 patients (23 percent).[33] In 14 patients, the phlebitis was minor and resolved with warm soaks; the catheters had to be removed from the remaining 6 patients (7 percent). Hoshal found that 6 of 36 catheters had to be removed because of local inflammation, including phlebitis.[34] The occurrence of phlebitis may be

---

Intrasil catheters are available from Vicra Division, Travenol Laboratories, Inc., Dallas, Texas.

related to the affinity of the silicone elastomer for particulate matter (for example, powder on surgical gloves) or to the improper location of the catheter tip in a small-caliber vessel (for example, the axillary vein). Consequently, x-ray confirmation of the proper location of the catheter in the superior vena cava before beginning TPN is important.[35] Catheter sepsis and subclavian vein thrombosis have also been reported with the silicone catheter.[33,35] Occasionally, this catheter cannot be introduced or cannot be advanced into the superior vena cava because of the small caliber of the peripheral vein or angulation at the shoulder. In other patients, placement is unsuccessful percutaneously but can be achieved with venous cut-down.

In summary, limited available data indicate that hypertonic nutrient solutions can be successfully infused through peripherally inserted silicone elastomer central venous catheters for at least several weeks, apparently with small risk of serious complications. Some freedom of mobility of the upper extremity is lost when such catheters are used, but the potential cardiothoracic complications of subclavian cannulation appear to be obviated. At the Los

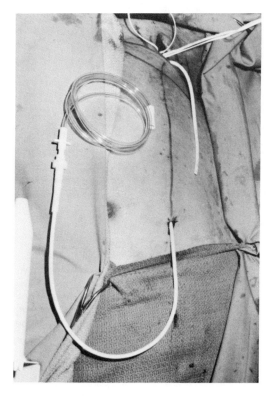

Figure 6-19. The catheter has been drawn through the tunnel and exits adjacent to the previously exposed internal jugular vein. The Dacron cuff lies within the tunnel in an intercostal space.

Angeles County–USC Medical Center, these catheters are used when a sub-clavian catheter cannot or should not be inserted.

Arteriovenous Shunts and Fistulas

Application of the vascular access techniques so useful in dialysis patients to nonuremic patients requiring parenteral nutrition has generally been unsatis-factory, although the experience has been limited.

The standard external Teflon–Silastic arteriovenous shunt (Scribner shunt) may be difficult to insert in patients requiring TPN. For example, Bro-viac found that in a series of patients with severe bowel disease, insertion of the shunt was extremely difficult because these patients invariably had tiny, fragile veins or the superficial veins were thrombosed by prior intravenous therapy.[36] Even when shunts were successfully placed, they often clotted, de-spite the administration of coumadin or heparin.

Buselmeier and associates described a modification of the Scribner shunt designed for TPN in which the shorter length of the tubing employed results

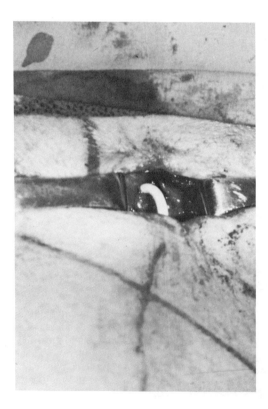

Figure 6-20. The catheter has been passed into the right atri-um through a venotomy in the internal jugular vein. The cath-eter is secured and hemosta-sis is obtained with a 7-0 pursestring suture in the vein.

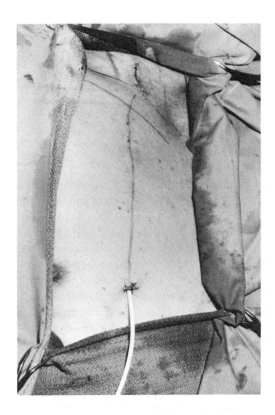

Figure 6-21. The procedure is completed by closing the neck incision with a subcuticular suture.

in much faster flow, evidently with less clotting.[37] Such a shunt was successfully used in four patients for 18 to 180 days.

Internal arteriovenous fistulas (Brecia–Cimino fistula[38]) may be useful for home hyperalimentation patients,[39,40] but this form of vascular access is generally not applicable to hospitalized patients because such fistulas require a maturation period of up to several months before they can be used successfully.[36] Internal arteriovenous shunts using prosthetic graft materials have occasionally been used in TPN patients. In a limited experience with bovine heterografts, Riella and Scribner encountered a high incidence of infection and thrombosis.[31] Buselmeier and associates reported successful use of a shunt created with an expanded polytetrafluoroethylene (PTFE) prosthesis in a patient with repeated infection of a central venous line.[41] TPN was successfully administered for 4 weeks by daily needle puncture of the graft, which remained uninfected despite the ongoing sepsis.

At the Los Angeles County–USC Medical Center, the percutaneously placed, infraclavicular subclavian catheter is the access route of choice for the administration of the glucose system of parenteral nutrition. In patients in whom a subclavian catheter cannot be placed for technical reasons or in whom it is contraindicated, a silicone elastomer central venous catheter is introduced peripherally. If this is unsatisfactory, a Broviac catheter is inserted. In patients in whom central venous access is a problem, the necessity for the glucose system is reassessed; the peripherally administered lipid system may be a satisfactory alternative (see Chapter 7).

ADMINISTRATION OF THE GLUCOSE SYSTEM

Because of the high concentration of glucose in this form of parenteral nutrition, therapy should be begun gradually to avoid hyperglycemia and allow for adaption. Therefore, on the first day of treatment, 1 liter of the nutrient solution is infused at a constant rate over the full 24 hour period. Blood and urine glucose levels are monitored frequently, and if this amount of glucose is well tolerated, 2 liters of nutrient solution are infused during the second day. Now the rate of infusion is adjusted so that the 2 liters are infused at a constant rate over the 24 hour period. Again, if this volume and amount of glucose are well tolerated, the patient receives 3 liters during the third day, again at a constant rate of infusion. The total volume of infusate is subsequently adjusted to meet the caloric requirements of the individual patient, the determination of which has been discussed in Chapter 3. Requirements for the average patient are usually met by 3 liters/day, providing 2550 nonprotein kcal. The nutrient solution is delivered to the patient through infusion apparatus consisting of infusion tubing (IV administration set), intravenous extension tubing, the indwelling venous cannula, and, when employed, infusion pumps and in-line filters. The intravenous tubing is changed with each new bottle of nutrient solution. The extension tubing, connected proximally to the infusion tubing and distally to the venous cannula, is changed only when the dressings overlying the venous cannula are changed, since the distal end of the extension tubing is incorporated in the dressings. Infusion of the glucose system at a constant rate is a critical feature of safe practice, since abrupt changes in the rate of delivery may be associated with marked alterations in blood sugar levels (see Chapter 8). Gravity infusion is usually successful, but infusion pumps may be required and, when available, provide a very efficient method of assuring a constant rate of infusion.

A variety of in-line filters are available for use in patients receiving intravenous infusions. Such filters may be inserted into the infusion apparatus between the intravenous tubing and the extension tubing or between the extension tubing and the venous cannula. Five micron filters may be used to trap particulate matter, including rubber, chemicals, glass, and cellulose fibers. Such particles may produce phlebitis and granulomas.[42] Bacterial filters are available in two pore sizes, $0.45\ \mu$ and $0.22\ \mu$. The former will block passage of all fungi and all bacteria except for some strains of Pseudomonas and aberrant bacterial forms; 0.22 μ filters will screen all bacteria, but an infusion pump may be required to overcome the resistance to flow introduced by the use of such a filter.[43-45] Both of these bacterial filters block particulate matter and air emboli, but not endotoxin.[43,44] Theoretically, these filters should reduce the hazard of infection caused by contaminated intravenous solutions. On the other hand, the manual insertion of any device into the infusion circuit increases the likelihood of contaminating the system.[43,45] Although the efficacy of bacterial filters in reducing the sepsis rate among patients receiving TPN is unestablished,[43,45-47] such filters are used in many institutions.[46,48,49]

At the Los Angeles County–USC Medical Center, the nutrient solution is passed through a 0.22 μ bacterial filter during preparation in the pharmacy, but in-line bacterial filters are not used. However, a 5 μ filter is used to screen particulate matter and is inserted between the intravenous tubing and the extension tubing. This filter is changed with each bottle of infusate.

Potential contamination of the TPN system is avoided by maintaining a closed system after the preparation of the nutrient solution and the attachment of the tubing. Thus no additions are made to the solution once it leaves the pharmacy, and the TPN system is not used to measure central venous pressure or to obtain blood samples; nor are blood products or medications given through the TPN infusion apparatus.

The management of the dressings overlying subclavian catheters has been discussed. The management of dressings is similar when other forms of vascular access have been employed.

At the completion of therapy, the rate of infusion of the glucose system should be tapered gradually over 2 to 3 days to avoid hypoglycemia. When the infusion must be abruptly terminated (for example, in patients undergoing surgery or requiring fluid resuscitation), a solution of 10 percent glucose is substituted for the nutrient solution (see Chapter 8).

COMPLICATIONS OF THE GLUCOSE SYSTEM

Complications can be classified as (1) those occurring during attempts to obtain vascular access (discussed previously), (2) metabolic complications (discussed in Chapter 8), and (3) TPN-related sepsis.

TPN-Related Sepsis
The development of sepsis attributable primarily to the administration of parenteral nutrition should be an infrequent complication in modern practice. However, when TPN-related sepsis does occur, it is a potentially serious, even life-threatening event.

A variety of factors may contribute to the development of sepsis in patients receiving intravenous feedings. Patients requiring this therapy are often inordinately susceptible to infection because of serious illness, malnutrition, or chronic debilitation, all conditions associated with impaired immune responses. Patients receiving immunosuppressive or cytotoxic drugs or corticosteroids are likewise susceptible to infection, and these drugs as well as the prolonged administration of broad-spectrum antibiotics may subject patients to sepsis from unusual or ordinarily saprophytic bacteria and fungi.

In addition to these patient-related factors, several specific TPN-related factors contribute to the pathogenesis of sepsis. The various components of the nutrient solution can become contaminated during manufacture, or contamination may occur at the time of component admixture in the hospital pharmacy. With present techniques of solution preparation, sepsis from these sources should be rare. Reported rates of solution contamination during admixture range from 0 to 3 percent.[27,50–52]

The ability of the nutrient solution to support microbial growth after contamination is in part dependent upon the protein source employed. *Candida albicans* proliferates rapidly at 25° or 37°C in TPN solutions prepared from protein hydrolysates,[53,54] whereas no significant proliferation occurs within 24 hours in solutions prepared from crystalline amino acids (Fig. 6-22).[53]

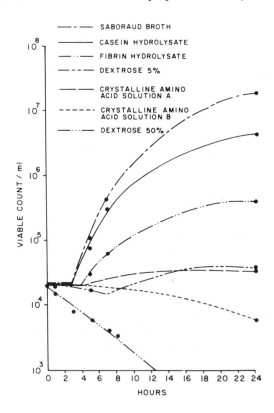

Figure 6-22. Growth of *Candida albicans* in various solutions at 37°C. The protein hydrolysate and amino acid solutions are TPN solutions with glucose. *(From Gelbart SM, et al: Appl Microbiol 26:874–879, 1973)*

TABLE 6-3
Growth of Fungi and Bacteria in Casein Hydrolysate–Glucose TPN Solution at Room Temperature (25°C)

Organism	Organisms/ml*				
	0 TIME	12 HR	24 HR	48 HR	7 DAYS
C. albicans	1	24.0	2.4×10^3	T‡	T
T. glabrata	1	15.0	1.7×10^3	T	T
S. marcescens	1	28.0	4.5×10^3	T	T
K. pneumoniae	1	12.0	2.2×10^3	T	T
Staph. aureus†	1	5.0	1.4×10^3	T	T
E. coli	1	3.0	1.1×10^3	1.7×10^6	T
E. cloacae	1	4.7	96.0	1.0×10^6	T
Pr. mirabilis	1	1.9	27.0	7.2×10^4	T
Ps. aeruginosa	1	2.7	1.6	1.1	0.13

*Mean concentration for five test strains of each organism, normalized to an inoculum of one organism/ml.
†Two strains failed to proliferate.
‡T = turbid.
From Goldmann DA, et al: Am J Surg 126:314–318, 1973.

Goldmann and associates found that *Klebsiella pneumoniae, Serratia marcescens,* and some strains of *Staphylococcus aureus* grew as rapidly at room temperature (25°C) as Candida in protein hydrolysates, but the other bacteria tested multiplied more slowly, and *Pseudomonas aeruginosa* slowly died (Table 6-3).[54] All of the bacterial strains tested either died or showed minimal growth in TPN solutions containing crystalline amino acids (Table 6-4). In contrast, Gelbart and associates found that none of the bacterial strains they tested at 37°C (*Staphylococcus aureus, Escherichia coli, Enterobacter aerogenes, Enterobacter cloacea, Enterobacter agglomerans, Serratia marcescens, Klebsiella pneumoniae, Pseudomonas cepacia,* and *Pseudomonas aeruginosa*) displayed significant multiplication in either protein hydrolysates or crystalline amino acids.[53]

Microbial proliferation is inhibited for at least 7 days in both types of TPN solutions during storage at 4°C.[54]

The infusion apparatus, especially the intravenous catheter, appears to be the most common source of TPN-associated sepsis. Contamination may take place when bottles of the nutrient solution are changed, during replacement of intravenous tubing, when in-line filters are inserted, and when the intravenous line is used for measurements of central venous pressure, blood drawing, or the infusion of medication or blood products. To and fro motion of a subclavian catheter due to inadequate fixation allows exposed portions of the catheter to enter the subcutaneous tract leading to the vein, which may

TABLE 6-4
Growth of Fungi and Bacteria in Synthetic Amino Acid–Glucose
TPN Solution at Room Temperature (25°C)

Organism	Organisms/ml*				
	0 TIME	12 HR	24 HR	48 HR	7 DAYS
C. albicans	1	8.5	49.0	1.7×10^2	1.7×10^3
T. glabrata	1	4.5	16.0	33.0	6.5×10^3
S. marcescens	1	2.5	3.0	0.77	1.5
K. pneumoniae	1	0.63	0.15	0.06	0.05
Staph. aureus	1	0.66	0.24	0.01	0.09
E. coli	1	0.89	0.67	0.46	0.18
E. cloacae	1	0.62	0.16	0.06	0.06
Pr. mirabilis	1	0.67	0.52	0.23	0.12
Ps. aeruginosa	1	0.30	0.12	0.02	0.06

*Mean concentration for five test strains of each organism, normalized to an inoculum of one organism/ml.
From Goldmann DA, et al: Am J Surg 126:314–318, 1973.

result in infection. Hematogenous seeding of the catheter may occasionally develop following bacteremia due to a focus of infection at a site distant to the catheter. More commonly, however, the catheter-related sepsis is due to contamination of the catheter by organisms colonizing the skin surrounding the catheter insertion site. Thus several studies have demonstrated the presence of organisms found on the skin to be the same as those causing septicemia or contaminating the catheter at the time of removal.[6,7,50,55–57]

Diagnosis of catheter-related sepsis. Catheter-related sepsis is defined as an episode of clinical sepsis due to contamination of the intravenous cannula, and it is diagnosed when sepsis occurs which is not attributable to the patient's underlying pathology and which resolves with removal of the catheter. Positive cultures obtained from the catheter tip or from blood aspirated from the catheter provide confirmatory evidence of catheter-related sepsis but generally are not required for the diagnosis.[27,57] Catheter-related sepsis is not diagnosed if catheter contamination is not associated with clinical evidence of sepsis. The diagnosis of catheter-related sepsis has proven to be more elusive than anticipated. Most of the catheters removed for suspected catheter-related sepsis are in fact removed unnecessarily, since 75 percent of the involved patients are eventually found to harbor a septic focus elsewhere.[27,48]

Incidence of TPN-related sepsis. The incidence of sepsis varies greatly in reported series (Table 6-5), but in recent years TPN has been administered with very low rates of infection. This improving trend is evidently due to increasing experience with this relatively recent modality of treatment, adherence to rigid protocols of practice, and the development of a multidisciplinary team approach to parenteral nutrition. Thus a 27 percent incidence of septicemia was reported by Curry and Quie in a group of patients who received nutrient solutions prepared at the nursing station and in whom the intravenous lines were used for the measurement of central venous pressure and the administration of albumin and blood.[65] Similarly, Sanders and Sheldon reported a sepsis rate of 28.6 percent before the initiation of a total parenteral nutrition service.[57] In contrast, the sepsis rate was 4.7 percent among the 172 patients most recently studied by these same investigators since the initiation of their TPN service and the development of protocols for solution preparation, administration, and infection control. Ryan and associates reported that 11 percent of 200 patients in whom 355 central venous catheters had been inserted developed catheter-related sepsis.[27] However, only 3 percent of the catheters managed "properly" became infected, whereas breaks in protocol were associated with a 20 percent incidence of catheter infection.

Gram-positive cocci and fungi are the predominant organisms causing TPN-related sepsis. *Staphylococcus epidermidis, Staphylococcus aureus,* and *Candida albicans* are the species most commonly isolated (Tables 6-6 and 6-7). Gram-negative bacteria are isolated relatively infrequently, especially in comparison to the frequency with which they cause septicemia due to primary infection at a site other than the TPN catheter.[50]

Clinical manifestations and management of TPN-related sepsis.   Fever is the hallmark of TPN-related sepsis; chills and tachycardia may also be prominent features. Increasing glucose intolerance with hyperglycemia and glucosuria, a manifestation of sepsis-induced insulin resistance, may be the earliest clue to impending sepsis.[57]

Serious manifestations of systemic Candidiasis include endocarditis,[87] osteomyelitis,[88,89] and endophthalmitis. Endophthalmitis may be diagnosed by the funduscopic appearance of "cotton wool" exudates.[90] The appearance of Candida in the urine may be an early manifestation of systemic fungal infection. These complications appear to have been more common in the early experience with TPN.

The TPN system becomes suspect immediately when fever develops which is not clearly attributable to the patient's underlying disease. The sequence of decisions in the management of TPN patients developing sepsis is detailed in Figure 6-23.

When shock or bacteremia supervene or cellulitis involves the catheter insertion site, TPN is discontinued and 10 percent glucose is infused through a peripheral vein to avoid reactive hypoglycemia. In the absence of cellulitis or these severe manifestations of sepsis, the TPN solution and the infusion apparatus (except the catheter) are changed, and the nutrient solution is cultured through the intravenous tubing. If fever persists for 12 to 24 hours,

TABLE 6-5
Incidence of TPN-Related Sepsis in Patients Receiving the Glucose System

Reference	Year	Number of Patients	Rate of Septicemia (%)			Comments
			BACTERIAL	FUNGAL	TOTAL	
Wilmore et al.[58]	1969	25	0	0	0	
Dudrick et al.[59]	1969	22	5	9	14	
Filler et al.[60]	1969	14	0	0	0	
Groff[61]	1969	18	—	17	17	
Filler and Erakis[62]	1970	53	6	11	17	
Boeckman and Krill[63]	1970	15	53	40	93	
Ashcraft and Leape[64]	1970	22	0	23	23	
Curry and Quie[65]	1971	49	10	16	27	
Owings et al.[66]	1972	66	0	0	0	
Helmuth et al.[67]	1972	4	0	25	25	
Peden and Karpel[68]	1972	13	23	0	23	
Driscoll et al.[69]	1972	9	0	11	11	
Johnson et al.[70]	1972	23	13	0	13	
Parsa et al.[71]	1972	307	7	2	9	Polyvinyl chloride catheter
		150	—	—	1	Silastic catheter
McGovern[72]	1972	25	8	4	12	
Asch et al.[73]	1972	51	8	4	12	
Freeman et al.[74]	1972	33	(12)*	21	21	Before starting TPN team
		78	0	1	1	After TPN protocol, nurse

Study	Year	Patients				Comments
CDC Survey[43]	1972	2078	3	4	7	Survey of 31 hospitals
Miller and Grogan[75]	1973	20	10	10	20	
Sanderson and Dietel[76]	1973	100	1	0	1	
Dillon et al.[77]	1973	122	2	2	4	
O'Neill et al.[78]	1974	19	0	0	0	
Freeman and Litton[79]	1974	105	11	3	14	Breaks in protocol observed
Copeland et al.[51]	1974	35	0	0	0	Catheter sepsis suspected in 11%
Copeland et al.[55]	1974	93	0	2	2	
Ryan et al.[27]	1974	200	7	4	11	Breaks in protocol observed
Abel et al.[80]	1974	64	0	0	0	
Myers et al.[81]	1974	212	0	2	2	
Popp et al.[82]	1974	26	31	23	54	14 episodes sepsis in 7 burn patients
		(15)	—	—	(7)	Catheter through unburned skin
		(11)	—	—	(118)	Catheter through burned skin
Skoutakis et al.[83]	1975	160	0	1	1	
Hoshal[34]	1975	35	0	0	0	
Heird and Winters[84]	1975	35	—	—	9	
Sanders and Sheldon[57]	1976	21	—	—	28.6	1970–72: Pre TPN team
		125	—	—	12	1972–74: With new TPN team
		172	—	—	4.7	1974–75: More experienced team
Reinhardt et al.[85]	1978	118	5.1	2.5	7.6	
Nehme[86]	1980	211	0.95	1.4	2.4	TPN team

*Patients had both gram-negative and Candida septicemia.
Adapted and updated from Allen JR: In Johnston IDA (ed): Advances in Parenteral Nutrition. Baltimore, University Park Press, 1978, pp 340–341.

TABLE 6-6
Microorganisms Causing TPN-Related Sepsis

Organism	Frequency of Isolation		Percentage	
Fungi	17		29	
Candida spp.		13		22
Torulopsis spp.		4		7
Gram-positive cocci	31		53	
Staphylococcus aureus		9		15
Staphylococcus epidermidis		18		31
Streptococcal species, alpha				
or nonhemolytic		3		5
Enterococcus		1		2
Gram-negative bacteria	10		17	
Klebsiella spp.		3		5
Pseudomonas spp.		3		5
Escherichia coli		2		3
Enterobacter spp.		1		2
Proteus rettgeri		1		2
Anaerobic bacteria	1		2	
Bacteroides spp.		1		2
Total	59			

From Allen JR: In Johnston IDA (ed): *Advances in Parenteral Nutrition.* Baltimore, University Park Press, 1978, p 348.

blood is aspirated through the intravenous catheter for culture, and the catheter is removed aseptically and its tip is also cultured.

Sepsis unrelated to TPN may occasionally produce hematogenous seeding of the TPN catheter. Such episodes of sepsis may not resolve, despite standard treatment, until the catheter is removed (Fig. 6-23, *pathway 5*). Sepsis usually resolves spontaneously when the offending nutrient solution, intra-

TABLE 6-7
Relative Frequency of Fungal Species Causing TPN-Related Sepsis

Fungal Species	Frequency of Isolation	Percentage
Candida albicans	33	59
Candida tropicalis	1	2
Candida parapsilosis	4	7
Candida parakrusei	2	4
Candida spp.	7	13
Torulopsis glabrata	9	16
Total	56	

From Allen JR: In Johnston IDA (ed): *Advances in Parenteral Nutrition.* Baltimore, University Park Press, 1978, p 348.

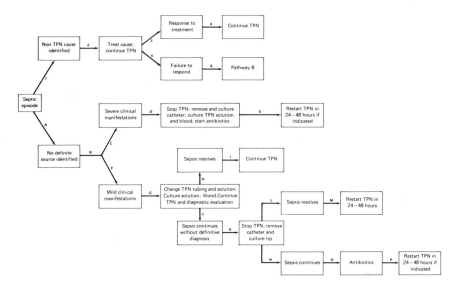

Figure 6-23. Sequence of decisions in the evaluation and management of sepsis occurring in patients receiving the glucose system of TPN.

venous tubing, or intravenous catheter is removed. However, severe manifestations must be treated empirically with antibiotics or antifungal agents as soon as appropriate cultures are obtained. Occasionally, lesser manifestations will require antimicrobial therapy, as well.

Prevention of TPN-related sepsis.   Strict adherence to a detailed clinical protocol under the supervision of experienced personnel appears to be the essential element contributing to the safe administration of intravenous feedings with minimal complications. Specific factors thought to contribute to the declining rate of TPN-related sepsis can be listed as follows:

1. Use of crystalline amino acids as a protein source.
2. Solution preparation under a laminar flow hood.
3. Aseptic catheter insertion.
4. Strict protocol for management of dressings and infusion apparatus.
5. Maintaining a closed infusion system used for nutrient solutions only.
6. Patient management under supervision of experienced personnel or a "team."

Periodic replacement of the subclavian catheter is not warranted, since there is no correlation between the incidence of catheter-related sepsis and the length of time that a catheter remains in place.[10,57] Burn patients represent an exception to this rule. It has been suggested that catheters in these patients be

TABLE 6-8
Monitoring Schedule for Patients Receiving the Glucose System:
Required Procedures

Procedure	Before TPN	Daily	Mondays	Tuesdays	Wednesdays	Thursdays	Fridays	Notes
Body weight	X	X						
Input/output record		X						
Fractional urine (sugar/acetone)		X						
CBC	X		X			X		Daily 1st 5 days
Chemistry panel*	X		X			X		Daily 1st 5 days
Liver panel†	X		X			X		
Prothrombin time	X					X		

*Serum glucose, urea, creatinine, sodium, potassium, chloride, bicarbonate, calcium, phosphate, magnesium, total protein, and albumin.
†Serum bilirubin, SGOT, SGPT, and alkaline phosphatase.

TABLE 6-9
Monitoring Schedule for Patients Receiving the Glucose System:
Optional Determinations

Procedure	Interval
Nutritional assessment*	Weekly
Skin tests	Biweekly
Cholesterol	Weekly
Triglycerides	Weekly
Serum B-12†	Initially and p.r.n.
Serum folate†	Initially and p.r.n.
Serum iron†	Initially and p.r.n.
Transferrin	Weekly
Zinc	Weekly
Copper	Weekly
24-hour urine nitrogen‡	1–7 times per week

*See Chapter 2.
†Essential if anemia present.
‡For nitrogen balance studies.

changed every 48 to 72 hours, especially if the catheter was introduced through burned tissues.[10-12]

MONITORING PROTOCOL

Patients receiving the glucose system require careful metabolic monitoring. Pre-TPN studies identify metabolic abnormalities requiring treatment prior to initiating or during nutritional therapy. Periodic evaluation of patients while receiving TPN permits early diagnosis of metabolic problems which may develop during the course of intravenous feedings. The most common metabolic complications include hyperglycemia, hypophosphatemia, hypokalemia, elevated liver transaminase values, and abnormalities of water balance, edema, or dehydration (see Chapter 8). The essential parameters measured during TPN are listed in Table 6-8. Other observations recommended but perhaps less important are outlined in Table 6–9.

SUMMARY

The glucose system of parenteral nutrition provides 850 nonprotein kcal and 6.5 gm of nitrogen per liter. Because of their hyperosmolality, glucose-based nutrient solutions must be infused into the vena cava, usually through a percutaneously inserted subclavian catheter. Complications during treatment can be minimized by strict adherence to proper technique in management of the venous cannula and by close metabolic monitoring.

REFERENCES

1. Duke JH, Dudrick SJ: Parenteral feedings, in Ballinger WF, Collins JA, Drucker WR, et al (eds): Manual of Surgical Nutrition. Philadelphia, WB Saunders Co, 1975, pp 285–317.
2. Shils ME: Parenteral nutrition, in Goodhart RS, Shils ME (eds): Modern Nutrition in Health and Disease. Philadelphia, Lea and Febiger, 1980, pp 1125–1152.
3. Giovanoni R: The manufacturing pharmacy solutions and incompatibilities, in Fischer JE (ed): Total Parenteral Nutrition. Boston, Little, Brown and Co, 1976, pp 27–53.
4. Turco SJ, Burke WA: Methods of ordering and use of intravenous phosphate (mEq vs mM). Hosp Pharm 10: 320–326, 1975.
5. Borja AR: Current status of infraclavicular subclavian vein catheterization. Ann Thorac Surg 13:615–624, 1972.
6. Banks DC, Cawdrey HM, Yates DB, et al: Infection from intravenous catheters. Lancet 1:443–445, 1970.
7. Goldmann DA, Maki DG: The problem of sepsis, in White PL, Nagy ME (eds):

Total Parenteral Nutrition. Acton, Mass, Publishing Sciences Group, Inc., 1974, pp 319–328.

8. Jarrard MM, Freeman JB: The effects of antibiotic ointments and antiseptics on the skin flora beneath subclavian catheter dressings during intravenous hyperalimentation. J Surg Res 22:521–526, 1977.

9. Jarrard MM, Olson CM, Freeman JB: Daily dressing change effects on skin flora beneath subclavian catheter dressings during total parenteral nutrition. JPEN 4:391–392, 1980.

10. Ryan JA Jr: Complications of total parenteral nutrition, in Fischer JE (ed): Total Parenteral Nutrition. Boston, Little, Brown and Co, 1976, pp 55–100.

11. Pruitt BA, McManus WF, Kim SH, Treat RC: Diagnosis and treatment of cannula-related intravenous sepsis in burn patients. Ann Surg 191:546–554, 1980.

12. Warden GD, Wilmore DW, Pruitt BA: Central venous thrombosis: A hazard of medical progress. J Trauma 13:620–626, 1973.

13. Bernard RW, Stahl WM: Subclavian vein catheterizations: A prospective study, I: Non-infectious complications. Ann Surg 173:184–190, 1971.

14. Parsa MH, Habif DV, Ferrer JM: Techniques for placement of long-term indwelling superior vena cava catheters. Film and pamphlet presented at the 56th annual Clinical Congress of the American College of Surgeons, Chicago, Ill, 1970 (revised 1972).

15. Mogil RA, DeLaurentis A, Rosemond GP: The infraclavicular venipuncture. Arch Surg 95:320–324, 1967.

16. Herbst CA: Indications, management, and complications of percutaneous subclavian catheters. Arch Surg 113:1421–1425, 1978.

17. Blackett RL: A prospective study of subclavian vein catheters used exclusively for the purpose of intravenous feeding. Br J Surg 65:393–395, 1978.

18. Armstrong RF, Peters JL, Cohen SL: Air embolism caused by fractured central-venous catheter. Lancet 1:954, 1977.

19. Feliciano DV, Mattox KL, Graham JM, et al: Major complications of percutaneous subclavian vein catheters. Am J Surg 138:869–874, 1979.

20. Peters JL, Armstrong R: Air embolism occurring as a complication of central venous catheterization. Ann Surg 187:375–378, 1978.

21. Durant TM, Long J, Oppenheimer MJ: Pulmonary (venous) air embolism. Am Heart J 33:269–281, 1947.

22. Green HL, Nemir P: Air embolism as a complication during parenteral alimentation. Am J Surg 121:614–616, 1971.

23. Oppenheimer MJ, Durant TM, Lynch P: Body position in relation to venous air embolism and the associated cardiovascular–respiratory changes. Am J Med Sci 225:362–373, 1953.

24. Hamby WB, Terry RN: Air embolism in operations done in the sitting position. Surgery 31:212–215, 1952.

25. Grace DM: Air embolism with neurologic complications: A potential hazard of central venous catheters. Can J Surg 20:51–53, 1977.

26. MacDonald AS, Master SKP, Moffitt E: A comparative study of peripherally inserted silicone catheters for parenteral nutrition. Can Anaesth Soc J 24:263–269, 1977.

27. Ryan A, Abel M, Abbott WM, et al: Catheter complications in total parenteral nutrition. N Engl J Med 290:757–761, 1974.

28. Jernigan WR, Gardner WC, Mahr MM, Milburn JL: Use of the internal jugular vein for placement of central venous catheter. Surg Gynecol Obstet 130:520–524, 1970.

29. Benotti PN, Bothe A Jr, Miller JDB, Blackburn GL: Safe cannulation of the internal jugular vein for long term hyperalimentation. Surg Gynecol Obstet 144:574–576, 1977.

30. Broviac JW, Cole JJ, Scribner BH: A silicone rubber atrial catheter for prolonged parenteral alimentation. Surg Gynecol Obstet 136:602–606, 1973.

31. Riella MC, Scribner BH: Five years' experience with a right atrial catheter for prolonged parenteral nutrition at home. Surg Gynecol Obstet 143:205–208, 1976.

32. Kirkemo A, Johnston MR: Percutaneous subclavian vein placement of the Hickman catheter. Surgery 91:349–351, 1982.

33. Bottino J, McCredie KB, Groschel DHM, Lawson M: Long-term intravenous therapy with peripherally inserted silicone elastomer central venous catheters in patients with malignant diseases. Cancer 43:1937–1943, 1979.

34. Hoshal VL Jr: Total intravenous nutrition with peripherally inserted silicone elastomer central venous catheters. Arch Surg 110:644–646, 1975.

35. Prian GW, VanWay CW III: The long-arm silastic catheter: A critical look at complications. JPEN 2:124–128, 1978.

36. Broviac J: Administration systems: Tubing, closures, infusion attachments, shunts. Proceedings of the AMA Symposium on Total Parenteral Nutrition, Nashville, Tenn, January 17–19, 1972, pp 160–170.

37. Buselmeier TJ, Najarian JS, Simmons RL, et al: An A–V shunt for long-term hyperalimentation in azotaemic patients. Proc Eur Dial Transplant Assoc 10:516–521, 1973.

38. Brescia MJ, Cimino JE, Appel K, Hurwich BJ: Chronic hemodialysis using venipuncture and a surgically created arteriovenous fistula. N Engl J Med 275:1089–1092, 1966.

39. Guba AM, Collins GJ, Rich NM, et al: Nondialysis uses for vascular access procedures. Ann Surg 190:72–74, 1979.

40. McGill DB: Long-term parenteral nutrition. Gastroenterology 67:195–197, 1974.

41. Buselmeier TJ, Kjellstrand CM, Sutherland DER, et al: Peripheral blood access for hyperalimentation: Use of expanding polytetrafluoroethylene arteriovenous conduit. JAMA 238:2399–2400, 1977.

42. Evans WE, Barker LF, Simone JV: Double-blind evaluation of 5-μm final filtration to reduce postinfusion phlebitis. Am J Hosp Pharm 33:1160–1163, 1976.

43. Goldmann DA, Maki DG: Infection control in total parenteral nutrition. JAMA 223:1360–1364, 1973.

44. Maki DG, Goldmann A, Rhame S: Infection control in intravenous therapy. Ann Intern Med 79:867–887, 1973.

45. Tenney JH, Dixon RE: What risk of Candidiasis from micropore filters in intravenous hyperalimentation? JAMA 229:467, 1974.

46. Jeejeebhoy KN: Total parenteral nutrition. Ann R Coll Phys Surg Can 9:287–300, 1976.

47. Miller RC, Grogan JB: Efficacy of inline bacterial filters in reducing contamination of intravenous nutritional solutions. Am J Surg 130:585–589, 1975.

48. Fleming CR, McGill DB, Hoffman HN II, Nelson RA: Total parenteral nutrition. Mayo Clin Proc 51:187–199, 1976.

49. Meng HC: Parenteral nutrition: Principles, nutrient, requirements, and techniques. Geriatrics 30:97–107, 1975.
50. Allen JR: The incidence of nosocomial infection in patients receiving total parenteral nutrition, in Johnston IDA (ed): Advances in Parenteral Nutrition. Baltimore, University Park, 1978, pp 339–377.
51. Copeland EM III, MacFadyen BV Jr, Dudrick SJ: Prevention of microbial catheter contamination in patients receiving parenteral hyperalimentation. South Med J 67:303–306, 1974.
52. Deeb EN, Natsios GA: Contamination of intravenous fluids by bacteria and fungi during preparation and administration. Am J Hosp Pharm 28:764–767, 1971.
53. Gelbart SM, Reinhardt GF, Greenlee HB: Multiplication of nosocomial pathogens in intravenous feeding solutions. Appl Microbiol 26:874–879, 1973.
54. Goldmann DA, Martin T, Worthington JW: Growth of bacteria and fungi in total parenteral nutrition solutions. Am J Surg 126:314–318, 1973.
55. Copeland EM III, MacFadyen BV Jr, McGown C, Dudrick SJ: The use of hyperalimentation in patients with potential sepsis. Surg Gynecol Obstet 138:377–380, 1974.
56. Mogensen JV, Frederiksen W, Jensen JK: Subclavian vein catheterization and infection: A bacteriologic study of 130 catheter insertions. Scand J Infect Dis 4:31–36, 1972.
57. Sanders RA, Sheldon GF: Septic complications of total parenteral nutrition: A five year experience. Am J Surg 132:214–220, 1976.
58. Wilmore DW, Groff DB, Bishop HC, Dudrick SJ: Total parenteral nutrition in infants with catastrophic gastrointestinal anomalies. J Pediatr Surg 4:181–189, 1969.
59. Dudrick SJ, Groff DB, Wilmore DW: Long term venous catheterization in infants. Surg Gynecol Obstet 129:805–808, 1969.
60. Filler RM, Eraklis AJ, Rubin VG, Das JB: Long-term total nutrition in infants. N Engl J Med 281:589–594, 1969.
61. Groff DB: Complications of intravenous hyperalimentation in newborns and infants. J Pediatr Surg 4:460–464, 1969.
62. Filler RM, Erakis AJ: Care of the critically ill child: Intravenous alimentation. Pediatrics 46:456–461, 1970.
63. Boeckman CR, Krill CE: Bacterial and fungal infections complicating parenteral alimentation in infants and children. J Pediatr Surg 5:117–126, 1970.
64. Ashcraft KW, Leape LL: Candida sepsis complicating parenteral feeding. JAMA 212:454–456, 1970.
65. Curry CR, Quie PG: Fungal septicemia in patients receiving parenteral hyperalimentation. N Engl J Med 285:1221–1224, 1971.
66. Owings JM, Bomar WE Jr, Ramage RC: Parenteral hyperalimentation and its practical applications. Ann Surg 175:712–719, 1972.
67. Helmuth WV, Adam PJ, Sweet AY: The effects of protein hydrolysate–monosaccharide infusion on low-birth-weight infants. J Pediatr 81:129–136, 1972.
68. Peden VH, Karpel JT: Total parenteral nutrition in premature infants. J Pediatr 81:137–144, 1972.
69. Driscoll JD, Heird WC, Schullinger JN, et al: Total intravenous alimentation in low-birth-weight infants: A preliminary report. J Pediatr 81:145–153, 1972.

70. Johnson JD, Albritton WL, Sunshine P: Hyperammonemia accompanying parenteral nutrition in newborn infants. J Pediatr 81:154–161, 1972.
71. Parsa MH, Habif DV, Ferrer JM, et al: Intravenous hyperalimentation: Indications, technique, and complications. Bull NY Acad Med 48:920–942, 1972.
72. McGovern B: Septic complications of hyperalimentation, in Cowan GSM Jr, Scheetz WL (eds): Intravenous Hyperalimentation. Philadelphia, Lea and Febiger, 1972, pp 165–174.
73. Asch MJ, Huxtable RF, Hays DM: High calorie parenteral therapy in infants and children. Arch Surg 104:434–437, 1972.
74. Freeman JB, Lemire A, MacLean LD: Intravenous alimentation and septicemia. Surg Gynecol Obstet 135:708–712, 1972.
75. Miller RC, Grogan JB: Incidence and source of contamination of intravenous nutritional infusion systems. J Pediatr Surg 8:185–190, 1973.
76. Sanderson I, Deitel M: Intravenous hyperalimentation without sepsis. Surg Gynecol Obstet 136:577–585, 1973.
77. Dillon JD Jr, Schaffner W, Van Way CW III, Meng HC: Septicemia and total parenteral nutrition: Distinguishing catheter-related from other septic episodes. JAMA 223:1341–1344, 1973.
78. O'Neill JA, Meng HC, Caldwell M, Otten A: Variations in intravenous nutrition in the management of catabolic states in infants and children. J Pediatr Surg 9:889–897, 1974.
79. Freeman JB, Litton AA: Preponderance of gram-positive infections during parenteral alimentation. Surg Gynecol Obstet 139:905–908, 1974.
80. Abel RM, Fischer JE, Buckley MJ, Austen WG: Hyperalimentation in cardiac surgery: A review of 64 patients. J Thorac Cardiovasc Surg 67:294–300, 1974.
81. Myers RN, Smink RD, Goldstein F: Parenteral hyperalimentation: Five years' clinical experience. Am J Gastroenterol 62:313–324, 1974.
82. Popp MB, Law EJ, MacMillan BG: Parenteral nutrition in the burned child: A study of 26 patients. Ann Surg 179:219–225, 1974.
83. Skoutakis VA, Martinez DR, Miller WA, Dobbie RP: Team approach to total parenteral nutrition. Am J Hosp Pharm 32:693–697, 1975.
84. Heird WC, Winters RW: Total parenteral nutrition. J Pediatr 86:2–16, 1975.
85. Reinhardt GF, Gelbart SM, Greenlee HB: Catheter infection factors affecting total parenteral nutrition. Am Surg 44:401–405, 1978.
86. Nehme AE: Nutritional support of the hospitalized patient. JAMA 243:1906–1908, 1980.
87. Gazzaniga AB, Mir-Sepasi MH, Jefferies MR, Yeo MT: Candida endocarditis complicating glucose total intravenous nutrition. Ann Surg 179:902–905, 1974.
88. Freeman JB, Wienke JW, Soper RT: Candida osteomyelitis associated with intravenous alimentation. J Pediatr Surg 9:783–784, 1974.
89. Noble HB, Layne ED: Candida osteomyelitis and arthritis from hyperalimentation therapy. J Bone Joint Surg 56A:825–829, 1974.
90. Freeman JB, Davis PL, MacLean LD: Candida endophthalmitis associated with intravenous hyperalimentation. Arch Surg 108:237–240, 1974.

7

Parenteral Nutrition:
The Lipid System

Fat emulsions safe for intravenous infusion have recently become available in the United States.* These fat emulsions have a high caloric density, provide essential fatty acids, and are, therefore, valuable components in intravenous feeding programs. In addition, fat emulsions are isotonic, and consequently, parenteral nutrition formulations in which lipids comprise the major calorie source can be infused safely through peripheral veins.

Many TPN formulations can be devised; these vary in the relative contribution of lipid and glucose to the total nonprotein calorie content and in the quantity of amino acids provided. In developing the lipid-based system described here, the aim was to maximize calorie and amino acid content without sacrificing safe peripheral venous administration.

A 10 percent emulsion of either soybean oil (Intralipid) or safflower oil (Liposyn) is used as the major calorie source. Each product provides 1.1 kcal/ml, 0.1 kcal of which is derived from glycerol. Both fat sources contain linoleic acid, but only the soybean oil provides significant amounts of linolenic acid, the human requirement for which, if any, is uncertain (see Table 5-3).

Because the addition of other substances to the fat emulsion may disturb the emulsion's stability, each liter-unit of the lipid system is prepared in two 500 ml containers, bottle A and bottle B (Table 7-1). Bottle A contains the fat

---

*The pharmacology of fat emulsions has been discussed in detail in Chapter 5.

emulsion as it is prepared by the manufacturer. Bottle B contains a 500 ml solution prepared in the hospital pharmacy which has a final concentration of 5.95 percent amino acids and 10 percent glucose. This small amount of glucose is added to the lipid system in part to supply additional calories, but primarily to provide the energy substrate for the glycolytic tissues (see p. 62). Bottle B also contains electrolytes, vitamins, trace elements, and a small amount of heparin to reduce the incidence of phlebitis.

The daily requirement for phosphorus is met in part by the phosphorus yielded by the metabolism of the phospholipid component of the fat emulsion. The phospholipid component of Intralipid 10 percent contains 14.8 mM (456 mg) of phosphorus per liter, and that of Liposyn 10 percent contains 13.9 mM (432 mg)/liter. The need for supplemental phosphate depends on the phosphate content of the preparation used to provide amino acids (Table 5-6). Thus routine supplementation is not required when FreAmine III is used, since this product contains 10 mM of phosphate (310 mg of phosphorus) per liter. This amino acid preparation and the metabolism of the phospholipids in the fat emulsion yield sufficient phosphorus to meet the needs of the anabolic state.[1,2]

Solution preparation. The fat emulsion (bottle A) is administered unaltered. However, the amino acid–glucose–additive solution (bottle B) must be prepared locally. Under a laminar flow air-filtered hood, a base solution consisting of 700 ml of 8.5 percent crystalline amino acids and 200 ml of 50 percent glucose is mixed in a 1 liter evacuated bottle. Then electrolytes and heparin are added and sterile, pyrogen-free water is used to bring the final volume to 1000 ml. At this point the solution is inspected for any precipitate and, if clear, is transferred into two 500 ml bottles through tubing connected to a 0.22 μ in-line membrane filter (Fig. 7-1). Vitamins and trace elements are added to 1 unit of bottle B daily for each patient. The nutrients provided in 1 liter-unit are presented in Table 7-2.

Administration. Therapy is initiated with the infusion of a 500 ml test dose of the fat emulsion during a 4 to 8 hour period in order to identify any adverse reactions. Fever, chills, a sensation of warmth, shivering, vomiting, and chest or back pain are among the few side-effects occasionally reported. Patients who tolerate the test dose thereafter receive equal volumes of the contents of bottles A and B in total amounts calculated to meet caloric requirements. The total volume infused is generally increased 1 liter each day until sufficient amounts are provided to meet calorie and protein requirements.

Bottles A and B are infused simultaneously at the same rate of infusion into the same peripheral vein (Fig. 7-2). This is accomplished by using intravenous tubing equipped with a side arm close to the infusion site. A special intravenous cannula is not required for administration of the lipid system. The fat emulsion should not be filtered.

Concurrent infusion of both bottles at the same rate is necessary because the contents of bottle B are so concentrated (approximately 1500 mOsm/liter) that infusion of this solution alone will always produce phlebitis. The feasibility of peripheral venous administration depends on the dilutional effect of the isotonic fat emulsion. When the contents of both bottles A and B are infused concurrently at the same rate, the vein is perfused with a solution containing about 900 mOsm/liter, which is usually well tolerated. If the contents of bottle A are inadvertently infused more rapidly than those of bottle B, the remaining contents of bottle B should be discarded and a fresh 1 liter-unit is begun.

Polyvinylchloride (PVC) intravenous tubing contains the plasticizer di-2-ethylhexyl phthalate (DEHP) which is sparingly soluble in lipid-containing materials, including fat emulsions. DEHP has been detected in the serum of patients receiving blood stored in PVC blood bags and in patients hemodialyzed across PVC tubing. [3-5] It would be anticipated, therefore, that DEHP

TABLE 7-1
The Lipid System: Preparation of 1 Liter-Unit

Bottle A	
10% Fat Emulsion[1]	500 ml
Bottle B	
8.5% Amino Acids[2,3]	350 ml
50% Glucose[4]	100 ml
Sodium (as acetate)	45 mEq
Potassium (as chloride)	40 mEq
Magnesium (as sulfate)	8 mEq
Calcium (as gluconate)	5 mEq
Heparin	1000 I.U.
Additives to one liter-unit per day [5]	
MVI-12[6]	10 ml
USC Trace Element Solution[7]	2 ml

[1]As Intralipid 10% which contains 7.4 mM phosphorus.
[2]Final concentration of amino acids in bottle B is 5.95%.
[3]As FreAmine III which provides sodium, 3.5 mEq, and phosphate, 7.0 mEq (3.5 mM).
[4]Final concentration in bottle B is 10%.
[5]All additives are in bottle B.
[6]Manufactured by USV Pharmaceutical Corporation.
[7]See Table 5-7.
Note: Vitamin K is supplied separately as needed.

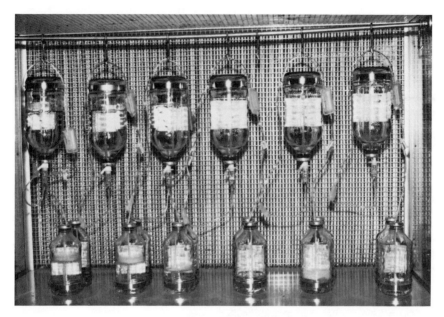

Figure 7-1. Preparation of "Bottle B" of the lipid system. Each liter of base solution, containing 5.95 percent amino acids, 10 percent glucose, and electrolytes, is filtered into 2 500 ml containers using a 0.22 μ in-line membrane filter. The solution is prepared under a laminar slow air-filtered hood.

TABLE 7-2
The Lipid System:
Nutrients Provided in 1 Liter-Unit

Non-protein calories	720 kcal
Caloric density	0.72 kcal/ml
Nitrogen	4.6 gm
Protein equivalent	28.4 gm
Calorie*/nitrogen ratio	157:1
Sodium	48.5 mEq
Potassium	40 mEq
Magnesium	8 mEq
Calcium	5 mEq
Chloride	40 mEq
Acetate	45 mEq
Sulfate	8 mEq
Phosphorus	10.9 mM

*Non-protein kcal.

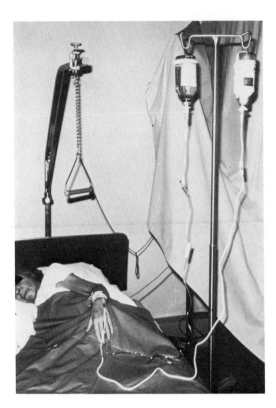

Figure 7-2. Patient receiving the lipid system. Bottles A and B are infused concurrently at the same rate through a peripheral vein.

extracted by fat emulsions during passage through PVC intravenous tubing would be detected in the serum of patients. Few data are available from humans, but evidently no adverse clinical effects have been observed to date among patients receiving fat emulsions. Cutter Laboratories supplies intravenous tubing which does not contain DEHP with each bottle of Intralipid, but use of such special tubing may be unnecessary.

The prescribed volume of the lipid system is infused over a 16 to 24 hour period each day. The 16 hour infusion schedule provides an 8 hour rest period, at the end of which the patient's serum can be observed for lipemia. Clear serum is taken to indicate the ability of the patient to clear the infused lipids. Nevertheless, infusion over 24 hours is more convenient and has not been associated with adverse clinical effects or marked hyperlipidemia at the University of Southern California.

In contrast to the glucose system, the lipid system can be terminated abruptly when treatment is to be discontinued.

Dosage. The volume of the lipid system prescribed is determined by caloric requirements, but according to the recommendations of the manufacturers, the daily dosage of intravenous lipids should not exceed 2.5 gm/kg in adults. However, the maximum elimination capacity of infused lipids varies widely with the clinical state of the patient (see Chapter 5), and several investigators have reported safe infusion of greater amounts of fat. Thus Blanchard and Gillespie treated 3 adult patients with 4.4 to 4.68 gm/kg for 16 to 46 days,[6] and Hadfield administered 12 gm/kg of Intralipid to 2 emaciated adult patients for 2 to 4 weeks with no adverse effects.[7] Daily administration of 3 to 4 liters (1.5 to 2 liters each of bottles A and B) meets the needs of most patients and has been uniformly well tolerated by patients at the University of Southern California.

Contraindications. The general contraindications to parenteral nutrition have been discussed in chapter 5. The lipid system in particular is not employed in patients with abnormalities of lipid metabolism. In addition, marked hepatic dysfunction may represent a contraindication to fat administration, since the liver is the most important organ in the uptake and metabolism of chylomicron triglyceride fatty acids and plasma free fatty acids. [1,8] The ability of septic or hypermetabolic patients to utilize lipids is controversial (see Chapter 9).

Metabolic effects. Lipid-based systems of parenteral nutrition are associated with nutritional repletion, weight gain, and positive nitrogen balance in a variety of clinical settings [9,10] (see Chapter 9).

Serum lipid levels may rise during treatment with the lipid system. During the infusion for 7 to 43 days of a lipid system in which 83 percent of nonprotein calories were provided as lipid, Jeejeebhoy and associates[10] observed elevations in the blood levels of the ketone bodies, β-hydroxybutyrate and acetoacetate; marked elevations of free fatty acids; and elevated levels of triglycerides and cholesterol. Mean cholesterol levels rose from 134 to 423 mg/dl, and mean triglyceride levels rose from 127 to 199 mg/dl. In both cases, values returned to normal within 2 weeks of discontinuing infusion. None of the changes observed were associated with adverse clinical effects.

Adverse reactions. Adverse reactions attributable to the lipid system have been very uncommon. Minor phlebitis at the infusion site occurs with little more frequency than that associated with infusion of isotonic solutions. Occasionally, phlebitis can be traced to the infusion of the amino acid–glucose–additive solution (bottle B) unaccompanied by the fat emulsion. Phlebitis is regarded as an indication for change in the infusion site but not for cessation of treatment. Rarely, suppurative phlebitis requiring venectomy has been observed.

Septicemia related to the peripherally infused lipid system is rare. No cases were observed among 426 patients studied in 6 reported series analyzed by Allen (Table 7-3).[11] However, sepsis from contamination of the fat emulsion is of the liver, and hepatic mitochondrial changes similar to those seen in mice

TABLE 7-3
Incidence of Septicemia Complicating TPN with the Lipid System

Reference	Year	Number of Patients	Rate of Septicemia (%)		
			BACTERIAL	FUNGAL	TOTAL
O'Neill et al.[12]	1974	4	0	0	0
Cashore et al.[13]	1975	23	0	0	0
Puri et al.[14]	1975	15	0	0	0
Filler and Coran[15]	1976	80	0	0	0
Hansen et al.[16]	1976	292	0	0	0
Allardyce and Williams[17]	1977	12	0	0	0

Adapted from Allen JR: In Johnston IDA (ed): Advances in Parenteral Nutrition. Baltimore, University Park Press, 1978, p 346.

a potential hazard, since Melly and associates demonstrated that soybean emulsion is capable of supporting the growth of several species of microorganisms, including *E. coli, Staph. aureus, Candida albicans, Enterobacter cloacae,* and *Pseudomonas aeruginosa.*[18]

Potential adverse effects of lipid infusions *per se* have been presented in Chapter 5. Metabolic complications associated with intravenous feedings in general are discussed in Chapter 8.

TABLE 7-4
Monitoring Schedule for Patients Receiving the Lipid System:
Required Procedures

	Before TPN	Daily	Mondays	Tuesdays	Wednesdays	Thursdays	Fridays	Notes
Body weight	X	X						
Input/output record		X						
Fractional urine (sugar/acetone)		X						
CBC	X		X			X		Daily 1st 5 days
Chemistry panel*	X		X			X		Daily 1st 5 days
Liver panel†	X		X			X		
Serum cholesterol	X					X		
Serum triglycerides	X					X		
Prothrombin time	X					X		

Serum glucose, urea, creatinine, sodium, potassium, chloride, bicarbonate, calcium, phosphate, magnesium, total protein, albumin.
†Serum bilirubin, SGOT, SGPT, alkaline phosphatase.

TABLE 7-5
Monitoring Schedule for Patients Receiving the Lipid System:
Optional Determinations

Procedure	Interval
Nutritional assessment*	Weekly
Skin tests	Bi-weekly
Serum B-12†	Initially and p.r.n.
Serum folate†	Initially and p.r.n.
Serum iron†	Initially and p.r.n.
Transferrin	Weekly
Zinc	Weekly
Copper	Weekly
24-hour urine nitrogen	1–7 times per week

*See Chapter 1.
†Essential if anemia present.

Monitoring patients receiving the lipid system. Patients receiving the lipid system require the same careful metabolic monitoring as patients receiving the glucose system. The required and optional determinations are presented in Tables 7-4 and 7-5.

The relative indications and comparative efficacy of the lipid and glucose systems are discussed in Chapter 9.

SUMMARY

The recently available fat emulsions for intravenous use provide a rich calorie source for patients requiring parenteral nutrition. The isotonic property of these emulsions allows the formulation of a lipid-based system of parenteral nutrition which can be infused safely through peripheral veins. The formulation described here, providing 720 nonprotein kcal/liter and 4.6 gm of nitrogen per liter, can supply sufficient nutrients to meet the needs of patients with a wide variety of clinical conditions with few adverse reactions.[19]

REFERENCES

1. Hallberg D: Therapy with fat emulsions. Acta Anesthesiol Scand [Suppl] 55:131–136, 1974.
2. Lee HA: Intravenous nutrition. Br J Hosp Med 11:719–728, 1974.
3. Gibson TP, Briggs WA, Boone BJ: Delivery of di-2-ethylhexyl phthalate to patients during hemodialysis. J Lab Clin Med 87:519–524, 1976.
4. Lewis LM, Flechtner TW, Kerkay J, et al: Bis (2-ethylhexyl) phthalate concentrations in the serum of hemodialysis patients. Clin Chem 24:741–746, 1978.

5. Jaeger RJ, Rubin RJ: Migration of a phthalate ester plasticizer from polyvinyl chloride blood bags into stored human blood and its localization in human tissues. N Engl J Med 287:1114–1118, 1972.

6. Blanchard RJ, Gillespie DJ: Some comparisons between fat emulsion and glucose for parenteral nutrition in adults at the Winnipeg Health Sciences Center, in Meng HC, Wilmore DW (eds): Fat Emulsions in Parenteral Nutrition. Chicago, American Medical Association, 1976, pp 63–64.

7. Hadfield JIH: High calorie intravenous feeding in surgical patients. Clin Med 73:25–30, 1966.

8. Meng HC: Fat emulsions in parenteral nutrition, in Fischer JE (ed): Total Parenteral Nutrition. Boston, Little, Brown and Co, 1976, pp 305–334.

9. Deitel M, Kaminsky V: Total nutrition by peripheral vein: The lipid system. Can Med Assoc J 111:152–154, 1974.

10. Jeejeebhoy KN, Anderson GH, Nakhooda AF, et al: Metabolic studies in total parenteral nutrition with lipid in man: Comparison with glucose. J Clin Invest 57:125–136, 1976.

11. Allen JR: The incidence of nosocomial infection in patients receiving total parenteral nutrition, in Johnston IDA (ed): Advances in Parenteral Nutrition. Baltimore, University Park Press, 1978, pp 339–377.

12. O'Neill JA Jr, Meng HC, Caldwell M, Otten A: Variations in intravenous nutrition in the management of catabolic states in infants and children. J Pediatr Surg 9:889–897, 1974.

13. Cashore WJ, Sedaghatian MR, Usher RH: Nutritional supplements with intravenously administered lipid, protein hydrolysate, and glucose in small premature infants. Pediatrics 56:8–16, 1975.

14. Puri P, Guiney EJ, O'Donnell B: Total parenteral feeding in infants using peripheral veins. Arch Dis Child 50:133–136 1975.

15. Filler RM, Coran AG: Total parenteral nutrition in infants and children: Central and peripheral approaches. Surg Clin North Am 56:395–412, 1976.

16. Hansen LM, Hardie WR, Hidalgo J: Fat emulsion for intravenous administration. Ann Surg 184:80–88, 1976.

17. Allardyce DB, Williams BJ: Parenteral solutions for nutritional support in surgical patients. Am J Surg 133:315–318, 1977.

18. Melly MA, Meng HC, Schaffner W: Microbial growth in lipid emulsions used in parenteral nutrition. Arch Surg 110:1479–1481, 1975.

19. Silberman H, Freehauf M, Fong G, Rosenblatt N: Parenteral nutrition with lipids. JAMA 238: 1380–1382, 1977.

8

Parenteral Nutrition: Nonnutritional Effects and Metabolic Complications

When nutrients are provided exclusively by vein, the salutary impact on nutritional status may be accompanied by a variety of nonnutritional morphologic and functional changes affecting the alimentary tract, liver, pancreas, and respiratory system. In addition, a wide range of metabolic derangements have been observed during the course of parenteral feedings.

EFFECTS ON THE STOMACH

Gastric acid secretion is significantly increased during the initial period of treatment with the glucose system of parenteral nutrition,[1] but the duration of this effect is unknown. The acid secretory response observed is due primarily to the infusion of crystalline amino acids, since the addition of glucose does not alter the response and the effect is not seen when protein hydrolysates are infused.[1,2] In addition, the stimulation is evidently due to a direct effect on the parietal cells, since serum gastrin levels are not increased.[1,3]

This effect of amino acids on gastric acid secretion is virtually abolished by the concurrent intravenous infusion of a fat emulsion. Circulating fat evidently is as potent an inhibitor of gastric acid secretion as intraduodenal fat.[4]

Psaila and associates compared the acid secretory effects of an amino acid infusion in normal subjects with those in patients with duodenal ulcers. The acid secretory response was twice as high in the ulcer patients. However this effect was completely inhibited after vagotomy or following the administration of cimetidine.[3]

The effect of chronic TPN on gastric secretory function is less clear. Studies in laboratory animals treated with TPN for prolonged periods have disclosed variable results. In dogs receiving TPN for 1 month, basal serum gastrin levels fell 50 percent, and acid secretion from denervated gastric pouches was significantly decreased in response to both a meal and pentagastrin. However, the secretory response to exogenous pentagastrin by innervated stomach remained normal.[5] In rats, parenteral nutrition was associated with decreased antral gastrin levels and atrophy of the parietal mass.[6] This latter observation is consistent with the gastric hyposecretion reported by Kotler and Levine in a patient who had received TPN for 2 years.[7] Pentagastrin-stimulated output in this patient was lowest during TPN, as compared to values obtained several months after oral alimentation was resumed. These authors postulated reduced secretory stimulating and trophic factors due to a lack of luminal contents.

MacGregor and associates found that gastric emptying of solid food was retarded during the administration of the glucose system.[8] The increment in plasma glucose produced by TPN was significantly correlated with the degree of slowed gastric emptying, which suggests that hyperglycemia may play a role in the observed results. This is consistent with the finding that acute hyperglycemia slows gastric emptying.[9] Acid entering the duodenum also retards gastric emptying;[10] therefore, if gastric acid output is stimulated by TPN, this provides another possible mechanism for delayed emptying.[8] The occurrence of delayed gastric emptying may explain the anorexia that some patients experience with TPN.

EFFECTS ON THE INTESTINAL TRACT

Morphologic and functional changes occur in the small intestine and the colon when nutrition is maintained exclusively by vein. A significant reduction in the mass of the small and large intestine occurs, and there is a marked decrease in mucosal enzyme activity.[6,11-13] Enzymes affected include maltase, sucrase, lactase, and peroxidase.[12,13]

These changes are not a response to intravenous nutrition *per se* but reflect the need for luminal nutrients for maintenance of normal intestinal mass and function (see Chapter 4). The mechanism by which food exerts a trophic effect appears to be 2-fold: (1) a direct effect related to utilization of luminal nutrients to meet the metabolic needs of the absorptive cells and (2) an indirect effect related to release of enteric hormones which have a trophic effect on the proliferative cells.[14] Thus supplemental gastrin can restore and maintain intestinal mass in animals receiving TPN,[15] and cholecystokinin and secretin have similar trophic effects.[16] The action of the last two hormones may be related to their stimulation of pancreatic and biliary secretions, both of which stimulate intestinal hypertrophy.[14]

EFFECTS ON THE PANCREAS

Dudrick and associates observed a marked reduction in the output of traumatic pancreaticoduodenal fistulas during treatment with total parenteral nutrition.[17] To elucidate the mechanisms responsible for the reduction in fistulous output, Johnson and associates studied the effects of TPN on the pancreas in experimental animals.[15,18] In rats, nutrition exclusively by vein for 2 weeks was associated with a 50 percent reduction in pancreatic weight, an effect averted by low-dose pentagastrin.[15] Studies in dogs receiving TPN for 6 weeks disclosed that bicarbonate secretion was significantly decreased in response to endogenous secretin and that pancreatic enzyme secretory capacity was significantly reduced.[18] These findings are consistent with the pancreatic insufficiency observed by Kotler and Levine in a patient receiving TPN for 2 years.[7] This patient had abnormally low values for peak bicarbonate concentration and volume when secretin was given intravenously. Pancreatic function returned to normal 9 months after the resumption of oral alimentation.

Grundfest and associates found that pancreatic fistula volume and the concentration of amylase and lipase in fistulous drainage decreased in 1 of 3 patients with pancreatic fistulas receiving the glucose system.[19] Similar decreases were observed when 500 to 1000 kcal/day were provided as 10 percent fat emulsion instead of glucose. Each of the parameters measured remained the same in the remaining 2 patients when either form of TPN was infused. Thus the intravenous lipids did not stimulate pancreatic secretion.

EFFECTS ON THE LIVER

Abnormalities in 1 or more liver function tests have been observed in 60 to 93 percent of adult patients without antecedent liver disease during the course of parenteral nutrition with the glucose system[20–23] (Table 8-1). The etiology of these biochemical changes is uncertain, but the abnormal findings are generally transient despite continued treatment and they evidently have not been associated with adverse clinical sequelae in adults.

After 8 to 10 days of glucose-based TPN, Grant and associates observed a 5-fold rise in the mean level of serum glutamic-pyruvic transaminase (SGPT) in 89 percent of patients and a nearly 3-fold rise in serum glutamic-oxalacetic transaminase (SGOT) in 93 percent, and serum bilirubin rose to levels averaging 2.3 times pre-TPN levels in 26 percent of patients (Table 8-

TABLE 8-1
Liver Indices During Parenteral Nutrition

Author	TPN System	Proportion of Patients with Elevated Values			
		SGOT	SGPT	BILIRUBIN	ALKALINE PHOSPHATASE
Grant, et al[20]	Glucose	93% (8 days)**	89% (10 days)	26% (8 days)	16% (32 days)†
Lindor, et al[21]*	Glucose	68% (9–12 days)	—	21% (6–12 days)	54% (9–12 days)
Lowry, et al[23]*	Glucose	87% (11 days)	87% (13 days)	33% (18 days)	64% (14 days)
	Lipid	60% (12 days)	36% (14 days)	13% (18 days)	33% (15 days)

*Reported patients having abnormal values at least 50% above baseline.
**Days in parentheses indicate interval to peak elevation after starting TPN.
†Of patients receiving TPN for more than 20 days 56% had elevations.

1).[20] These elevations were transient, lasting 4 to 10 days. Biopsies of the liver taken during maximal elevations demonstrated marked periportal fatty change. No early elevation in alkaline phosphatase levels were observed by these investigators, but increased values, averaging 2.4 times baseline, were noted in 56 percent of patients receiving TPN for more than 20 days. In addition, a second, more prolonged elevation of SGPT and SGOT also occurred in from one-third to one-half of patients receiving TPN for periods exceeding 20 days.

A survey of TPN patients receiving the glucose system at the Mayo Clinic generally confirms the frequent incidence of liver function derangements (Table 8-1).[21] Seventy-eight percent of the patients had abnormal levels of SGOT, alkaline phosphatase, or bilirubin that were at least 50 percent above the pre-TPN baseline. In contrast to the report of Grant and associates, the Mayo Clinic group frequently observed elevated alkaline phosphatase levels early in the course of TPN.

Lowry and Brennan also measured alkaline phosphatase, SGOT, and SGPT during glucose-based TPN.[22] Elevations above the normal range in at least 2 of the tests occurred in 83 percent of their patients at a mean interval of 14 days from the onset of parenteral feeding. Values usually returned to normal even with continued intravenous feeding. Histologic changes observed in the liver during treatment included glycogen deposition, cholestasis, and, perhaps most commonly, fatty infiltration.

Lowry, Wagner, and Silberman analyzed liver indices in 15 patients receiving the glucose system and compared the results with those obtained from 25 patients receiving the lipid system of TPN (Table 8-1).[23] Transient elevations of SGOT, SGPT, bilirubin, or alkaline phosphatase were observed in 87 percent of the patients receiving the glucose system and in 60 percent of the patients receiving the lipid system.

Various hypotheses have been advanced to explain the biochemical and histologic derangements: (1) glucose and protein infusions providing amounts exceeding requirements for energy and nitrogen balance,[22] (2) excessive calorie:nitrogen ratios, [24] (3) relative deficiencies of individual amino acids due to imbalances in amino acid solutions,[24] (4) toxic tryptophan degradation products resulting from the action of the antioxidant sodium bisulfite present in amino acid preparations,[20] and (5) essential fatty acid deficiency.[25,26]

Various laboratory and clinical investigations bear on the validity of these hypotheses. For example, studies in rats disclose that protein-free infusions of hypertonic glucose providing excessive calories (130 to 341 kcal/kg) are associated with gross fatty infiltration of the liver.[27] Rats receiving a protein-free but otherwise complete diet likewise develop fatty infiltration, which can be successfully treated with intravenous protein repletion.[28]

Richardson and Sgoutas reported two patients in whom EFA deficiency was associated with marked elevations of SGOT and SGPT, fatty infiltration of the liver, and hepatic mitochondrial changes similar to those seen in mice with advanced EFA deficiency. Safflower oil supplement corrected the fatty acid deficiency, and the levels of SGOT and SGPT simultaneously returned to normal.[26] In addition, reports from the University of Toronto indicate that fatty infiltration of the liver occurring in patients receiving glucose-based TPN can be reversed by supplemental fat infusions.[25,29] However, the frequent abnormalities in liver indices observed by Lowry, Wagner, and Silberman in patients who received the lipid system, which provides essential fatty acids in amounts far exceeding requirements, indicate that while EFA deficiency may be an etiologic factor in some TPN patients it is not the sole cause of these laboratory derangements in all of the affected patients.[23]

In summary, derangements of liver function indices, often transient, are frequently observed during TPN; the etiology is uncertain and probably multifactorial, but the clinical course associated with such dysfunction is generally benign. Nevertheless, certain precautions appear worthwhile. Calories and protein should be administered in the appropriate ratio and in amounts necessary to meet but not exceed demands. Providing the glucose calories over a 14 to 16 hour period rather than by a 24 hour continuous infusion ("cyclic hyperalimentation") has been proposed as a means of averting liver dysfunction, presumably by lowering insulin levels during the rest period, thereby allowing lipolysis and fat mobilization from the liver.[30] Rowlands and associates, however, were unable to confirm the efficacy of this method.[31,32] Essential fatty acids should be provided regularly to patients receiving glucose-based TPN. Finally, when liver abnormalities do develop, causes unrelated to TPN should be considered.

EFFECTS ON THE RESPIRATORY SYSTEM

Studies by Askanazi and associates disclosed that the administration of glucose calories in amounts exceeding requirements is associated with increased energy expenditure, CO_2 production, O_2 consumption, tidal volume, and respiratory rate.[32-34] The magnitude of these changes is dependent upon the metabolic status of the patient (Figs. 8-1 and 8-2).

Nutritionally depleted patients receiving excess glucose calories have a respiratory quotient (RQ) exceeding 1.0, reflecting lipogenesis. This lipogenesis is associated with a marked increase in CO_2 production and modest increases in resting energy expenditure and O_2 consumption.[33]

In contrast, lipogenesis is limited in hypermetabolic patients, presumably because of insulin resistance. In these patients receiving large amounts of glucose, the RQ rises, indicating a shift in energy source from endogenous fat ($RQ=0.7$) to glucose ($RQ=1.0$), but remains less than 1.0. Energy expenditure and O_2 consumption markedly increase, and the latter may produce a cardiovascular stress. Increased CO_2 production is also observed and is secondary to increases in both the RQ and O_2 consumption.[32]

In both groups of patients, the increased CO_2 produced would be expected to stimulate a compensatory increase in minute ventilation. However, the risk of CO_2 retention is present in patients with decreased sensitivity to CO_2 or impaired pulmonary function.[34] In addition, weaning patients from mechanical ventilators may be hampered by increased CO_2 production.[32]

On the basis of these observations, excessive glucose loads should be avoided. In addition, Askanazi and associates suggested that CO_2 production can be reduced by replacing a portion of the glucose load with an isocaloric infusion of a fat emulsion which is oxidized with an RQ of 0.7.[32,34] The clinical relevance of these considerations was emphasized recently by Covelli and associates.[35] They described three seriously ill patients with significant underlying pulmonary disease and a relatively fixed ventilatory response who developed acute respiratory failure, manifested by hypercapnea and acidosis,

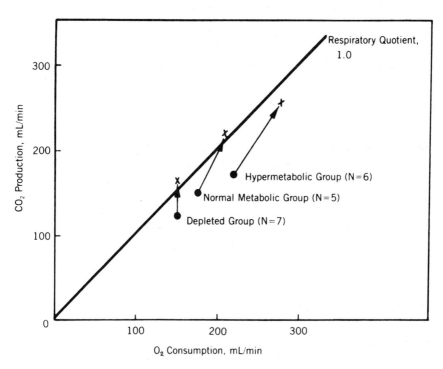

Figure 8-1. Gas exchange prior to (circle) and during (X) TPN. *(From Askanazi J, et al: JAMA 243:1444–1447, 1980)*

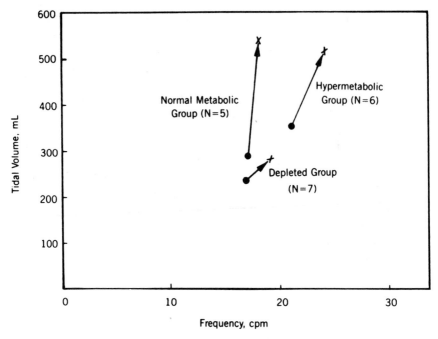

Figure 8-2. Tidal volume and respiratory frequency relationships prior to (circle) and during (X) TPN. Depleted patients increase both tidal volume and frequency, while the other two groups increase primarily tidal volume. *(From Askanazi J, et al: JAMA 243:1444–1447, 1980 Copyright 1980, American Medical Association.)*

within 12–24 hours after glucose-based TPN was begun. In each case the PCO_2 fell when the carbohydrate load was reduced; in one patient a fat emulsion was used to replace glucose, and hypercapnea did not occur.

An additional respiratory effect of fat emulsions has been observed by Greene and associates.[36] These investigators reported diminished pulmonary diffusion capacity unaccompanied by changes in PO_2 during intravenous fat infusions. However, this observation could not be confirmed by Wilmore and associates (see p. 123).[37]

METABOLIC COMPLICATIONS

Abnormalities of Blood Sugar

Derangements of serum glucose levels are the most common metabolic complications observed in patients receiving total parenteral nutrition. Ryan observed a 15 percent incidence of marked hyperglycemia (glucose > 400 mg/dl) and a 9.5 percent incidence of hypoglycemia (glucose < 50 mg/dl) among 200 consecutive patients receiving the glucose system.[38] These abnormalities are most commonly associated with administration of the glucose system, rather than the lipid system, since the latter provides substantially less glucose.

Hyperglycemia. Sanderson and Deitel found that relatively healthy patients were able to maintain normal glucose levels even when TPN was given at full dosage initially and later when rates of infusion were increased modestly.[39] Nevertheless, many patients manifest hyperglycemia when the glucose load is abruptly increased. Such glucose intolerance may be a manifestation of overt or latent diabetes mellitus, or it may reflect the reduced pancreatic insulin response to a glucose load which is routinely observed during starvation, stress, pain, major trauma, infection, and shock.[38] Hyperglycemia also may be a reflection of the peripheral insulin resistance observed during sepsis and acute stress, conditions which are accompanied by high levels of circulating catecholamines and glucocorticoids.[38,39] Decreased tissue sensitivity to insulin is also associated with hypophosphatemia,[40] and hyperglycemia has been observed in patients with a deficiency of chromium.[41] The latter trace metal probably acts as a cofactor for insulin.[42]

Hyperglycemia is avoided by initiating therapy with the glucose system gradually. Full dosage is achieved over a 3 day period, during which time adaption to the glucose load takes place, and metabolic monitoring will disclose any tendency to hyperglycemia. Subsequently, a constant rate of infusion is maintained around the clock. Inadvertent decreases in the rate of infusion should not be compensated by abrupt increases in the rate; such "catching up" is not allowed.

When hyperglycemia supervenes despite these precautions, the etiology is sought. A common cause of hyperglycemia after a period of stability is emerging sepsis, the overt manifestations of which may not appear for 18 to 24 hours after the development of elevated glucose levels.[43]

Uncomplicated moderate hyperglycemia is controlled initially by subcutaneous or intravenous administration of crystalline zinc insulin; the TPN infusion is continued at the usual rate. Subsequently, the TPN pharmacist adds the appropriate amount of insulin to the TPN solution during its aseptic preparation in the pharmacy. Supplements of insulin required on a given day are on the following days added to the TPN solution. In this way, glucose levels less than 200 mg/dl are eventually achieved with insulin administered exclusively in the TPN solution. Providing insulin in the TPN solution has the advantage that inadvertent alterations in the rate of glucose delivery are automatically accompanied by appropriate adjustments in the amount of insulin administered.

Patients with hyperglycemia which is complicated by massive diuresis, dehydration, neurologic manifestations (confusion, disorientation, lethargy), or the syndrome of hyperosmolar nonketotic coma are managed by immediate termination of the TPN infusion, fluid resuscitation, and insulin administration.

Hypoglycemia.   Blood sugar levels decrease when the rate of infusion of the glucose system is abruptly reduced. Symptomatic hypoglycemia is most likely to occur when the reduction in infusion rate was recently preceded by an increased rate of infusion.[39] When the glucose system is to be discontinued electively, the rate of delivery should be tapered gradually over 2 to 3 days. Patients who are hemodynamically unstable or who are undergoing surgery should not receive TPN, since fluid resuscitation may be inadvertently carried out using the TPN solution. Therefore, the TPN infusion is discontinued in such patients, and hypoglycemia is averted by infusing a solution of 10 percent glucose.

Hypoglycemia may also reflect an excessive dosage of exogenous insulin. This most commonly occurs as a result of failure to recognize the fact that improvement or resolution of a condition associated with peripheral insulin resistance results in a decreased insulin requirement. For example, as sepsis responds to antibiotics or surgical drainage, insulin resistance resolves and the exogenous insulin requirement falls. Hypoglycemia on this basis is best avoided by reconsidering insulin dosage on a daily basis rather than having a standing order for insulin administration for the duration of TPN therapy.

Deficiencies of Potassium, Phosphate, and Magnesium

In the catabolic state, the protein structure of cells is metabolized as energy sources, intracellular ions are lost, and the total body concentrations of these ions, including potassium, magnesium, and phosphate, are decreased.[38] In contrast, during nutritional repletion, these ions, derived from the serum, are deposited or incorporated in newly synthesized cells. When supplementation of these ions in nutrient solutions is insufficient, hypokalemia, hypomagnesemia, and hypophosphatemia ensue. Recommended daily allowances for these major intracellular ions have been presented in Chapters 3 and 5. The serum levels of these substances should be measured regularly during TPN, since such monitoring will disclose deficiencies before the clinical manifestations described below develop.

Hypokalemia.   Symptoms are unusual when serum levels of potassium are 3.0 mEq/liter or greater. The cardiac effects of symptomatic hypokalemia are among the most important, and the electrocardiographic changes are the most prominent manifestations. These changes, shown in Figure 8-3, include flattened T-waves, the presence of U-waves, S–T segment depression, and ar-

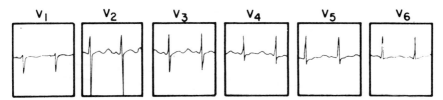

Figure 8-3. Electrocardiogram demonstrating the flattened T-waves and U-waves seen in patients with severe hypokalemia. *(From Gabow P, Peterson LN: In Schrier RW (ed): Renal and Electrolyte Disorders, ed 2. Boston, Little, Brown and Co, 1980)*

rhythmias. The arrhythmias are predominantly atrial and ventricular premature beats.[44] Digitalis toxicity is aggravated or provoked by hypokalemia.

Neuromuscular disturbances associated with hypokalemia include weakness, hyporeflexia, and paresthesias. Nausea, paralytic ileus, and metabolic alkalosis may also occur.

Asymptomatic hypokalemia can be managed by increasing the potassium supplements added to the nutrient solution at the time of preparation. When cardiac arrhythmias or other significant symptoms develop, the rate of TPN infusion should be tapered promptly while serum glucose levels are monitored closely, and an intravenous infusion of potassium chloride should be administered through a peripheral vein—10 mEq/hr can be safely infused. More rapid rates, rarely necessary, require close monitoring of the electrocardiogram and serum potassium level.[44]

Hypophosphatemia. The intracellular consumption of inorganic phosphate during the synthesis of proteins, membrane phospholipids, DNA, and ATP may produce a striking deficit in serum phosphate level after only several days of intravenous feedings which are devoid of or deficient in phosphate supplements.[45] Evidently, available phosphate is sequestered by cells undergoing rapid turnover as nutritional repletion is initiated in malnourished patients, and nondividing cells, such as red cells, white cells, platelets, and brain cells, are at a competitive disadvantage and rapidly become phosphate-depleted.[38,46]

Patients requiring parenteral support may have conditions besides nutritional depletion which predispose to hypophosphatemia. These conditions include chronic antacid consumption, alcoholism, liver disease, and the use of diuretics.[47,48]

Symptoms may occur when serum phosphate levels fall to 2 mg/dl or less. However, severe manifestations are particularly apt to occur as levels fall below 1 mg/dl. These include acute respiratory failure from marked muscle weakness,[49] impaired myocardial contractility,[50] severe congestive cardiomyopathy,[51] acute hemolytic anemia,[52] coma,[53] and death (Table 8-2).

TABLE 8-2
Manifestations of Hypophosphatemia

System and Syndrome	Abnormality or Mechanism
Neuromuscular[53,54]	
Muscle weakness	Decreased CNS ATP*
Anorexia	Inhibition of muscle
Intention tremor	glycolytic pathways
Paresthesia	
Coma	
Convulsions	
Anisocoria	
Ballismus	
Rhabdomyolysis	
Hyporeflexia	
Ataxia	
Death	
Hematologic[45,46,52,55–57]	
Erythrocytes	
Hemolytic anemia	Decreased ATP
Decreased oxygen release	Decreased 2,3-DPG*
	? Abnormal membrane lipids
Leukocytes	
Decreased chemotaxis	Decreased ATP
Decreased phagocytosis	? Abnormal membrane lipids
Decreased killing	
Platelets	
Decreased clot retraction	Decreased ATP
Decreased survival in vivo	
Hepatic[58]	
? Failure of compensatory	
2,3-DPG→hepatic hypoxia	
Correlation with hepatic coma	
Cardiac[50,51]	
Impaired myocardial contractility	? Decreased ATP
Congestive cardiomyopathy	? Decreased ATP
Respiratory[49]	
Respiratory failure	Muscle weakness
Skeletal[59]	
Osteomalacia	Negative calcium balance
Arthritis	with reabsorption

*CNS, central nervous system; ATP, adenosine triphosphate; 2,3-DPG, 2,3 diphospho-glycerate.
Adapted and updated from Fitzgerald FT: West J Med 122:482–489, 1975.

Hypophosphatemic patients who are asymptomatic or whose serum levels exceed 1 mg/dl can be managed by increasing the phosphate supplement to 20 to 30 mM/1000 kcal.[45] Calcium supplements must be continued to avoid hypocalcemia, but as additional phosphate is added in the presence of calcium, the solutions must be inspected for precipitates. Alternatively, patients able to tolerate oral phosphate supplements can receive 5 to 10 ml of Fleets phosphosoda three times per day until repleted. Each milliliter of this preparation provides 129 mg (4.2 mM) of phosphorus and 4.8 mEq of sodium.

Symptomatic patients or those with serum phosphate levels less than 1 mg/dl should be repleted intravenously through a separate line. TPN should be stopped and a 10 percent glucose solution should be infused to avert hypoglycemia. Since intracellular phosphate consumption is dependent on caloric intake, withdrawing TPN alone often results in increasing serum phosphate levels within 24 hours.[60] Satisfactory repletion can usually be achieved with a phosphate infusion containing 20 to 30 mM (620 to 930 mg) of elemental phosphorous as KH_2PO_4–K_2HPO_4 diluted in 1 liter of 5 percent glucose. The solution is administered over an 8 hour period and can be repeated as indicated by serum phosphate levels.[47,48,51] Careful monitoring during repletion is mandatory since hyperphosphatemia due to overenthusiastic therapy may lead to widespread metastatic calcification and severe hypocalcemia. Hyperkalemia may also develop because of the large quantities of potassium present in the phosphate infusion.

Hypomagnesemia. The clinical manifestations of magnesium deficiency may include lethargy, weakness, increased central nervous system and neuromuscular irritability, muscle fasciculation, tremors, Chvostek's and Trousseau's signs, tetany, convulsions, and personality changes.

Magnesium deficiency also impairs calcium and potassium metabolism. Thus hypomagnesemia may be associated with hypocalcemia that is resistant to calcium administration alone; magnesium repletion is required.[61,62]

Magnesium is a necessary metallocoenzyme of adenosine triphosphatase which is required for the normal function of the sodium–potassium pump. Consequently, hypomagnesemia is associated with intracellular potassium deficiency. This may be the mechanism by which magnesium deficiency facilitates digitalis toxicity.[63]

Additional magnesium can be added to the nutrient solution when asymptomatic patients develop low serum magnesium levels. However, TPN should be stopped in symptomatic patients. Twelve milliliters of 50 percent magnesium sulfate (49 mEq mg) are added to 1 liter of 10 percent glucose solution and infused over 3 hours. Two additional liters, each containing 10 ml of magnesium sulfate (40 mEq mg) may be infused over the next 24 hours.[62]

Essential Fatty Acid Deficiency

Individuals, healthy or malnourished, who receive a constant parenteral (or enteral) infusion of a fat-free but otherwise complete diet develop clinical and biochemical manifestations that are completely reversed by the administration of linoleic acid. Thus the syndrome of essential fatty acid (EFA) deficiency in man is due principally, if not exclusively, to a lack of linoleic acid. Exogenous linolenic acid is required by some species, but its essentiality for man is unproven.

In addition to dietary sources, linoleic acid can ordinarily be derived from adipose tissue stores, except in severely malnourished patients. This endogenous source is, however, apparently rendered unavailable during TPN because of the antilipolytic effect of high insulin levels associated with continuous glucose-based feedings.[64,65]

Biochemical changes may occur within several days and eventually are observed in nearly all patients after starting TPN regimens devoid of fat.[65,66] In the presence of linoleic acid deficiency, the enzyme system which normally converts linoleic to arachidonic acid (C20:4) instead elongates and desaturates oleic acid. The result is the production of eicosatrienoic (C20:3) rather than arachidonic acid. Thus the appearance of normally undetectable eicosatrienoic acid, the production of which is competitively inhibited by linoleic acid, is the biochemical hallmark of essential fatty acid deficiency.[65] This observation led Holman to define essential fatty acid deficiency by means of the triene:tetraene ratio (20:3/20:4).[67] A triene:tetraene ratio greater than 0.4 is taken as evidence of EFA deficiency.[68]

The clinical manifestations occur later than the biochemical changes. Perhaps the most commonly recognized manifestation is an eczematous, desquamative dermatitis, largely but not always confined to the body folds.[64,66] Riella and associates described three patients who developed the characteristic dermatitis 46 days, 6 months, and 2 years, respectively, after beginning fat-free TPN.[69] Other clinical findings include hepatic dysfunction (pp. 195–196), anemia,[66] thrombocytopenia,[70] hair loss,[70,71] and possibly impaired wound healing.[70] Growth retardation has been observed in infants.[72]

Freund and associates found a significant decrease in intraocular pressure in a series of patients who developed EFA deficiency while receiving fat-free TPN; pressure measurements returned to normal with fat supplementation.[73] Prostaglandin levels, presumably affecting catecholamine turnover and, therefore, intraocular pressure, were reduced, evidently reflecting the reduced levels of essential fatty acids, which are precursors of prostaglandins. These authors therefore suggested measurement of intraocular pressure as a diagnostic test for EFA deficiency.

EFA deficiency is treated by the administration of linoleic acid, usually by infusing one of the currently available fat emulsions. Riella and associates cured their patients in 2 to 6 weeks with a daily infusion of approximately 500 ml of 10 percent fat emulsion (Intralipid).[69]

Cures have also been effected by the daily topical application of 120 to 150 mg of linoleic acid in the form of sunflower seed oil or safflower oil.[71,74]

Deficiencies of Trace Elements

Deficiencies of zinc, copper, and chromium have been associated with characteristic clinical syndromes in humans.

Zinc deficiency. Decreased serum levels of zinc and increased urinary excretion have been observed in patients receiving nutrient solutions devoid of the trace elements. Blood and urine zinc levels, however, provide only partial information about zinc status. Hair or red blood cell zinc analysis may be more reliable than serum levels in detecting a deficiency state, and tests of taste acuity have also been useful in diagnosis.[75]

Evidently, tissue demand for zinc during anabolism rapidly depletes plasma stores, leading to the clinical deficiency syndrome.[76] Manifestations of acute zinc deficiency may include anorexia, diarrhea, abnormalities of taste and smell, mental depression, cerebellar dysfunction, alopecia, and a characteristic dermatitis. The syndrome observed in TPN patients closely resembles acrodermatitis enteropathica of infants, which consists of a vesiculopustular dermatitis involving body orifices, head, and extremities, with diarrhea and hair loss.[75,76] The rash often starts as a moist eczematoid area in the nasolabial folds and progresses to crusting. This is followed by bullous or pustular lesions on other parts of the face, in the groin, and on the hands and feet which in some cases coalesce to form large erosive areas.[77] Zinc-deficient patients may also have impaired wound healing[75,78] and abnormal humoral and cellular immune responses, including impaired reactivity to delayed hypersensitivity skin test antigens.[79,80]

Kay and Tasman-Jones observed prompt resolution of symptoms when zinc sulfate was given intravenously in a dose providing 32 mg of elemental zinc daily for 5 days and 16 mg/day thereafter.[81]

Copper deficiency. Serum copper levels routinely decline in patients receiving TPN without copper supplements.[78] Clinical manifestations have been observed in such patients, and these include anemia, leukopenia, and neutropenia.[78,82,83] Wound healing may also by impaired.[78]

The anemia of copper deficiency, often microcytic and hypochromic,[75,82] is thought to result from reduced red cell synthesis, shortened erythrocyte survival, and impaired transferrin formation from ferrous iron due to inadequate concentrations of ceruloplasmin, a feroxidase enzyme. Iron stores are normal, but iron utilization is poor. This is consistent with a defect in the release of iron from tissue stores.[78,83]

Copper deficiency can be treated with an intravenous copper solution providing 1 mg elemental copper daily until a rise in hematocrit is observed and then with maintenance therapy of 0.4 mg/day.[84]

Chromium deficiency.   Chromium deficiency has been documented in several patients receiving TPN.[41,85] Manifestations have included severe glucose intolerance, mental confusion suggestive of a metabolic encephalopathy, and a peripheral sensory neuropathy with ataxia. In patients reported by Jeejeebhoy and associates and Freund and associates[41,85] symptoms resolved within 2 weeks after starting treatment with intravenous chromium, 150 to 250 μg/day. As previously noted (p. 72), chromium, probably acting as a cofactor for insulin, is required for maintaining normal glucose metabolism.

Vitamin-Related Derangements

The fat-soluble vitamins—A, D, E, and K—are adequately stored, and therefore the development of a deficiency state is usually a late phenomenon. Since turnover is slow and urinary excretion is not prominent, toxicity can be produced by indiscriminant loading. In contrast, the water-soluble vitamins are stored in small amounts or not at all, and constant supplementation is required to avert deficiency syndromes.[86] Toxic manifestations due to excessive administration are rare.[87] Vitamin supplements in TPN solutions are designed to prevent vitamin-related abnormalities.

Vitamin A-related abnormalities.   Manifestations of vitamin A toxicity include headache, epistaxis, dry skin, exfoliative dermatitis, extraosseous calcium deposits, and skeletal defects.[38,86]

Howard and associates reported low vitamin A levels in four patients receiving TPN at home for more than 6 months.[88] One of the patients developed night blindness, which resolved with vitamin A administration. Each of the patients was receiving premixed nutrient solutions which were stored in the dark at 4°C. Investigation revealed that vitamin A activity was lost over time. Activity was decreased 77 percent after 2 weeks of storage, with approximately 30 percent of the "missing" vitamin A found adsorbed to the polyvinyl plastic bags. This problem is avoided by using freshly prepared solutions.

TPN solutions inadequate in vitamin A may precipitate an acute vitamin A deficiency in patients with low liver stores, since high-quality protein is known to stimulate the release of vitamin A from the liver.[87]

Vitamin D toxicity.   Hypercalcemia and metastatic calcification occur with vitamin D intoxication. Such manifestations have been associated with intravenous feedings containing excessive vitamin D supplements.[87] Hypercalcemia was observed in 11 of 200 patients at the Massachusetts General Hospital while receiving TPN. The high serum levels were thought to be due to excessive vitamin D.[38]

Thiamine (vitamin B1) deficiency.   Thiamine deficiency is usually associated with chronic alcoholism, but it has also been reported with starvation and during repletion of malnourished patients.[89] Thiamine functions as a coenzyme in carbohydrate metabolism; therefore, its requirement is directly proportional to the amount of carbohydrate in the diet. Thus a carbohydrate load can precipitate manifestations of thiamine deficiency in a moderately thiamine-depleted individual, because the remaining vitamin is promptly consumed during carbohydrate metabolism.[90]

Manifestations of thiamine deficiency include the high-output cardiac failure of beriberi and Wernicke's encephalopathy. The latter is characterized by peripheral neuropathy, ataxia, oculomotor abnormalities, and amnestic psychosis. Both conditions have been described during high-carbohydrate TPN with inadequate thiamine supplementation. Response to thiamine administration is usually rapid and dramatic[86,89,90] and perhaps represents the most important diagnostic test of deficiency.[91] The neurologic findings of thiamine deficiency must be distinguished from those associated with hypophosphatemia.[89]

Folate deficiency. Megaloblastic anemia responsive to folate administration has been observed in patients receiving parenteral feedings without folate or vitamin B12 supplementation.[92-94] Intravenous preparations of these vitamins are currently available (see Table 5-9), and routine supplementation should avert deficiency states.

Biotin deficiency. Biotin deficiency has recently been described in a 12-month-old child who had received TPN for 7 months following extensive small bowel resection and short gut syndrome.[95] Clinical manifestations included an erythematous, exfoliative rash; loss of body hair; waxy pallor of the skin; irritability; lethargy; and mild hypotonia. These findings were associated with reduced plasma, whole blood, and urine biotin levels. All of the clinical and biochemical features resolved after 2 weeks of biotin administration. This syndrome must be distinguished from syndromes produced by essential fatty acid deficiency and zinc deficiency.

Metabolic Bone Disease

Shike and associates and Klein and associates have observed abnormalities in bone metabolism in patients receiving TPN for prolonged periods.[96,97] Shike and associates described a disease occurring in 16 patients receiving parenteral nutrition at home for 7 to 89 months which was characterized by osteomalacia, hypercalciuria, intermittent hypercalcemia, reduced skeletal calcium, and low circulating parathormone levels.[96] Although vitamin D (25-hydroxyvitamin D) levels were normal, the features of the disease greatly improved when vitamin D was withdrawn.

In the 11 patients studied by Klein and associates, intense periarticular and lower extremity pain was a striking feature.[97] Hypercalciuria and osteomalacia were present, but serum levels of calcium and parathormone were normal.

The pathogenesis of this syndrome is obscure.

Abnormalities of Calcium Metabolism

Hypercalcemia may be associated with excessive administration of calcium or vitamin D, or with the metabolic bone disease previously discussed. Hypercalciuria has also been associated with the latter.

Adelman and associates reported the development of hypercalciuria and nephrolithiasis in an immobilized patient receiving TPN and corticosteroids.[98] The stones rapidly dissolved and urinary calcium returned to normal when calcium was removed from the nutrient solution. It is suggested that immobilized patients are at especial risk, and calcium metabolism should be monitored closely.

Hypercalcemia developing during TPN has been associated with the development of acute pancreatitis.[99,100] These findings resolved when TPN was discontinued.

Prerenal Azotemia

Elevated blood urea nitrogen levels may be due to hypovolemia. The latter can occur in TPN patients—for example, when hyperglycemia produces an osmotic diuresis.

Prerenal azotemia also may occur during excessive amino acid infusion,[101] and when insufficient nonprotein calories are provided and the infused amino acids are used to meet immediate energy needs rather than for replenishing body protein.[102,103]

Hyperammonemia

Hyperammonemia may occur during the infusion of protein hydrolysates, especially in infants and patients with hepatic disorders. These solutions contain significant amounts of free ammonia.[101]

Hyperammonemia has also been observed during the infusion of crystalline amino acids, solutions which contain no free ammonia. This abnormality appears to correlate with the dosage of amino acids and apparently is associated with a serum arginine deficiency. Thus the hyperammonemia is corrected by reducing the rate of infusion or, alternatively, by adding more arginine to the nutrient solution.

A possible explanation for this disorder is that the relative deficiency of arginine, developing as a consequence of the low content of arginine in the early crystalline amino acid preparations, impairs the efficiency of the urea cycle for the metabolism of endogenously produced ammonia.[101] To avoid this problem, current amino acid preparations have an increased content of arginine.

REFERENCES

1. Isenberg JI, Maxwell V: Intravenous infusion of amino acids stimulates gastric acid secretion in man. N Engl J Med 298:27–29, 1978.
2. Mariano EC, Beloni A, Landor JH: Some properties shared by amino acids and entero-oxyntin. Ann Surg 188:181–185, 1978.
3. Psaila JV, Wheeler MH, Bradley D, Newcombe R: Effect of an intravenous infusion of aminoacids (Aminoplex 14) on gastric secretion in healthy subjects and patients with duodenal ulcers. Ann Surg 194:18–25, 1981.
4. Varner AA, Isenberg JI, Elashoff JD, et al: Effect of intravenous lipid on gastric acid secretion stimulated by intravenous amino acids. Gastroenterology 79:873–876, 1980.
5. Thor PJ, Copeland EM, Dudrick SJ, Johnson LR: Effect of long-term parenteral feeding on gastric secretion in dogs. Am J Physiol 232:E39–E43, 1977.
6. Johnson LR, Copeland EM, Dudrick SJ, et al: Structural and hormonal alterations in the gastrointestinal tract of parenterally fed rats. Gastroenterology 68:1177–1183, 1975.
7. Kotler DP, Levine GM: Reversible gastric and pancreatic hyposecretion after long-term total parenteral nutrition. N Engl J Med 300:241–242, 1979.
8. MacGregor IL, Wiley ZD, Lavigne ME, Way LW: Slowed rate of gastric emptying of solid food in man by high caloric parenteral nutrition. Am J Surg 138:652–654, 1979.
9. MacGregor IL, Gueller R, Watts HD, Meyer JH: The effect of acute hyperglycemia on gastric emptying in man. Gastroenterology 70:197–202, 1976.
10. Hunt JN, Knox MT: The slowing of gastric emptying by nine acids. J Physiol 201:161–179, 1969.
11. Cameron IL, Pavlat WA, Urban E: Adaptive responses to total intravenous feeding. J Surg Res 17:45–52, 1974.
12. Castro GA, Copeland EM, Dudrick SJ, Johnson LR: Intestinal disaccharidase and peroxidase activities in parenterally nourished rats. J Nutr 105:776–781, 1975.
13. Levine GM, Deren JJ, Steiger E, Zinno R: Role of oral intake in maintenance of gut mass and disaccharide activity. Gastroenterology 67:975–982, 1974.
14. Tilson MD: Pathophysiology and treatment of short bowel syndrome. Surg Clin North Am 60:1273–1284, 1980.
15. Johnson LR, Litchtenberger LM, Copeland EM, et al: Action of gastrin on gastrointestinal structure and function. Gastroenterology 68:1184–1192, 1975.
16. Hughes C, Bates T, Dowling RM: The trophic effect of cholecystokinin/secretin stimulated pancreatobiliary secretions on dog intestine. Eur J Clin Invest 6:320, 1976.
17. Dudrick SJ, Wilmore DW, Steiger E, et al: Spontaneous closure of traumatic pancreatoduodenal fistulas with total intravenous nutrition. J Trauma 10:542–553, 1970.
18. Johnson LR, Schanbacher LM, Dudrick SJ, Copeland EM: Effect of long-term parenteral feeding on pancreatic secretion and serum secretin. Am J Physiol 233:E524–E529, 1977.
19. Grundfest S, Steiger E, Selinkoff P, Fletcher J: The effect of intravenous fat emulsions in patients with pancreatic fistula. JPEN 4:27–31, 1980.

20. Grant JP, Cox CE, Kleinman LM, et al: Serum hepatic enzyme and bilirubin elevations during parenteral nutrition. Surg Gynecol Obstet 145:573–580, 1970.
21. Lindor KD, Fleming CR, Abrams A, Hirschkorn MA: Liver function values in adults receiving total parenteral nutrition. JAMA 241:2398–2400, 1979.
22. Lowry SF, Brennan MF: Abnormal liver function during parenteral nutrition: Relation to infusion excess. J. Surg Res 26:300–307, 1979.
23. Lowry, AC, Wagner W, Silberman H: Liver indices in patients receiving lipid-based parenteral nutrition. JPEN 5:576, 1981.
24. Sheldon GF, Petersen SR, Sanders R: Hepatic dysfunction during hyperalimentation. Arch Surg 113:504–508, 1978.
25. Jeejeebhoy KN, Zohrab WJ, Langer B, et al: Total parenteral nutrition at home for 23 months, without complication, and with good rehabilitation. Gastroenterology 65:811–820, 1973.
26. Richardson TJ, Sgoutas D: Essential fatty acid deficiency in four adult patients during total parenteral nutrition. Am J Clin Nutr 28:258–263, 1975.
27. Chang S, Silvis SE: Fatty liver produced by hyperalimentation of rats. Am J Gastroenterol 62:410–418, 1974.
28. Steiger E, Daly JM, Vars HM, et al: Animal research in intravenous hyperalimentation, in Cowan G Jr, Scheetz W (eds): Intravenous Hyperalimentation. Philadelphia, Lea and Febiger, 1972, pp 186–194.
29. McDonald ATJ, Phillips MJ, Jeejeebhoy KN: Reversal of fatty liver by Intralipid in patients on total parenteral nutrition. Gastroenterology 64:885, 1973.
30. Maini B, Blackburn GL, Bistrian BR, et al: Cyclic hyperalimentation: An optimal technique for preservation of visceral protein. J Surg Res 20:515–525, 1976.
31. Rowlands BJ, MacFadyen BV, DeJong P, Dudrick WJ: Monitoring hepatic dysfunction during intravenous hyperalimentation. J Surg Res 28:471–478, 1980.
32. Askanazi J, Carpentier YA, Elwyn DH, et al: Influence of total parenteral nutrition on fuel utilization in injury and sepsis. Ann Surg 191:40–46, 1980.
33. Askanazi J, Elwyn DH, Silverberg PA, et al: Respiratory distress secondary to a high carbohydrate load: A case report. Surgery 87:596–598, 1980.
34. Askanazi J, Rosenbaum SH, Hyman AI, et al: Respiratory changes induced by the large glucose loads of total parenteral nutrition. JAMA 243:1444–1447, 1980.
35. Covelli HD, Black JW, Olsen MS, Beekman JF: Respiratory failure precipitated by high carbohydrate loads. Ann Intern Med 95:579–581, 1981.
36. Greene HL, Hazlett D, Demaree R: Relationship between Intralipid-induced hyperlipemia and pulmonary function. Am J Clin Nutr 29:127–135, 1976.
37. Wilmore DW, Moylan JA, Helmkamp GM, Pruitt BA Jr: Clinical evaluation of a 10 percent intravenous fat emulsion for parenteral nutrition in thermally injured patients. Ann Surg 178:503–513, 1973.
38. Ryan JA Jr: Complications of total parenteral nutrition, in Fischer JE (ed): Total Parenteral Nutrition. Boston, Little, Brown and Co, 1976, pp 55–100.
39. Sanderson I, Deitel M: Insulin response in patients receiving concentrated infusions of glucose and casein hydrolysate for complete parenteral nutrition. Ann Surg 179:387–394, 1974.
40. DeFronzo RA, Lang R: Hypophosphatemia and glucose tolerance: Evidence for tissue insensitivity to insulin. N Engl J Med 303:1259–1263, 1980.

41. Jeejeebhoy KN, Chu RC, Marliss EB, et al: Chromium deficiency, glucose intolerance, and neuropathy reversed by chromium supplementation in a patient receiving long-term total parenteral nutrition. Am J Clin Nutr 30:531–538, 1977.
42. Recommended Daily Allowances, ed 9, Food and Nutrition Board of the National Research Council, Washington, DC, National Academy of Sciences, 1980.
43. Fischer JE: Nutritional support in the seriously ill patient. Curr Probl Surg 17:466–532, 1980.
44. Gabow P, Peterson LN: Disorders of potassium metabolism, in Schrier RW (ed): Renal and Electrolyte Disorders, ed 2. Boston, Little, Brown and Co, 1980, pp 183–221.
45. Grzyb S, Jelinek, Scheldon GF: The phosphate depletion syndrome: Relation to caloric intake and phosphate infusion. Surg Forum 24:103–104, 1973.
46. Craddock PR, Yawata Y, VanSanten L, et al: Acquired phagocyte dysfunction: A complication of the hypophosphatemia of parenteral hyperalimentation. N Engl J Med 290:1403–1407, 1974.
47. Fitzgerald F: Clinical hypophosphatemia. Annu Rev Med 29:177–189, 1978.
48. Fitzgerald FT: Hypophosphatemia—Medical staff conference, University of California, San Francisco. West J Med 122:482–489, 1975.
49. Newman JH, Neff TA, Ziporin P: Acute respiratory failure associated with hypophosphatemia. N Engl J Med 296:1101–1103, 1977.
50. O'Connor LR, Wheeler WS, Bethune JE: Effect of hypophosphatemia on myocardial performance in man. N Engl J Med 297:901–903, 1977.
51. Darsee JR, Nutter DO: Reversible severe congestive cardiomyopathy in three cases of hypophosphatemia. Ann Intern Med 89:867–870, 1978.
52. Yawata Y, Hebbel RP, Silvis S, et al: Blood cell abnormalities complicating the hypophosphatemia of hyperalimentation: Erythrocyte and platelet ATP deficiency associated with hemolytic anemia and bleeding in hyperalimented dogs. J Lab Clin Med 84:643–653, 1974.
53. Silvis SE, Paragas PD Jr: Paresthesias, weakness, seizures, and hypophosphatemia in patients receiving hyperalimentation. Gastroenterology 62:513–520, 1972.
54. Weintraub MI: Hypophosphatemia mimicking acute Guillain–Barre–Strohl syndrome: A complication of parenteral hyperalimentation. JAMA 235:1040–1042, 1976.
55. Jacob HS, Amsden T: Acute hemolytic anemia with rigid red cells in hypophosphatemia. N Engl J Med 285:1446–1450, 1971.
56. Lichtman MA, Miller DR, Cohen J, Waterhouse C: Reduced red cell glycolysis, 2,3-diphosphoglycerate and adenosine triphosphate concentration, and increased hemoglobin–oxygen affinity caused by hypophosphatemia. Ann Intern Med 74:562–568, 1971.
57. Travis S, Sugerman HJ, Ruberg RL, et al: Alterations of red cell glycolytic intermediates and oxygen transport as a consequence of hypophosphatemia in patients receiving intravenous hyperalimentation. N Engl J Med 285:763–768, 1971.
58. Rajan KS, Levinson R, Leevy EM: Hepatic hypoxia secondary to hypophosphatemia. Clin Res 21:521, 1973.
59. Moser CR, Fessel WJ: Rheumatic manifestations of hypophosphatemia. Arch Intern Med 134:674–678, 1974.

60. Ruberg R, Allen T, Goodman M, et al: Hypophosphatemia with hypophosphaturia in hyperalimentation. Surg Forum 22:87–88, 1971.
61. Shils ME: Magnesium, in Goodhart RS, Shils ME (eds): Modern Nutrition in Health and Disease, ed 6. Philadelphia, Lea and Febiger, 1980, pp 310–323.
62. Alfrey AC: Disorders of magnesium metabolism, in Schrier RW (ed): Renal and Electrolyte Disorders, ed 2. Boston, Little, Brown and Co, 1980, pp 299–319.
63. Seller RH, Cangiano J, Kim KE, et al: Digitalis toxicity and hypomagnesemia. Am Heart J 79:57–68, 1970.
64. Connor WE: Pathogenesis and frequency of essential fatty acid deficiency during total parenteral nutrition. Ann Intern Med 83:895–896, 1975.
65. Wene JD, Connor WE, DenBesten L: The development of essential fatty acid deficiency in healthy men fed fat-free diets intravenously and orally. J Clin Invest 56:127–134, 1975.
66. Fleming CR, McGill DB, Hoffman HN II, Nelson RA: Total parenteral nutrition. Mayo Clin Proc 51:187–199, 1976.
67. Holman RT: The ratio of trienoic:tetraenoic acid in tissue lipids as a measure of essential fatty acid requirement. J Nutr 70:405–410, 1960.
68. Goodgame JT, Lowry SF, Brennan MF: Essential fatty acid deficiency in total parenteral nutrition: Time course of development and suggestions for therapy. Surgery 84:271–277, 1978.
69. Riella MC, Broviac JW, Wells M, Scribner BH: Essential fatty acid deficiency in human adults during total parenteral nutrition. Ann Intern Med 83:786–789, 1975.
70. O'Neill JA, Caldwell MD, Meng HC: Essential fatty acid deficiency in surgical patients. Ann Surg 185:535–542, 1977.
71. Skolnick P, Eaglstein WH, Ziboh VA: Human essential fatty acid deficiency. Arch Dermatol 113:939–941, 1977.
72. Caldwell MD, Jonsson HT, Othersen HB Jr: Essential fatty acid deficiency in an infant receiving prolonged parenteral alimentation. J Pediatr 81:894–898, 1972.
73. Freund H, Floman N, Schwartz B, Fischer JE: Essential fatty acid deficiency in total parenteral nutrition: Detection by changes in intraocular pressure. Ann Surg 190:139–143, 1979.
74. Press M, Hartop PJ, Prottey C: Correction of essential fatty acid deficiency in man by the cutaneous application of sunflower-seed oil. Lancet 1:597–598, 1974.
75. Lowry SF, Goodgame JT Jr, Smith JC Jr, et al: Abnormalities of zinc and copper during total parenteral nutrition. Ann Surg 189:120–128, 1979.
76. Kay RG, Tasman-Jones C, Pybus J, et al: A syndrome of acute zinc deficiency during total parenteral alimentation in man. Ann Surg 183:331–340, 1976.
77. Kay RG, Tasman-Jones C: Zinc deficiency and intravenous feeding. Lancet 2:605–606, 1975.
78. Fleming CR, Hodges RE, Hurley LS: A prospective study of serum copper and zinc levels in patients receiving total parenteral nutrition. Am J Clin Nutr 29:70–77, 1976.
79. Beisel WR, Edelman R, Nauss K, Suskind RM: Single nutrient effects on immunologic functions. JAMA 245:53–58, 1981.
80. Golden MHN, Harland PSEG, Golden BE, Jackson AA: Zinc and immunocompetence in protein–energy malnutrition. Lancet 1:1226–1228, 1978.

81. Kay RG, Tasman-Jones C: Acute zinc deficiency in man during intravenous alimentation. Aust NZ J Surg 45:325–330, 1975.
82. Karpel JT, Peden VH: Copper deficiency in long-term parenteral nutrition. J Pediatr 80:32–36, 1972.
83. Vilter RW, Bozian RC, Hess EV, et al: Manifestations of copper deficiency in a patient with systemic sclerosis on intravenous hyperalimentation. N Engl J Med 291:188–191, 1974.
84. Dunlap WM, James GW, Hume DM: Anemia and neutropenia caused by copper deficiency. Ann Intern Med 80:470–476, 1974.
85. Freund H, Atamian S, Fischer JE: Chromium deficiency during total parenteral nutrition. JAMA 241:496–498, 1979.
86. Gann DS, Robinson HB Jr: Salt, water and vitamins, in Ballinger WF, Collins JA, Drucker WR, et al (eds): Manual of Surgical Nutrition. Philadelphia, WB Saunders Co, 1975, pp 73–90.
87. Greene HL: Vitamins in total parenteral nutrition. Drug Intell Clin Pharm 6:355–360, 1972.
88. Howard L, Chu R, Freman S, et al: Vitamin A deficiency from long-term parenteral nutrition. Ann Intern Med 93:576–577, 1980.
89. Baughman FA Jr, Papp JP: Wernicke's encephalopathy with intravenous hyperalimentation: Remarks on similarities between Wernicke's encephalopathy and the phosphate depletion syndrome. Mt Sinai J Med (NY) 43:48–52, 1976.
90. Nadel AM, Burger PC: Wernicke encephalopathy following prolonged intravenous therapy. JAMA 235:2403–2405, 1976.
91. Kramer J, Goodwin JA: Wernicke's encephalopathy: Complication of intravenous hyperalimentation. JAMA 238:2176–2177, 1977.
92. Denburg J, Bensen W, Ali MAM, et al: Megaloblastic anemia in patients receiving total parenteral nutrition without folic acid or vitamin B12 supplementation. Can Med Assoc J 117:144–146, 1977.
93. Green PJ: Folate Deficiency and intravenous nutrition. Lancet 1:814, 1977.
94. Shah PC, Zafar M, Patel AR: Folate deficiency during intravenous hyperalimentation. J Med 8:383–392, 1977.
95. Mock DM, DeLorimer AA, Liebman WM, et al: Biotin deficiency: An unusual complication of parenteral alimentation. N Engl J Med 304:820–823, 1981.
96. Shike M, Harrison JE, Sturtridge WC, et al: Metabolic bone disease in patients receiving long-term parenteral nutrition. Ann Intern Med 92:343–350, 1980.
97. Klein GL, Ament ME, Bluestone R, et al: Bone disease associated with total parenteral nutrition. Lancet 2:1041–1044, 1980.
98. Adelman RD, Abern SB, Halsted CH, Hodges RE: Nephrolithiasis in a patient on total parenteral nutrition. Am J Clin Nutr 28:420, 1975.
99. Izsak EM, Shike M, Roulet M, Jeejeebhoy RN: Pancreatitis in association with hypercalcemia in patients receiving total parenteral nutrition. Gastroenterology 79:555–558, 1980.
100. Manson RR: Acute pancreatitis secondary to iatrogenic hypercalcemia. Arch Surg 108:213–215, 1974.
101. Dudrick SJ, MacFadyen BV Jr, Van Buren CT, et al: Parenteral hyperalimentation: Metabolic problems and solutions. Ann Surg 176:259–264, 1972.
102. Ausman RK, Hardy G: Metabolic complications of parenteral nutrition, in

Johnston IDA (ed): Advances in Parenteral Nutrition. Baltimore, University Park Press, 1978, pp 403–410.

103. Chen WJ, Ohashi E, Kasai M: Amino acid metabolism in parenteral nutrition: With special reference to the calorie:nitrogen ratio and the blood urea nitrogen level. Metabolism 23:1117–1123, 1974.

9

Nutrition Therapy: Comparison of Methods

The choice of the most appropriate form of nutritional therapy for a given patient who is unable to eat is dependent upon a variety of factors. Many of the specific indications and contraindications to the available methods of parenteral and enteral nutrition have already been discussed. Other considerations include relative nutritional value, comparative physiologic effects, ease and safety of nutrient preparation and administration, and cost-effectiveness.

ENTERAL VS. PARENTERAL NUTRITION

Nitrogen balance. Only limited data are available comparing the relative effects of nutrients provided enterally and those provided parenterally. Although some studies suggest that enterally administered nutrients have a greater impact on nitrogen balance than parenteral feedings,[1,2] the preponderance of data indicates that a comparable degree of nitrogen retention is achieved when the same nutrients are infused intravenously or by continuous infusion into the gastrointestinal tract[3-9] (see p. 67). This is not to imply, however, that all metabolic events are the same when comparing parenteral and enteral administration. Differences in insulin levels and in specific areas of amino acid and fat metabolism have been observed in studies designed to compare the impact of the two different routes of nutrient delivery[4,9], but the clinical consequences of these differences, if any, are unknown.

Recently, McArdle and associates reported the results of a prospective randomized study in which the metabolic effects of enteral and parenteral nutrition were compared.[4] Malnourished surgical patients received equal volumes of either a TPN solution providing 3.5 percent crystalline amino acids and 25 percent glucose or an enteral formulation also containing 3.5 percent amino acids and an identical carbohydrate load provided as the glucose polymer, Polycose. Significant positive nitrogen balance was achieved to the same extent and in the same period of time in both groups of patients. However, blood insulin and cortisol levels were significantly elevated and free fatty acid levels were significantly decreased in the patients receiving TPN. These changes were not observed in the enterally fed patients.

Effects on the alimentary tract. Involutional changes are observed in the gastrointestinal tract and pancreas when all nutrients are provided intravenously (see Chapter 8). Evidently, luminal nutrition is needed to maintain the structural and functional integrity of these organs, and this can be preserved by feeding enteral formulations providing intact protein or protein isolates and, to a lesser extent, by feeding elemental diets (see Chapter 4).[10,11] In most clinical situations, the involutional changes occurring during parenteral nutrition are of little relevance, since they apparently are reversed when oral alimentation is resumed.[12] In certain conditions, however, these changes are of clinical importance. For example, the pancreatic hyposecretion associated with TPN is thought to be beneficial in cases of acute pancreatitis or pancreatic fistula. On the other hand, in the short bowel syndrome the involutional changes associated with TPN are undesirable, and maximal compensatory villous hypertrophy is achieved only when enteral nutrition is part of the therapeutic regimen (see Chapter 10).[13]

Preparation and administration. Enteral nutrition has the advantage that the preparation of the nutrient solutions does not require special facilities or specially trained personnel. In addition, the stringent requirements for asepsis necessary for the safe administration of intravenous feedings are not applicable to enteral feedings. Thus nursing care is simplified, since dressing changes and catheter care are not involved.

Complications. Patients receiving either enteral or parenteral nutrition may develop similar metabolic derangements. However, those receiving the glucose system of parenteral nutrition are subject to the potentially serious complications associated with introducing and maintaining the central venous catheter necessary for vascular access. These potential problems, including pneumothorax and catheter sepsis, are averted in patients fed enterally. On the other hand, pulmonary aspiration is a major complication that may occur in enterally fed patients. In general, the enteral technique, when used for appropriate indications, is associated with fewer serious complications than

TPN using the centrally administered glucose system.[10,14] Serious complications are very rare in patients receiving the lipid system through peripheral veins.

Cost-effectiveness.   Feeding products which are formulated for intravenous administration are significantly more expensive than products of equivalent nutritional value that are designed for enteral feeding. Parenteral preparations may be 5 to 25 times more expensive.[10,14] Unlike enteral feeding products, solutions for total parenteral nutrition must be prepared from individual ingredients just prior to administration by highly trained personnel using specialized equipment. This, of course, further increases the expense of this form of nutritional support.

In summary, medical evaluation of some patients may indicate that parenteral or enteral feedings would be equally suitable therapeutic methods of nutritional support. Under these circumstances, enteral feedings are generally preferred because of comparable nutritional value, greater ease and safety of preparation and administration, and lesser cost.

THE GLUCOSE SYSTEM VS. THE LIPID SYSTEM OF PARENTERAL NUTRITION

Factors to be considered in comparing the glucose and lipid systems of parenteral nutrition include the composition and nutrient value of the two methods, the relative efficacy of glucose and lipid calories, ease and safety of administration, and cost-effectiveness.

Composition of the standard glucose and lipid systems.   The glucose system described in Chapter 6 provides 850 nonprotein kcal/liter exclusively of carbohydrate origin, whereas the lipid system, described in Chapter 7 supplies 720 nonprotein kcal/liter, of which nearly 70 percent are of lipid origin. The glucose system also provides 40 percent more nitrogen per liter, but its much greater osmolarity (2000 mOsm/liter) requires that this system be infused into a central vein. The lesser concentration of the lipid system (900 mOsm/liter) permits safe peripheral venous administration (Table 9-1).

When comparing nutrients provided a 70 kg man receiving the glucose or lipid system at various rates of infusion, it can be seen that 4 liters/day of the lipid system provide about the same nutrients as 3 liters/day of the glucose system (Table 9-2).

Glucose vs. lipid as a caloric source.   The relative impact of glucose and lipid calories on nitrogen retention or body composition is the subject of current controversy. Analysis of available data is confounded because much of the in-

TABLE 9-1
Nutrients in the Lipid and Glucose Systems*

	Lipid System	Glucose System
Carbohydrate calories	220 kcal/liter	850 kcal/liter
Lipid calories	500 kcal/liter	—
Total nonprotein calories	720 kcal/liter	850 kcal/liter
Nitrogen provided	4.6 gm/liter	6.5 gm/liter
Protein equivalent	28.4 gm/liter	40.6 gm/liter
Calorie: nitrogen ratio	157:1	131:1
Concentration (approximate)	900 mOsm/liter	2000 mOsm/liter

*Based on protocols outlined in Tables 6-1 and 7-1.

formation has been derived from uncontrolled, retrospective studies of subjects with a variety of illnesses of varying severity.

Carbohydrate has a characteristic protein-sparing effect in patients in whom dietary protein is withheld that is not observed with fat administration. The alterations in nitrogen excretion that do occur in such patients during fat administration have been attributed to adjustments in nitrogen loss secondary to starvation adaption.[9] In addition, the protein-sparing effect seen when one of the currently available fat emulsions is given to an otherwise fasting patient is evidently due exclusively to the carbohydrate (glycerol) component of the emulsion.[9,15]

The pertinent studies necessary to evaluate the relative efficacy of glucose and lipid calories are those in which isocaloric exchanges of glucose and lipid are evaluated in patients or experimental animals receiving adequate nitrogen and at least the minimum amount of carbohydrate necessary to supply the glycolytic tissues. Many of the available data are summarized in Table 9-3.

TABLE 9-2
Nutrients Provided for a 70 kg Man

Infusion Rate	Lipid System	Glucose System
3 liters/day	30.9 nonprotein kcal/kg 1.2 gm protein/kg 157 kcal/gm nitrogen	36.4 nonprotein kcal/kg 1.7 gm protein/kg 131 kcal/gm nitrogen
4 liters/day	41.1 nonprotein kcal/kg 1.6 gm protein/kg 157 kcal/gm nitrogen	48.6 nonprotein kcal/kg 2.3 gm protein/kg 131 kcal/gm nitrogen

Wolfe and associates studied the effect of various intravenously administered nutrients on nitrogen balance in normal fasting male volunteers (Fig. 9-1).[20] In particular, these investigators compared the effect of a lipid system providing 86 percent of nonprotein calories as lipid and a glucose system providing all nonprotein calories as glucose. Eight patients received one or the other regimen for 8 days. There was no statistically significant difference between the two systems in either daily or cumulative nitrogen balance.

The major study suggesting the comparable efficacy of both systems in sick individuals is that of Jeejeebhoy and associates.[22] Twenty-four chronically ill patients each received in random sequence 1 week of a lipid system providing 83 percent of nonprotein calories as lipid and 1 week of a glucose system providing 100 percent of nonprotein calories as glucose. Each system provided 40 nonprotein kcal/kg and 1 gm/kg of protein as casein hydrolysate daily. Patients with systemic infections with septicemia, insulin-dependent diabetes, or hepatic, renal, or cardiac insufficiency were excluded from the study group. The data indicated that the mean daily nitrogen balance over the entire 7 day study period was significantly higher with the glucose system than with the lipid system (Table 9-4). However, the greater nitrogen retention observed with the glucose system was entirely due to its greater effect during the first 4 days of treatment. No significant difference in nitrogen balance was observed when the last 3 days (days 5 through 7) of treatment with each system were compared. The authors concluded that optimal nitrogen retention with the lipid system requires a period of about 4 days to establish equilibrium, after which nitrogen balance is positive to a comparable degree with both systems.

In contrast, the major study suggesting the superiority of the glucose system is that of Long and associates.[21] These investigators studied three burn patients and two patients with gastrointestinal disease who were clinically stable. Thirteen intravenous diets providing a constant amount of nitrogen (11.7 gm/m²/day) but different combinations of carbohydrate (110 to 2300 kcal/m²/day) and fat (0–1100 kcal/m²/day) were evaluated by measuring urea nitrogen excretion. Three of the diets were isocaloric, including one providing all nonprotein calories as glucose and two providing 76 percent and 40 percent of nonprotein calories as lipid, respectively. There were 34 three day study periods, during which each of the five patients received at least three different diets assigned in a random sequence. The data, presented in Tables 9-5 and 9-6, led the authors to conclude that urea nitrogen excretion is inversely related to carbohydrate intake, and the addition of intravenous fat does not significantly influence nitrogen excretion at any level of carbohydrate administration.

One may speculate that the apparent discrepancy between the conclusions of Jeejeebhoy and associates and Long and associates relates to the dif-

TABLE 9-3
Relative Effectiveness of Glucose and Lipid as Caloric Sources in Total Parenteral Nutrition

Investigator	Subjects	Duration and Type of Study
Macfie et al. 1981[16]	2 groups of 16 matched patients with GI disease	14 days
Kirkpatrick et al. 1981[17]	45 stable patients, including 23 with sepsis	12–15 days (mean); randomized
Elwyn et al. 1980[18]	6 nutritionally depleted patients	7 days; crossover
Shizgal and Forse 1980[19]	204 malnourished patients	2 weeks; randomized
Wolfe et al. 1977[20]	8 fasting male volunteers	8 days
Long et al. 1977[21]	5 patients stable after injury or operation	3 days; crossover
Jeejeebhoy et al. 1976[22]	24 chronically ill patients	7 days; crossover
Bark et al. 1976[23]	9 patients postgastric resection	6 days
Gazzaniga et al. 1975[24]	18 surgical patients	4–38 days
Freund et al. 1980[25]	Rats, postlaparotomy	4 days
Buzby et al. 1979[26]	Rats, protein-depleted	6 days
Steiger et al. 1977[27]	Rats, protein-depleted	7 days

Nonprotein kcal in Glucose (G) and Lipid (L) Systems	Criterion of Efficacy	Conclusions
G = 100% glucose L = 60% lipid, 40% glucose	Total body nitrogen	Lipid superior
G = 100% glucose L = 56% lipid, 44% glucose	Nitrogen balance	Both systems comparable
G = 100% glucose L = 33% lipid, 67% glucose	Nitrogen balance	Both systems comparable
G = 100% glucose L = 54% lipid, 46% glucose	Restoration of body cell mass	Glucose system more efficient
G = 100% glucose L = 86% lipid, 14% glucose	Nitrogen balance	Both systems comparable
G = 100% glucose L 1 = 76% lipid, 24% glucose L 2 = 40% lipid, 60% glucose	Urea nitrogen excretion (UNE)	UNE inversely related to glucose intake; lipid had no effect
G = 100% glucose L = 83% lipid, 17% glucose	Nitrogen balance	Glucose superior first 4 days; then glucose and lipid equivalent
G = 100% glucose L = 71% lipid, 29% carbohydrate	Nitrogen balance	Both systems comparable
G = 66% glucose, 34% fructose L = 79% lipid, 21% glucose	Days of nitrogen balance	Both systems comparable
G = 100% L = 90% lipid, 10% carbohydrate	Nitrogen balance	Glucose system superior
G = 100% glucose L 1 = 25% lipid, 75% glucose L 2 = 50% lipid, 50% glucose L 3 = 75% lipid, 25% glucose L 4 = 90% lipid, 10% carbohydrate	Nitrogen balance	L2 superior to other regimens
G = 100% glucose L = 40% lipid, 60% glucose	Nitrogen balance	Both systems comparable

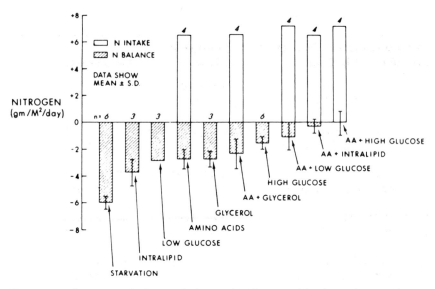

Figure 9-1. Summary of nitrogen balance data in normal fasting volunteers in response to various nutritional regimens. There was no statistically significant difference between the lipid system (AA + Intralipid) and the glucose system (AA + high glucose); AA = amino acids. *(From Wolfe BM, et al: Ann Surg 186:518–540, 1977)*

TABLE 9-4

Mean Daily Nitrogen Balance in Patients Receiving the Glucose and Lipid Systems in Random Sequence

	Days 1–7	*Days 1–4*	*Days 5–7*
Lipid followed by glucose			
Lipid*	2.27 ± 0.20	2.15 ± 0.34	2.41 ± 0.34
Glucose*	2.99 ± 0.20	3.44 ± 0.28	2.78 ± 0.30
P†	<0.005	<0.005	NS‡
Glucose followed by lipid			
Glucose*	2.49 ± 0.21	2.55 ± 0.28	2.40 ± 0.33
Lipid*	1.89 ± 0.21	1.46 ± 0.28	2.52 ± 0.31
P†	<0.001	<0.001	NS

*Values are gm/day of nitrogen retained expressed as mean ± SEM for each study period.
†P-value is that for significance of difference between means by paired t test.
‡NS = Not significant.
Data from Jeejeebhoy KN, et al: J Clin Invest 57:127–136, 1976, by copyright permission of the American Society for Clinical Investigation.

TABLE 9-5
Urea Nitrogen Excretion During Administration of Isonitrogenous Feeding Regimens Providing Varying Proportions of Carbohydrate and Fat*

Patient	Nonprotein Caloric Intake (kcal/m²/day)		Urea Nitrogen Excretion (gm/m²/day)	Plasma Insulin (μU/ml)
	CARBOHYDRATE	FAT		
1	1450	0	6.1	—
	875	575	6.2	34
	350	1100	9.6	22.5
	1450	0	6.8	75
	875	575	7.5	34
	350	1100	9.0	21.5
	350	1100	10.0	29.5
	875	1100	7.5	34.7
	1450	1100	4.7	52†
2	1450	0	7.0	—
	875	575	8.5	—
	350	1100	9.1	—
3	1450	0	6.8	82
	875	575	6.3	57
	350	1100	8.8	22
4	350	0	10.2	12
	350	1100	10.7	12
	875	0	9.1	16.5
	875	1100	8.5	26
	1450	0	7.6	30
	1450	1100	7.8	28
	1450	1100	8.1	28
	1450	0	7.6	27
	1850	0	8.0	30.5
	2300	0	7.6	53
	110	0	12.0	15.5
	110	1000	11.6	18.5
5	350	0	8.4	17
	875	0	7.0	49
	875	575	7.5	33
	1450	575	5.4	35†
	2050	0	4.5	94†
	2050	575	3.9	30†
	2050	0	3.5	19†

*All patients received 11.7 gm/m²/day of nitrogen.
†Patients receiving intermittent doses of exogenous insulin.
Data from Long JM III, et al: Ann Surg 185:417–422, 1977.

TABLE 9-6

Mean Nitrogen Excretion During Administration of Various Isonitrogenous Feeding Regimens Providing Varying Proportions of Carbohydrate and Fat*

Fat Intake (kcal/m²/day)	Carbohydrate Intake (kcal/m²/day)			
	110	350	875	1450
0	12.0†	9.3	8.0	7.0
575	—	—	7.2	5.4
1100	11.6	9.5	8.0	6.7

*Nitrogen intake was 11.7 gm/m²/day.
†Mean urea nitrogen excretion (gm/m²/day) on third day of each infusion period.
Data from Long JM III, et al: Ann Surg 185:417–422, 1977.

ference in the types of patients evaluated in the two studies and a difference in the duration of the study period. Jeejeebhoy and associates demonstrated that the comparable efficacy of the glucose and lipid systems becomes evident only after a 4 day period of equilibration.[22]

While the preponderance of evidence supports the conclusion that the glucose and lipid systems are of comparable value in their effect on nitrogen retention in normal or chronically ill malnourished patients, the equivalent efficacy of the lipid system in critically ill septic or hypermetabolic patients remains controversial and unestablished. Studies evaluating the impact of oral diets in patients with hypermetabolic disease processes, such as typhoid fever and burns, suggest that carbohydrate intake exerts the dominant effect on nitrogen retention.[9]

Woolfson and associates evaluated the protein-sparing effects of three isocaloric, isonitrogenous intravenous feeding regimens in patients who were catabolic following injury.[28] These authors found that a regimen providing glucose plus insulin produced a strikingly greater inhibition of protein breakdown than glucose alone and that glucose alone was marginally more protein-sparing than a regimen containing mainly fat. The protein-sparing effect of insulin seen in these severely ill, traumatized patients was not observed in noncatabolic patients.

O'Donnell and associates evaluated endogenous fat metabolism in peripheral tissues in previously well nourished, acutely ill patients with severe gram-negative sepsis.[29] Whereas the metabolic events in normal fasting man are characterized by a progressive increase in the uptake of free fatty acids and ketone bodies as the primary source of energy for peripheral tissues, in the septic patients fat metabolism was abnormal. Arterial free fatty acid levels were significantly reduced, uptake of free fatty acids was also reduced, and ketogenesis was completely suppressed. In this study O'Donnell and associates examined the effect of gram-negative sepsis on *endogenous* fat metabolism in *normally nourished* individuals, and therefore the conclusions are not necessarily applicable to malnourished septic patients,[30] to patients with other forms of sepsis, or to the metabolism of exogenously administered lipids.

The clearance of exogenously infused lipids from the blood stream during sepsis has been studied by Robin and associates and Kaufmann and associates[31,32] The former investigators found that infected patients had a greater capacity for lipid clearance than normal volunteers. In contrast, the latter investigators observed that Rhesus monkeys with gram-negative sepsis had a reduced clearance of intravenously administrated lipid, but intravenous lipid clearing was unimpaired during pneumococcal sepsis. These latter findings are consistent with those of Wannemacher and associates, who observed that the addition of lipid calories to a glucose-based intravenous feeding regimen resulted in an increment in body protein in Rhesus monkeys with pneumococcal sepsis.[33]

Askanazi and associates studied fuel utilization in injured and septic patients receiving the glucose system of parenteral nutrition (see p. 196).[34,35] In contrast to its effect in chronically ill, nutritionally depleted patients, the administration of glucose to acutely ill patients in quantities exceeding energy expenditure was accompanied by ongoing utilization of endogenous fat for energy, resulting in a respiratory quotient significantly less than 1.0. Contrary to data suggesting that there is decreased fat utilization during infection, these authors concluded that septic and injured man appears to utilize fat preferentially as an energy source. Jeejeebhoy concurred in the latter view and, furthermore, observed superior protein synthesis with the lipid system in severely stressed patients.[36]

In summary, glucose and lipid are effective caloric sources in normal persons and chronically ill patients. Lipid is probably effective in patients with gram-positive sepsis, but equivalent efficacy in patients with gram-negative sepsis remains unproven.

Ease and safety of administration. The glucose system requires central venous administration. Acquiring vascular access is associated with certain complications not seen with the peripherally administered lipid system (see pp. 151–158). Once vascular access is obtained, however, managing the infusion of the glucose system is rather simple. The solution, prepared in a single container, is administered at a constant rate over the prescribed time period. On the other hand, the lipid system, infused through a simply cannulated peripheral vein, is provided in two containers which must be infused concurrently at the same rate.

The lipid system is not associated with the septic complications which may occur during administration of the glucose system, and special attention to dressings at the infusion site is unnecessary. In addition, abnormalities of glucose metabolism are less common in patients receiving the lipid system.

Cost-effectiveness.   At present, materials required for preparation of the lipid system are about twice as costly as those required for isocaloric volumes of the glucose system. In addition, the glucose system can be more rapidly prepared by the TPN pharmacist.

Choosing between the glucose and lipid systems.   Patients requiring intravenous nutritional support often have associated or concurrent medical conditions which influence the choice of treatment.

Because of its greater caloric density, the glucose system is usually preferred for patients with conditions requiring fluid restriction. Thus, for any given tolerable fluid volume, more calories can be provided by the glucose system. In patients requiring marked fluid restriction, as in severe congestive heart failure, the glucose system can be modified to increase caloric density from 850 nonprotein kcal/liter to 1190 nonprotein kcal/liter (see p. 266).

In patients with disorders of lipid metabolism, the infusion of exogenous lipids is avoided and the glucose system is recommended. In addition, the glucose system is presently recommended for patients with gram-negative sepsis in view of the data previously presented.

One of the major advantages of the lipid system is that it can be given through peripheral veins. When the use of the latter is precluded by thrombosed or otherwise unsuitable peripheral veins and a subclavian catheter is required primarily to obtain vascular access the glucose system is generally preferred because of its greater caloric density, greater ease of preparation, and lesser cost. However, under certain limited circumstances it may be desirable to infuse the lipid system through a central vein. Occasionally, the tip of the subclavian catheter is inadvertently advanced into the internal jugular vein or the contralateral subclavian vein rather than into the superior vena cava. In such cases, the less concentrated lipid system can be safely infused into the smaller vein eliminating the need to reposition the catheter or recannulate the subclavian vein. Patients with inaccessible peripheral veins and marked glucose intolerance may also receive the lipid system centrally (infra vide). Finally, fluid-restricted patients with glucose intolerance may receive a more concentrated, modified lipid system which requires central venous administration (see p. 267).

Use of the glucose system may be associated with additional risk factors in certain patients with pulmonary disease. Patients with a tracheostomy who receive the glucose system are at increased risk of subclavian catheter sepsis because of the close proximity of the inevitably purulent secretions around the tracheostomy stoma and the subclavian catheter and its overlying dressings. Consequently, the lipid system is generally recommended in such patients. Alternatively, the glucose system could be infused through a Broviac catheter or a peripherally inserted silicone elastomer catheter (see Chapter 6). In addition, percutaneous subclavian catheterization is best avoided in patients in whom the risk of pneumothorax is significantly increased or in whom the consequences of pneumothorax may be severe morbidity or even mortality. Patients in the former group include those with bullous emphysema, and patients in the latter category include those with severe pulmonary dysfunction or respiratory failure. In these two groups of patients, the glucose system may be infused through an alternative route of vascular access, or the lipid system may be prescribed.

The administration of excess glucose calories should be avoided, since it is associated with increased oxygen consumption and increased carbon dioxide production, and the latter may aggravate the condition of patients with little pulmonary reserve. Since carbon dioxide production can be reduced by providing fat calories (see pp. 196–198), the lipid system should be considered in such patients.

Finally, the glucose system has been used successfully in patients with diabetes mellitus and other forms of glucose intolerance, but the metabolic management of such patients should be simpler with the infusion of less glucose, as in the lipid system.[22,37] However, controlled studies are not available on this point.

REFERENCES

1. Blackburn GL, Bistrian BR: Nutritional care of the injured and/or septic patient. Surg Clin North Am 56:1195–1224, 1976.
2. Lickley HL, Track NS, Vranic M, Bury KD: Metabolic response to enteral and parenteral nutrition. Am J Surg 135:172–176, 1978.
3. Anderson GH, Patel DG, Jeejeebhoy KN: Design and evaluation by nitrogen balance and blood aminograms of an amino acid mixture for total parenteral nutrition of adults with gastrointestinal disease. J Clin Invest 53:904–912, 1974.
4. McArdle AH, Palmason C, Morency I, Brown RA: A rationale for enteral feeding as the preferable route for hyperalimentation. Surgery 90:616–623, 1981.
5. Freeman JB, in discussion, Lickley HLA, Track NS, Vanic M, Bury KD: Metabolic response to enteral and parenteral nutrition. Am J Surg 135:172–176, 1978.
6. Kihlberg R, Levin G, Roos KA: A comparison of enteral and parenteral nutrition in rats. Acta Chir Scand [Suppl] 466:42–43, 1976.
7. Munro HN: Basic concepts in the use of amino acids and protein hydrolysates for parenteral nutrition. Proceedings of the AMA Symposium on Total Parenteral Nutrition, Nashville, Tennessee, January 17–19, 1972, pp 7–35.
8. Munro HN: Carbohydrate versus fat versus protein calories (panel discussion), in Greep JM, Soeters PB, Wesdorp RIC, et al (eds): Current Concepts in Parenteral Nutrition. The Hague, Martinus Nijoff Medical Division, 1977, p 357.

9. Wilmore DW: Energy requirements for maximum nitrogen retention, in Greene HL, Holliday MA, Munro HN (eds): Clinical Nutrition Update: Amino Acids. Chicago, American Medical Association, 1977, pp 47–58.

10. Heymsfield SB, Bethel RA, Ansley JD, et al: Enteral hyperalimentation: An alternative to central venous hyperalimentation. Ann Intern Med 90:63–71, 1979.

11. Levine GM, Deren JJ, Steiger E, Zinno R: Role of oral intake in maintenance of gut mass and disaccharidase activity. Gastroenterology 67:957–982, 1974.

12. Kotler DR, Levine GM: Reversible gastric and pancreatic hyposecretion after long-term total parenteral nutrition. N Engl J Med 300:241–242, 1979.

13. Sheldon GF: Role of parenteral nutrition in patients with short bowel syndrome. Am J Med 67:1021–1029, 1979.

14. Hoover HC Jr, Ryan JA, Anderson EJ, Fischer JE: Nutritional benefits of immediate postoperative jejunal feeding of an elemental diet. Am J Surg 139:153–159, 1980.

15. Brennan MF, Fitzpatrick GF, Cohen KH, Moore FD: Glycerol: Major contributor to the short-term protein-sparing effect of fat emulsions in normal man. Ann Surg 182:386–394, 1975.

16. Macfie J, Smith RC, Holl GL: Glucose or fat as a non-protein energy source? A controlled clinical trial in gastroenterological patients requiring intravenous nutrition. Gastroenterology 80:103–107, 1981.

17. Kirkpatrick JR, Dahn M, Lewis L: Selective versus standard hyperalimentation. Am J Surg 141:116–121, 1981.

18. Elwyn DH, Kinney JM, Gump FE, et al: Some metabolic effects of fat infusions in depleted patients. Metabolism 29:125–132, 1980.

19. Shizgal HM, Forse RA: Protein and caloric requirements with total parenteral nutrition. Ann Surg 192:562–569, 1980.

20. Wolfe BM, Culebras JM, Sim AJW, et al: Substrate interaction in intravenous feeding: Comparative effects of carbohydrate and fat on amino acid utilization in fasting man. Ann Surg 186:518–540, 1977.

21. Long JM III, Wilmore DW, Mason AD Jr, Pruitt BA Jr: Effect of carbohydrate and fat intake on nitrogen excretion during total intravenous feeding. Ann Surg 185:417–422, 1977.

22. Jeejeebhoy KN, Anderson GH, Nakhooda AF, et al: Metabolic studies in total parenteral nutrition with lipid in man: Comparison with glucose. J Clin Invest 57:127–136, 1976.

23. Bark S, Holm I, Hakansson I, Wretlind A: Nitrogen-sparing effect of fat emulsion compared with glucose in the post-operative period. Acta Chir Scand 142:423–427, 1976.

24. Gazzaniga AB, Bartlett RH, Shobe JB: Nitrogen balance in patients receiving either fat or carbohydrate for total intravenous nutrition. Ann Surg 182:163–168, 1975.

25. Freund H, Yoshimura N, Fischer JE: Does intravenous fat spare nitrogen in the injured rat? Am J Surg 140:377–383, 1980.

26. Buzby GP, Mullen JL, Stein TP, et al: Optimal TPN caloric substrate for correction of protein malnutrition. Surg Forum 30:64–67, 1979.

27. Steiger E, Naito HK, Cooperman AM, O'Neill M: Effect of lipid calories on weight gain, nitrogen balance, liver weight, and composition in total parenteral nutrition (TPN). Surg Forum 28:83–85, 1977.

28. Woolfson AMJ, Heatley RV, Allison SP: Insulin to inhibit protein catabolism after injury. N Engl J Med 300: 14–17, 1979.

29. O'Donnell TF, Clowes GHA Jr, Blackburn GL, et al: Proteolysis associated with a deficit of peripheral energy fuel substrates in septic man. Surgery 80:192–200, 1976.

30. Beisel WR, Wannemacher RW Jr: Gluconeogenesis, ureagenesis, and ketogenesis during sepsis. JPEN 4:277–285, 1980.

31. Robin AP, Nordenstrom J, Askanazi J, et al: Plasma clearance of fat emulsion in trauma and sepsis: Use of a three-stage lipid clearance test. JPEN 4:505–510, 1980.

32. Kaufmann RL, Matson CR, Rowberg AH, Beisel WR: Defective lipid disposal mechanisms during bacterial infection in Rhesus monkeys. Metabolism 25:615–624, 1976.

33. Wannemacher RW Jr, Kaminski MV, Dinterman RE, McCabe TR: Use of lipid calories during pneumococcal sepsis in Rhesus monkeys. JPEN 3:22, 1979.

34. Askanazi J, Carpentier YA, Elwyn DH, et al: Influence of total parenteral nutrition on fuel utilization in injury and sepsis. Ann Surg 191:40–46, 1980.

35. Askanazi J, Elwyn DH, Silverberg PA, et al: Respiratory distress secondary to a high carbohydrate load: A case report. Surgery 87:596–598, 1980.

36. Jeejeebhoy KN, in discussion, Kirkpatrick JR, Dahn M, Lewis L: Selective versus standard hyperalimentation. Am J Surg 141:116–121, 1981.

37. Kleinberger G, Druml W, Laggner A, Lenz K: Parenteral nutrition of diabetic patients with fat. JPEN 5:579, 1981.

10

Nutrition Therapy: Clinical Applications

Special nutrition therapy with enteral or parenteral feedings is indicated for malnourished patients who are unresponsive to conventional dietary therapy, for depleted patients in whom oral feedings are contraindicated, and for patients in whom malnutrition is anticipated because oral intake will be inadequate or contraindicated for periods exceeding 7 to 10 days. Besides these general indications, enteral or parenteral nutrition has been advocated as primary or adjunctive therapy for patients with such specific conditions as gastrointestinal fistula, short bowel syndrome, inflammatory bowel disease, burns, renal failure, cancer, and pancreatitis, and for malnourished patients in the perioperative period.

In addition, special techniques or modified nutrient solutions have been described for fluid-restricted patients, postoperative patients, minimally catabolic patients, and patients with renal failure or liver failure.

GASTROINTESTINAL FISTULAS

Major factors contributing to mortality in patients with gastrointestinal fistulas include fluid and electrolyte disturbances, sepsis, and malnutrition. The impact of improved methods of nutritional support on the management of fistulas is obscured to some extent by lack of controlled clinical studies and concomitant advances in other aspects of supportive care, including antibiotic

230

therapy, fluid and electrolyte management and monitoring, enterostomal therapy, and respiratory care.

Nevertheless, retrospective analyses suggest that nutrition therapy is of significant value in the management of patients with gastrointestinal fistulas (Table 10-1). Thus mortality rates in major series range from 8 to 29 percent for patients receiving special nutrition therapy, whereas mortality rates were between 15 and 60 percent for those not receiving this therapy. However, published series of patients with fistulas are not strictly comparable, since the fistulas studied have varied in etiology and anatomic distribution. In addition, in some series only the most seriously ill patients received special nutritional support.[11] The studies of Chapman et al.,[2] Himal et al.,[7] Dietel,[8] and Thomas[13] are of particular interest, since in each case two groups of patients managed within the same institution were analyzed: those who had received nutritional support and those who had not. These investigators each found that nutritional support had a significant salutary effect on the outcome of patients with fistulas in their respective institutions. Data from these studies reveal a 2 to 4-fold reduction in mortality and about a 2-fold increase in the overall rate of fistula closure, including a substantial increase in the rate of spontaneous (nonoperative) closure, in patients receiving enteral or parenteral nutrition.

The value of special nutrition therapy in patients with fistulas is multifold. Regular oral diets are generally contraindicated in these patients because such diets frequently are not absorbed and they tend to increase fistulous output, thereby aggravating fluid and electrolyte disturbances and impairing wound healing. Thus parenteral nutrition, or, in certain circumstances, enteral feedings, is prescribed to avert or reverse malnutrition and consequently stimulate wound healing, improve immunocompetence, and increase resistance to infection. In addition, fistulous output frequently decreases sharply during this treatment, thus simplifying fluid and electrolyte management and wound care. The ability to maintain nutrition despite the presence of the fistula eliminates the urgency to restore gastrointestinal continuity, and consequently, operative repair is not indicated in the early stage of therapy. Instead, fluid balance is restored, nutrition is supported, and sepsis is controlled. This program allows the inflammatory process within the abdomen to subside and, ideally, promote spontaneous closure of the fistula. However, if surgical repair is ultimately required, it can be carried out electively after nutrition has been repleted and the operative field has become quiescent. This delayed, elective approach to operative management is of significant benefit to patients, since early attempts at surgical closure are associated with a high mortality rate and a low rate of successful fistula closure. Himal and associates reviewed the courses of 17 patients with small intestinal fistulas in whom surgical repair was attempted within 48 hours of diagnosis.[7] The fistulas recurred promptly in ten patients, eight of whom died, resulting in a mortality rate of 47 percent.

TABLE 10-1
Gastrointestinal Fistulas: Treatment, Closure Rate, and Mortality*

Investigator	Nutrition Protocol	Period of Study	Number of Fistulas In Series†
Edmunds et al[1]	NS§	1946–1959	157
Chapman et al[2]	I. NS (< 1600 kcal/day, usually < 1000)	1953–1963	38
	II. Enteral, (≥ 1600–2000 kcal/day, usually 3000)	1953–1963	18
	I and II	1953–1963	56
Sheldon et al[3]	TPN initially, then enteral	1964– ?	51
Rocchio et al[4]	Enteral (elemental) (glucose TPN initially in 26 patients)	1968–1972	37
Voitk et al[5]	Enteral (elemental)	—	36
MacFadyen et al[6]	TPN (glucose)	1970–1972	78
Himal et al[7]	I. NS	—	66
	II. TPN (glucose) in 22 patients; enteral in 3 patients	—	25
Dietel[8]	I. NS	1965–1969	32
	II. TPN (glucose or lipid) or enteral	1969–1975	100
Graham[9]	TPN (lipid)	—	39
Reber et al[10]	TPN (glucose) or enteral	1968–1977	186
Soeters et al[11]	I. NS	1960–1970	119
	II. NS	1970–1975	55
	III. TPN (glucose)¶	1970–1975	73
Silberman et al[12]	TPN (glucose or lipid)	1975–1978	35
Thomas[13]	I. NS	1968–1971	35
	II. TPN (glucose)	1975–1978	42

*The retrospective series analyzed here are not strictly comparable, since the fistulas in the various groups vary widely in etiology and anatomic distribution.
†Some patients had more than one fistula.

Spontaneous Closure Rate (%)	Days (Mean) of Nutritional Support Till Spontaneous Closure	Successful Operative Closure (%)	Overall Closure Rate (%)	Mortality (%)‡
24.8	—	29.3	54.1	43.3
—	—	—	37	58
—	—	—	89	16.7
32.1	—	21.4	53.5	45
29.4	—	52.9	82.4	12
64.8	—	16.2	81	16.2
75	—	0	75	28
70.5	34.9	21.8	92.3	6.5
27	—	32	59	33
56	—	36	92	8
34.4	—	25	59.4	40
81	39.1	8	89	9.3
89.7	31.0	2.6	92.3	7.7
32	—	45	77	22
10.1	—	68.1	78.2	15
5.5	—	60.0	65.5	16.3
23.2	—	45.2	68.4	24.7
51	31.2	14.3	65.3	29
—	—	—	31	60
—	20.0	—	71	26

‡Includes mortality from all causes temporally related to the presence of the fistula.
§NS=No special nutrition therapy offered.
¶TPN only offered to patients with major complications.

The salutary impact of nutritional support on the outcome of patients with gastrointestinal fistulas is not due exclusively to intravenous feedings. Prior to the advent of total parenteral nutrition, maintaining nutrition by intensive enteral feedings produced a favorable effect on mortality and a rate of spontaneous closure comparable to that subsequently observed in series of patients managed with TPN.[10] Nevertheless, parenteral nutrition simplifies management. For example, fistulous output is more effectively controlled with TPN than with enteral feedings.[10,14,15] In addition, proper placement of a nasal feeding tube distal to a small bowel fistula is difficult and surgical placement is undesirable. However, enteral feedings may be satisfactory in the management of very proximal or very distal fistulas, and even oral diets may be satisfactory in patients with low-output chronic fistulas. For the remaining lesions, parenteral nutrition is the preferred modality of nutritional support.[6,10,14]

Initial management is aimed at restoring hemodynamic stability and electrolyte balance with crystalloid infusions and blood transfusions, if necessary. Fistulous output is controlled by withholding all oral intake and by placing suction catheters within and about the fistulous tract to reduce the corrosive effect of the enteric contents on the surrounding tissues. Subsequently, a collection bag is fashioned with the assistance of an enterostomal therapist. Sepsis is managed with antibiotics and operative drainage of any purulent collections. At a later date, after the patient is stabilized, the anatomy of the fistulous tract is determined radiographically.

After fluid and electrolyte balance has been achieved, generally within 24 to 48 hours, TPN is begun using either the lipid or the glucose system.[12] Oral feedings are withheld, and TPN is continued for as long as 4 to 5 weeks or more to allow every opportunity for nutritional repletion, wound healing, and spontaneous closure of the fistula. Nutritional support is generally continued for 4 to 7 days following spontaneous closure of a fistula to prevent recurrence. Thereafter oral alimentation is begun gradually as parenteral nutrition is tapered.

Reber and associates found that 90 percent of fistulas destined to close spontaneously did so within 1 month after control of sepsis.[10] Various investigators have reported that the mean duration of nutritional support until spontaneous closure was 20, 31, 31.2, 34.9, and 39.1 days, respectively (Table 10-1).[6,8,9,12,13] Consequently, an operative approach to fistula closure is considered after 30 to 40 days of nutritional support following control of sepsis.

Certain circumstances mitigate against spontaneous closure. These include the presence of Crohn's disease, radiation enteritis, residual tumor, epithelialization of the fistulous tract, short fistulous tract (less than 2 cm between bowel and skin), discontinuity of the gastrointestinal tract (as in complete anastomotic disruption), and persistent distal intestinal obstruction. In these cases, an operative approach to the fistula may be considered as soon as fluid and electrolyte balance has been restored, sepsis has been controlled, nutrition has been repleted, and maximal resolution of the intra-abdominal inflammatory process has been achieved by conservative means.

In summary, intensive nutritional support has had a major impact on the prognosis of gastrointestinal fistulas and consequently should be an inherent part of primary therapy for these lesions.

SHORT BOWEL SYNDROME

The short bowel syndrome is a constellation of gastrointestinal symptoms and metabolic abnormalities due to the severely impaired or absent enteric digestive and transport functions associated with extensive disease or massive resection of the small intestine (Fig. 10-1).[16] The syndrome is seen when more than 70 to 75 percent of the small intestine has been removed. Such massive resections may be required in the treatment of small bowel infarction secondary to mesenteric arterial or venous occlusion or strangulated obstruction, Crohn's disease, radiation enteritis, neoplasm, or trauma.

Fluid and electrolyte disturbances, due to disabling diarrhea, and protein–calorie malnutrition are the major life-threatening consequences of this syndrome. Other manifestations may include megaloblastic anemia, osteomalacia, calcium oxalate renal calculi, cholelithiasis, and a variety of findings associated with the malabsorption of micronutrients. The occurrence and severity of the various clinical and laboratory manifestations are dependent upon the extent and site of resection; the presence of the ileocecal valve and colon; the functional condition of the remaining small bowel, colon, and other digestive organs; and the adaptive response of the residual enteric segment.[17]

Ileal resection is clinically and metabolically more significant than loss of jejunum. The transit time is slower in the ileum, and this segment has a significantly greater potential for adaption than the jejunum.[18] In addition, the ileum is the specialized site for absorption of vitamin B12 and conjugated bile salts. While the jejunum may partially compensate by increased diffusion of these substances across the mucosa, conjugated bile salts are actively transported only by the ileal mucosa.[17,18] Loss of this ileal function leads to a reduction in the enterohepatic circulation of bile salts and excess entry of bile salts into the large bowel. These events are associated with increasing diarrhea, steatorrhea, and malabsorption of fat-soluble vitamins.[17]

When the ileocecal valve is intact, shorter lengths of remaining small intestine are better tolerated with fewer symptoms and metabolic consequences. Resection of the ileocecal valve permits extensive colonization of the shortened small bowel by coliform organisms. The bacteria may deconjugate bile salts, alter fatty acids, and metabolize vitamin B12, thus aggravating diarrhea, steatorrhea, and B12 deficiency. In addition, experimental data indicate that an intact ileocecal valve prolongs the transit time of luminal contents within the small bowel. Extensive colon resection further seriously aggravates diarrhea and fluid and electrolyte disturbances.[17,19,20]

The adaptive response to enterectomy involves morphologic and functional changes. Compensatory growth principally involves villous enlargement due to epithelial hyperplasia. Increased villous height and crypt depth are accompanied by dilatation and lengthening of the intestinal remnant. The magnitude of this response is greater after proximal than after distal small bowel resection, and the intensity of epithelial hyperplasia is directly propor-

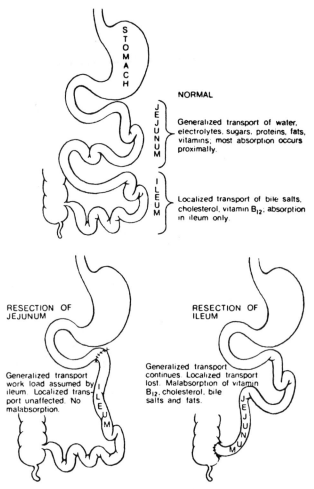

Figure 10-1. The normal transport functions of the jejunum and ileum. The consequences of resection are predictable in part from the loss of regionally localized transport processes. *(From Schrock TR: In Dunphy JE, Way LW (eds): Current Surgical Diagnosis and Treatment, ed. 5. Los Altos, CA, Lange Medical Publications, 1981. Reproduced with permission).*

tional to the length of intestine resected. Functional changes accompanying these adaptive increments in villous height include increased intestinal uptake of substances absorbed throughout the small bowel (water, electrolytes, mono- and disaccharides, calcium, and amino acids) as well as of those substances with localized transport mechanisms (bile acids and vitamin B12). Such functional adaption is the result of mucosal hyperplasia producing an increased number of epithelial cells, the individual absorptive capacity, of which however, is not increased. Villous hyperplasia and improving intestinal absorption generally continue for more than a year.[21] Ninety percent of ultimate villous height is reached in approximately 1 year.[18]

The stimuli to these adaptive responses are complex and incompletely understood. Food and the enteric secretions and hormones, regulated by the presence of food, play a dominant role. Consequently, luminal nutrition provided as oral or enteral feedings is required to achieve the maximal adaptive response. The latter cannot be achieved with total parenteral nutrition despite restoration and maintenance of normal nutritional status (see pp. 94–96, and 192).[17] Feldman and associates found no evidence of adaption in jejunectomized dogs fed exclusively by vein; in fact, a decrease in mean villous height was observed.[22] However, Levine and Deren found that the adaptive response was blunted in enterectomized rats receiving TPN, but it was not completely eliminated.[23]

The nutritional management of the short bowel syndrome includes an appropriate combination of intravenous and oral or enteral feedings. In the period immediately following massive small bowel resection, therapy is directed to controlling massive diarrhea, correcting fluid and electrolyte disturbances, and providing nutrition exclusively by vein. Often after 1 to 3 weeks massive diarrhea is controlled and fecal output is less than 2 liters/day. At this point parenteral nutrition is continued, but, in addition, a trial of enteral feedings is undertaken by providing a diluted formulation in small volumes infused continuously through a feeding tube. If tolerance is demonstrated, these feedings are continued, and subsequently, volume and concentration are gradually increased. Elemental diets are useful in initiating luminal feedings, since they are devoid of or low in long-chain triglycerides, they are predigested, and they are more easily absorbed. Elemental diets may be less effective, however, than other enteral preparations in stimulating compensatory hyperplasia.[18] The aim during this transitional stage of therapy is to make sure that nutritional requirements are met by providing nutrients intravenously and that the adaptive response is stimulated by introducing luminal nutrients. As adaption proceeds, oral nutrition, initially providing carbohydrates and protein, is substituted for tube feedings. Fat is limited to less than 30 gm/day, but medium-chain triglycerides may be added as a useful calorie source. Diet is slowly advanced, and by trial and error a suitable diet for the individual is determined.[16]

After about 6 months, complete dependence on oral intake may be anticipated in many patients and parenteral nutrition may be discontinued. Full adaption, however, may take as long as 2 years.[16]

After parenteral nutrition is discontinued, dietary supplements of calcium and fat-soluble vitamins are prescribed for life. In addition, patients with extensive ileal resection should receive a diet low in fat and oxalate. This regimen is required, since steatorrhea is associated with malabsorption of fat-soluble vitamins and the precipitation of calcium in insoluble soaps. When steatorrhea is further aggravated by ileal resection, the intraluminal concentration of calcium may be insufficient to bind oxalate, which is therefore absorbed in abnormal amounts. Unabsorbed fatty acids and bile acids also increase the permeability of the colon to oxalate.[16] Pancreatic enzyme supplements may be useful in reducing steatorrhea. Since ileal resection also results in vitamin B12 malabsorption, vitamin B12 must be given parenterally at regular intervals.

In some patients the extent of small bowel resection or insufficient compensatory hyperplasia precludes the resumption of adequate oral nutrition indefinitely or permanently. Such patients are therefore placed on permanent parenteral nutrition at home.

INFLAMMATORY BOWEL DISEASE

Use of parenteral or enteral nutrition in patients with Crohn's disease or ulcerative colitis may be indicated for the treatment of malnutrition and certain nonnutritional complications, such as enterocutaneous fistulas, short bowel syndrome, and early or partial small bowel obstruction. In addition, parenteral nutrition has been advocated as a form of primary therapy for patients with inflammatory bowel disease who have been unresponsive to conventional nonoperative therapeutic modalities.

Nutritional deficiencies are common in patients with inflammatory bowel disease (Table 10-2). Deficits arise from a variety of causes, including inadequate oral intake, an element of malabsorption, protein-losing enteropathy, and increased metabolic demands associated with an active inflammatory process.[24] Consequently, significant weight loss, anemia, vitamin and mineral deficiencies, and depressed levels of visceral protein are frequently observed. Protein–calorie malnutrition is present in approximately 50 percent of these patients requiring hospital admission.[24,25] When malnutrition is unresponsive to optimal dietary therapy, enteral or parenteral feedings are advisable. Several studies attest to the effectiveness of elemental diets in achieving nutritional repletion.[26–29] For example, Voitk and associates reported weight gain in each of 11 patients treated with an elemental diet, Flexical.[29] However, enteral feedings often aggravate symptoms, and florid gastrointestinal manifestations preclude a trial of an elemental diet. Consequently, parenteral nutrition is more frequently prescribed.

TABLE 10-2
Frequency of Nutritional Deficiencies Reported
in Inflammatory Bowel Disease

	Crohn's Disease (%)	Ulcerative Colitis (%)
Weight loss	65–75	18–62
Hypoalbuminemia	25–80	25–50
Intestinal protein loss	75	*
Negative nitrogen balance	69	*
Anemia	60–80	66
Iron deficiency	39	81
Vitamin B12 deficiency	48	5
Folic acid deficiency	54	36
Calcium deficiency	13	*
Magnesium deficiency	14–33	*
Potassium deficiency	6–20	*
Vitamin A deficiency	11	NR†
Vitamin C deficiency	*	NR
Vitamin D deficiency	75	*
Vitamin K deficiency	*	NR
Zinc deficiency	*	*
Copper deficiency	*	NR
Metabolic bone disease	*	*

*Reported but incidence not described.
†NR = Not reported.
From Driscoll RH Jr, and Rosenberg IH: Med Clin North Am 62:185-201, 1978.

Many series indicate that nutritional status is improved in the great majority of patients with inflammatory bowel disease receiving parenteral nutrition (Tables 10-3 and 10-4). It is generally believed that this improvement in nutrition contributes to a reduction in the risk of subsequently required operative procedures.[30,38,39] In a recent study, Rombeau and associates found that patients who had received preoperative TPN for at least five days had significantly fewer postoperative complications than those who did not.[39] A significant reduction in the incidence of sepsis was also observed. All patients with postoperative complications had severe preoperative deficiencies in serum albumin or serum transferrin levels.

Nutritional repletion has an additional advantage in children with Crohn's disease. These patients are subject to growth arrest and delayed onset of puberty. Layden and associates found that when the additional nutritional requirements imposed by the demands of growth were met with parenteral feedings, growth could be reestablished and sexual maturation stimulated in some of the affected children.[40] Similar results were reported by Strobel and associates.[41]

Enteric fistulas commonly develop in patients with Crohn's disease, and

TABLE 10-3
Total Parenteral Nutrition in Crohn's Disease*

Series	No. of Patients	Successful Nutritional Repletion	Clinical Remission in Hospital	Sustained Improvement (> 3 mos)
Anderson and Boyce[30]	4	4 (100%)	4 (100%)	1 (25%)
Cohen et al.[31]	3	3	2	2
Franklin and Grand[32]	2	2	1	—
Marshall[33]	2	2	2	2
Vogel et al.[34]	8	8 (100%)	8 (100%)	3 (37.5%)
Reilly et al.[35]	21	—	14 (67%)	—
Elson et al.[36]	16	16 (100%)	12 (75%)	7 (44%)
TOTALS	56	35/35 (100%)	43/56 (77%)	15/33 (45%)

*Table considers patients who have failed medical treatment but excludes those with fistulas.
Adapted from Driscoll RH Jr, and Rosenberg IH: Med Clin North Am 62:185–201, 1978.

although they may close spontaneously during treatment with parenteral nutrition, this favorable outcome apparently occurs less frequently than when the fistula arises from other causes. Reber and associates observed spontaneous closure in only 8 percent of fistulas (1 of 12) due to Crohn's disease.[10] However, Eisenberg et al.,[42] Mullen et al.,[38] and Dudrick et al.[43] reported long-term spontaneous closure rates of 20 percent (4 of 20), 27 percent (10 of 37), and 55 percent (17 of 31), respectively. Dudrick et al. observed spontaneous closure of 75 percent of small bowel fistulas (12 of 16) and only 33 percent of large bowel fistulas (5 of 15).[43]

The concept of total parenteral nutrition as a primary therapy for inflammatory bowel disease is based on the hypothesis that intravenous nutritional repletion and "bowel rest" will have a salutary effect on the course of

TABLE 10-4
Total Parenteral Nutrition in Ulcerative Colitis*

Series	No. of Patients	Successful Nutritional Repletion	Clinical Remission in Hospital	Sustained Improvement (> 3 mos)
Stanchev[37]	10	9 (90%)	4 (40%)	—
Franklin and Grand[32]	5	5 (100%)	2 (40%)	1 (20%)
Reilly et al.[35]	11	6 (55%)	1 (9%)	—
Mullen et al.[38]	24	20 (83%)	9 (38%)	—
Elson et al.[36]	10	9 (90%)	4 (40%)	3 (30%)
TOTALS	60	49/60 (82%)	20/60 (33%)	4/15 (27%)

*Table considers patients who have failed medical treatment.
Adapted and updated from Driscoll RH Jr, Rosenberg IH: Med Clin North Am 62:185–201, 1978.

inflammatory bowel disease. The bowel rest consequent to withholding all nutrients from the gastrointestinal tract is thought to have the following benefits: (1) elimination of mucosal trauma due to roughage and food particles, (2) reduction in the irritation of the inflamed enteric surface as a result of markedly diminished peristaltic activity, (3) marked diminution of the caustic effect of gastrointestinal secretions (hydrochloric acid, bile, pancreatic juice, and succus entericus) on the inflamed or denuded bowel because of decreased hormonal and autonomic stimuli to production and flow of these secretions, and (4) redirection of the primary function of the damaged mucosa toward healing processes rather than digestive or absorptive processes.[43]

The value of TPN and bowel rest as primary therapy in inflammatory bowel disease has not been thoroughly evaluated by long-term, controlled, prospective studies. However, various retrospective series have been reported (Tables 10-3 and 10-4). This form of treatment is deemed successful if a prolonged clinical remission (for more than 3 months) is induced or if clinical improvement is achieved which allows prolonged or indefinite postponement of surgical intervention.

Mullen and associates recently reported the course of 50 patients with Crohn's disease, including 20 with gastrointestinal fistulas, who were managed at the University of Pennsylvania with total parenteral nutrition.[38] Thirty-seven patients (74 percent) gained weight, and 19 patients (38 percent), all of whom had previously failed on a conventional medical regimen, had a clinical remission which allowed hospital discharge without operation.

When patients with Crohn's disease uncomplicated by fistulas are analyzed separately, clinical remission has been observed in 67 to 100 percent of patients. However, these remissions are often short-lived; sustained remission exceeding 3 months has been reported in 25 to 44 percent of patients (Table 10-3).

In one of the few available prospective studies, Dickinson and associates randomly assigned 36 patients with acute colitis, including 27 with ulcerative colitis and 9 with Crohn's disease, to receive either TPN and total bowel rest or a normal hospital diet.[44] In addition, patients in both groups received prednisone. No salutary effect on the colitis *per se* was observed. Thus there was no difference in outcome in the two patient groups with regard to the frequency of surgery or the time required to taper the prednisone dosage. In contrast, there was severe erosion of the body protein mass in the orally fed group, and this was prevented in patients treated with TPN. The findings in this study are consistent with those of others indicating that patients with ulcerative colitis are less likely to experience either transient or sustained clinical remission (Table 10-4). Thus Reilly and associates found that in patients with ulcerative colitis in whom conventional medical therapy failed to control the disease, it was usually not possible to avoid surgery by parenteral nutrition and bowel rest.[35]

In summary, available data based largely on retrospective analyses of heterogenous series of patients indicate that parenteral nutrition is a highly effective therapy for malnutrition occurring in patients with inflammatory bowel disease. Enteral feedings may also be effective. In addition, it appears that a sustained clinical remission can be induced with parenteral nutrition and bowel rest in about half of the patients with intractable Crohn's disease and in a smaller proportion of patients with ulcerative colitis.

Patients for whom parenteral nutrition is indicated generally receive this therapy for 4 to 5 weeks.[35,36,38] However, long-term, home parenteral nutrition may be advisable for some patients, including those with short bowel syndrome, jejunoilietis, or other conditions not amenable to surgical intervention.[41,45]

BURNS

Major thermal injury is characterized by a hypermetabolic response which is mediated primarily by an increased elaboration of catecholamines. Increased adrenergic activity results in a metabolic rate which increases in curvilinear fashion in proportion to the extent and severity of the burn until a plateau is reached corresponding to approximately twice the normal caloric expenditure

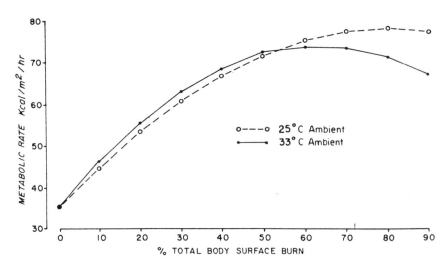

Figure 10-2. Metabolic rate is a curvilinear function of burn size, with ambient temperatures between 25°C and 33°C exerting no significant effect on metabolic rate in patients with burns of less than 40 to 50 percent of the total body surface. In patients with more extensive burns a consistent but modest decrease in metabolic rate was observed at 33°C, but metabolic rate remained significantly greater than "normal" even in those patients. *(From Pruitt BA Jr: In Ballinger WF, et al (eds): Manual of Surgical Nutrition. Philadelphia, WB Saunders, 1975)*

at about 50 percent total body surface area (BSA) burn (Fig. 10-2). This prodigious energy expenditure begins to taper as normal healing or grafting takes place but does not return to normal until the entire burn wound is covered with autogenous skin. Thus the metabolic rate varies with the amount of time postburn. Energy expenditure may be near normal during resuscitation, then rise and peak between the sixth and tenth postburn days and subsequently decrease in a curvilinear manner to return to predicted basal levels when satisfactory coverage of the burn wound is achieved.[47]

In the absence of aggressive nutritional support, this hypermetabolic state may be associated with a dramatic degree of tissue breakdown, loss of protoplasmic mass, and erosion of body reserves that will eventually lead to the morbid consequences associated with acute starvation.[46-50] Retrospective studies have shown that mean body weight may decrease 25 percent within 6 to 7 weeks in patients with burns exceeding 40 percent of total body surface. The acute loss of more than 10 percent of preburn weight is often associated with severe complications, including impaired wound healing and immunologic deficits. Death usually ensues when weight loss exceeds 30 percent of preinjured levels.[49]

Weight loss is not an obligatory component of the response to thermal injury but rather reflects the difference between energy requirements of the patient and the ability to meet these requirements from exogenous sources. Energy demands may be reduced by control of infection, pain, anxiety, and cold stress, but the cornerstone of metabolic support is intensive nutritional therapy until burn wound closure has been accomplished.[47,49]

Caloric requirements can be determined by indirect calorimetry, or they can be estimated by an upward adjustment of the basal metabolic rate for a normal person to account for the increase known to occur following burn injury. Various methods of estimating caloric requirement are listed in Table 10-5. Protein requirements are likewise substantially increased and are also directly related to the extent of the burn. Protein needs parallel the changes in oxygen consumption and energy utilization, and the requirements have usually been calculated as 2 to 4 times those of normal persons (Table 10-5).[46]

A program designed to meet these nutritional requirements should be initiated before the fourth postburn day. Oral diets may meet the needs of patients with limited injury, but patients with burns involving more than 30 percent of the total body surface are often unable to achieve the goals of nutritional support if voluntary ingestion of oral diets is the sole means of alimentation.[49] Since the alimentary tract generally functions normally in patients who have sustained extensive thermal injury, an enteral feeding program is usually prescribed. When tube feedings are contraindicated or unsuccessful in meeting the nutritional goals, parenteral nutrition is administered to supplement the enteral program or to provide all required nutrients. When parenteral nutrition is required, fat emulsions are well utilized and are of value in providing part of the caloric requirements.[53] Wilmore and associates studied 10 critically ill burn patients.[53] Six patients received a fat emulsion administered along with other parenteral nutrients to supplement enteral feedings, and the remaining 4 patients received a fat emulsion in combination with glucose and a protein hydrolysate to provide all required nutrients. The fat emulsion contributed 38 percent of the total caloric intake in this group of ten patients. The nitrogen and caloric support resulted in improved nitrogen economy in each of the patients.

Burn patients receiving parenteral nutrition through a subclavian catheter are at increased risk of catheter sepsis, and special precautions are required to minimize this danger. When obtaining vascular access, every effort should be made to avoid cannulating through burned tissue. Subclavian catheter care is provided either on a daily basis or more frequently, and some authors have recommended that the catheter itself be changed prophylactically every 72 hours in patients with extensive burns.[54,55]

Larkin and Moylan evaluated an oral feeding program in 15 patients who had burn wounds which ranged from 25 to 76 percent of BSA and averaged 43 percent.[56] After initial intravenous fluid resuscitation, these patients received a high-caloric, high-protein oral diet supplemented by Meritene or Vivonex-HN to provide a total of 46.0 kcal/kg/day and 1.6 gm protein/kg. One patient required supplemental tube feedings to achieve this nutrient intake. The maximal weight loss averaged only 2.1 percent of preburn weight and ranged from a loss of 7.2 percent to a gain of 4.6 percent. Moreover, no mortality or stress ulcers were observed.

TABLE 10-5
Nutritional Requirements of Burn Patients

Author	Patients	Caloric Requirement	Protein or Nitrogen Requirement
Curreri and Luterman[49,51]	Adults	25 kcal/kg + 40 kcal/%BSA*	Provide 1 gm of nitrogen for each 150 kcal required (calorie: nitrogen = 150:1)
	Child (< 8 yr)	60 kcal/kg + 35 kcal/%BSA	
Wilmore[47]	Adults with 30–60% BSA	2000–2200 kcal/m²	15 gm of nitrogen/m² (equivalent to approximately 2.3 gm protein/kg)
Alexander et al.[52]	Children	$(1 + \%BSA/100) \times$ 95th %ile RME†	Provide 25% of total calories as protein or amino acids (calorie‡: nitrogen = 100:1)

*BSA = Body surface area burned.
†RME = Resting metabolism expenditure.
‡Total calories.

Bartlett and associates studied 556 patients, 452 of whom had sustained burns involving 1 to 39 percent BSA, 38 of whom had sustained burns involving 40 to 59 percent BSA, and 20 of whom had burns involving 60 to 80 percent BSA.[48] These patients all received an oral or enteral diet which provided a caloric intake which matched predicted expenditure. If weight loss was recorded, caloric intake was adjusted to exceed actual expenditure, which was determined by indirect calorimetry. Continuous nasogastric tube feedings were required in most patients with burns involving more than 40 percent BSA. Patients with burns over more than 60 percent BSA were automatically started on a regimen of tube feeding. Parenteral nutrition was rarely employed. This feeding regimen achieved the goal of zero weight loss or actual weight gain in almost every patient except those requiring an amputation.

In addition to providing adequate nutrients, the continuous infusion of an elemental diet into the stomach appears to have a favorable effect on the incidence of gastrointestinal stress bleeding in burn patients. Choctaw and associates studied a group of 146 severely burned patients, 77 of whom received a balanced oral diet and 69 of whom received a continuous infusion of Vivonex-HN.[57] A significantly reduced incidence of all upper gastrointestinal bleeding, including major episodes requiring transfusion, was observed in the enterally fed group (see Fig. 4-1).

Hiebert and associates observed a definite association between nutritional status, diminished immune responses, and mortality in a series of 80 burn patients.[58] Results of sequential skin testing were correlated with nitrogen bal-

TABLE 10-6
Sequential Skin Testing in Burn Patients

Group	Skin Test Reactivity	N	Mortality (%)*	Nitrogen Balance Data
I	Initial and sustained reactivity	44	0	Mean daily nitrogen balance in group I patients ($+3.2$ gm) was significantly different ($P < 0.01$) than that in Group II patients (-3.8 gm)
II	Initial and sustained anergy	17	83	
III	Anergy → Reactivity	16	6	Sustained mean daily positive nitrogen balance (3–15 gm) observed for 6–14 days prior to conversion
IV	Reactivity → Anergy	3	100	Exaggerated mean daily negative nitrogen balance (-10 to -45 gm) observed for 5–9 days prior to conversion

*Mortality due to septic complications in 17 of 18 patients.
Based on data of Hiebert JM, et al: Surgery 86:242–247, 1979.

ance and mortality (Table 10-6). The data indicate that skin test reactivity was predictive of outcome. Furthermore, since nitrogen balance figures correlated with skin test results, this study suggests the potential value of aggressive nutritional therapy designed to promote anabolism and enhance immune responsiveness.

Alexander and associates evaluated the benefit of supplementing a diet adequate in energy with additional protein containing a high proportion of essential amino acids.[52] In a study designed to test the hypothesis that protein malnutrition can persist in severely burned patients despite consumption of a balanced diet meeting energy requirements, these investigators evaluated 18 children with burns involving 41 to 64 percent BSA for at least 6 weeks. The patients were randomized into 2 groups. The control group received a diet providing 16.5 percent of calories in the form of protein or amino acids, a normal distribution for the average American diet. The high-protein, experimental group received a similar diet which was, however, supplemented with ultrafiltered whey protein (Pro-Mix) to the extent that 23 percent of the caloric intake was from protein. The total calorie:nitrogen ratio of the control diet was 151:1, and the ratio for the high protein diet was 110:1. In both groups, caloric requirements were met orally, if possible, but tube feedings or parenteral nutrition were prescribed, if necessary.

The data, presented in Table 10-7, provide strong evidence that dietary supplementation with larger amounts of a high-quality protein is of benefit to seriously burned children.

TABLE 10-7
Comparison of Regular and Protein-Supplemented Isocaloric Diets in Seriously Burned Children

	Control (N-9)	High Protein (N-9)	P
Survival*	5/9 (56%)	9/9 (100%)	<0.03
Bacteremic days/total days at risk	27/254 (11%)	23/281 (8%)	<0.005
Percent weight change from preburn (average)	− 2.24 ± 1.70	4.01 ± 1.64	<0.009
Total serum protein (gm/dl)	5.5 ± 0.1	6.3 ± 0.2	<0.0002
Albumin (gm/dl)	2.93 ± 0.08	2.95 ± 0.08	NS†
Transferrin (mg/dl)	200 ± 10	283 ± 18	<0.0001
C3 (μg/ml)	1371 ± 55	1585 ± 64	<0.01
IgG (mg/dl)	805 ± 52	975 ± 56	<0.03
Factor B (μg/ml)	480 ± 38	559 ± 33	NS†
Opsonic index	0.42 ± 0.04	0.62 ± 0.05	<0.0007
Neutrophil bactericidal index	4.0 ± 0.6	3.6 ± 0.4	NS†

*All deaths were caused by septicemia or burn wound sepsis.
†Not significant.
Data from Alexander JW, et al: Ann Surg 192:505–517, 1980.

In summary, aggressive nutritional support of hypermetabolic burn patients is of value in maintaining body weight, enhancing immune functions, reducing septic complications, and improving survival.

RENAL FAILURE

Acute renal failure frequently develops against a background of severe illness or injury giving rise to a hypercatabolic state and a combination of abnormalities which, on the one hand, increase the nutrient requirements for homeostasis and, on the other, produce a state of protein and fluid intolerance. Oral feedings are frequently precluded in these patients because of anorexia, lethargy, or postoperative ileus. Patients with chronic renal failure may also be unable to meet nutritional requirements orally when serious intercurrent illness develops.

When such patients with acute or chronic renal failure require special nutritional support with enteral or parenteral feedings, the dosage and composition of the formulation provided must be modified to take into account the metabolic derangements associated with impaired or absent renal function and the nutritional demands imposed by renal failure, peritoneal dialysis or hemodialysis, and concurrent injury or illness.

Current concepts of enteral and parenteral nutrition for renal failure patients are based in part on the independent observations of Giordano[59] and Giovannetti and Maggiore.[60] These investigators treated uremic patients with low-protein diets containing a high percentage of essential amino acids together with adequate calories. There was clinical improvement of uremic symptoms, stabilization or a decrease in blood urea concentration, an increase in lean body mass, and a decrease in total body urea production. Two mechanisms have been advanced to explain the beneficial effects observed. First, urea recycling may occur, resulting in the synthesis of nonessential amino acids from nitrogen released by bacterial hydrolysis of urea in the gut.[59] This mechanism has been substantiated,[61,62] but the quantitative contribution of the urea-derived nitrogen may be of minor nutritional significance.[63-66] Alternatively, the diet recommended may decrease the rate of urea production as a result of decreased breakdown of lean body mass.[67]

Acute Renal Failure

Wilmore and Dudrick were the first to apply the concepts of Giordano and Giovannetti and Maggiore to intravenous feedings.[68] A solution containing pure crystalline essential L-amino acids in amounts designed to meet or exceed the minimum daily requirement was administered together with hypertonic glucose and vitamins to a patient with acute renal failure and severe abdominal injuries. Weight gain, wound healing, and positive nitrogen bal-

TABLE 10-8
Experience with Total Parenteral Nutrition in Acute Renal Failure

Investigators	Infusate	Number of Patients	Nitrogen Balance	Rate of Rise of BUN
Dudrick et al.[69]	EAA + G§	10¶	Positive	Stabilized or decreased
Abel et al.[70–74]	EAA + G	52	—	Stabilized or
	EAA + G as compared to G	53	—	decreased
Leonard et al.[75]	EAA + G as compared to G	20	Negative both groups	Stabilized or decreased
Baek et al.[76]	Fibrin-hydroly-sate + G as compared to G	129	—	No difference
Sofio and Nicora[77]	EAA + G	192	—	Decreased
Feinstein et al.[78]	EAA + G compared to EAA + NEAA + G compared to G alone	30	Negative	Lower in EAA + G than in EAA + NEAA + G

*Refers to duration of the time that patient had acute renal failure.
†Indicates patients who survived at least until they recovered from renal failure.
‡Indicates the percentage of patients who did not survive beyond the period of their hospitalization.

ance occurred, while the blood urea nitrogen level remained stable and other symptoms of uremia resolved.

The following year, Dudrick and associates reported their results using this renal failure formulation in 10 patients with acute or chronic renal failure (Table 10-8).[69] A greater than 50 percent reduction of blood urea nitrogen (BUN) was observed in all 10 patients, eliminating or decreasing significantly the need for dialysis. In addition, hyperphosphatemia, hypocalcemia, and acidosis were reversed spontaneously and positive potassium and nitrogen balance was achieved in 8 of the 10 patients.

In a similar uncontrolled study, Abel and associates also observed positive nutritional effects, including weight gain, improved wound healing, and stabilization of the BUN.[71] Additional favorable effects included lower serum concentrations of magnesium, phosphate, and potassium. Subsequently, these investigators subjected the value of intravenous essential amino acids for pa-

Serum Potassium	Serum Phosphate	Duration of Renal Failure*	Survival from Acute Renal Failure†	Overall Mortality‡
Decreased	Decreased	—	—	—
Stabilized or decreased	Stabilized or decreased	—	—	—
		Decreased	Improved	57
Stabilized or decreased	Stabilized	No difference	No difference	60
Stabilized or decreased	—	—	Improved	58
Decreased	Decreased	—	—	60
Decreased	Decreased	No difference	No difference	63

§EAA, essential amino acids; NEAA, nonessential amino acids; G, glucose.
¶Some patients had chronic renal failure.
Adapted and updated from Kopple JD, Blumenkrantz MJ: In Maxwell MH, Kleeman CR (eds): Clinical Disorders of Fluid and Electrolyte Metabolism, ed 3. New York, McGraw–Hill Book Co, 1980, pp 413–498.

tients with acute renal failure to a prospective, double-blind appraisal.[72] Twenty-eight patients randomized to the treatment group received a solution containing hypertonic glucose and eight essential amino acids in amounts providing at least twice the daily minimum requirement. The 25 patients in the control group received an isocaloric solution of glucose. The patients receiving both amino acids and glucose had increased survival from the episode of renal failure but overall hospital mortality including that from nonrenal causes was only slightly and not significantly improved in the treatment group (Fig. 10-3). However, in the patients with more severe renal failure, as indicated by the need for dialysis, and in those with serious complications, such as pneumonia, generalized sepsis, or gastrointestinal hemorrhage, survival was significantly greater in those receiving amino acids and glucose (Fig. 10-4). In addition, the data from this study suggest that the duration of renal failure was decreased in the patients in the treatment group. This finding is consistent with the experimental work of Toback, who found enhanced regeneration of renal cortical cells and lower maximum serum creatinine levels in rats with acute tubular necrosis that had received a mixture of essential and nonessential amino acids and glucose, as compared to those who had received isocaloric amounts of glucose alone.[79]

Available data do not permit firm conclusions concerning the optimal parenteral feeding regimen for patients with acute renal failure. The impressive results of Dudrick et al. and Abel et al. have not been consistently confirmed (Table 10-8). Uremic symptoms have often been stabilized or improved, but nutritional repletion has not been regularly observed with available regimens, and mortality rates remain high. In many studies, histidine, now known to be an essential amino acid,[80] was not provided.

In view of recent data suggesting that the capacity to reutilize urea to synthesize nonessential amino acids is limited even in azotemic man,[65,81] the quantity of amino acids necessary to promote nitrogen equilibrium or positive nitrogen balance in uremic patients may be greater than previously thought. Moreover, it is unclear whether there is any overall advantage to providing the infused nitrogen exclusively as essential amino acids.[81] While the infusions of small amounts of essential amino acids with glucose may produce less nitrogen waste and may be indicated for patients in whom dialysis is a particu-

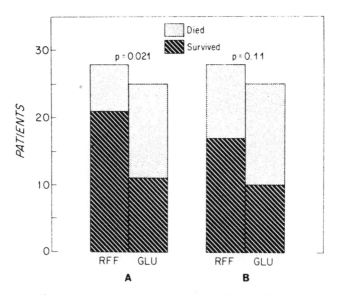

Figure 10-3 A: Survival rates from acute renal failure in 53 patients treated with either renal failure fluid (RFF) consisting of essential L-amino acids and hypertonic glucose or hypertonic glucose alone (GLU). **B:** Overall hospital mortality rates. (Analyses by Fisher Exact Test—One-tailed). *(From Abel RM, et al: N Engl J Med 288:695–699, 1973. Reprinted with permission of the New England Journal of Medicine).*

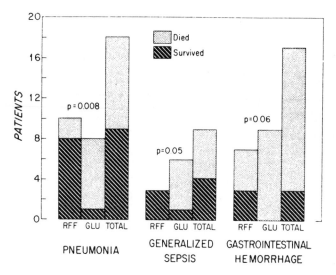

Figure 10-4. Effect of complications of acute renal failure on survival in patients treated with either essential L-amino acids and hypertonic glucose (RFF) or hypertonic glucose alone (GLU). *(From Abel RM. et al: N Engl J Med 288:695–699, 1973. Reprinted with permission of the New England Journal of Medicine).*

lar hazard, Kopple and Blumenkrantz prefer to use more nourishing solutions providing about 40 to 42.5 gm/day of approximately equal quantities of essential and nonessential amino acids and to control uremic symptoms and fluid imbalance with dialysis as frequently as necessary.[82] Recommended daily allowances for protein (or amino acids) are outlined in Table 10-9). These recommendations take into account the protein losses associated with dialysis.

The caloric requirements of patients with renal failure are similar to those of patients without renal failure and are dependent upon the associated nonrenal disease. Concentrated glucose solutions (50 to 70 percent), administered through a central line, are generally recommended in order to meet nonprotein caloric requirements within the fluid limitations imposed by the renal disease. A peripherally administered, lipid-based system may be useful in nonoliguric patients or in those with substantial gastrointestinal or other fluid losses. Lipid emulsions have been used safely in these patients,[83] but serum triglycerides and cholesterol should be monitored carefully, since uremic patients often have hypertriglyceridemia.[82]

Electrolytes are prescribed in accordance with the patient's clinical condition, including cardiovascular status, fluid balance, and serum electrolyte levels. Potassium, phosphate, and magnesium often must be withheld initially. However, when the anabolic state is achieved in response to nutritional support supplements are required; otherwise the serum levels of these major intracellular ions may fall precipitously. Vitamins are provided in accordance with the recommendations for intravenous administration for normal persons (see Table 3-8). However, supplements of folate (1 mg/day) and pyridoxine (5 mg/day) are recommended.[82] Trace element requirements are unestablished, but zinc and chromium should be withheld or the dosage should be reduced, since these elements are excreted in the urine (see p. 72).

Based on current information, the standard glucose system can be modified to provide formulations designed to meet the needs of patients with renal failure. Solutions used at the University of Southern California are outlined in Tables 10-10 and 10-11. These solutions can be further tailored as necessary to meet the specific caloric, protein, and fluid requirements of a given patient. For example, the concentration of the glucose solution employed may be reduced from 70 to 50 percent, or a 10 percent amino acid solution can be substituted for the 8.5 percent solution used in the formulation described in Table 10-11.

Two enteral feeding products, Amin-Aid and Travasorb Renal, have been formulated specifically for patients with renal failure (see Table 4-3). Favorable results using Amin-Aid, each liter of which provides 2000 kcal and 19 gm of essential amino acids, have been reported by Meng.[86]

Liquid feeding products with a high caloric density and containing addi-

TABLE 10-9
Guidelines for Protein Administration in Acute and Chronic Renal Failure

Daily Allowances for Patients Not Regularly Dialyzed

1. GFR* > 25 ml/min	No protein restriction
2. Dialysis undesirable or contraindicated	12–20 gm EAA†
3. Dialysis not contraindicated	40–42 gm (0.55–0.60 gm/kg)‡
4. Supplement per each hemodialysis	40–42 gm‡
5. Supplement for each day of peritoneal dialysis	40–42 gm‡

Daily Allowances for Patients Regularly Dialyzed

1. Hemodialysis	1.0–1.2 gm/kg‡
2. Peritoneal dialysis	1.2–1.5 gm/kg‡

*GFR = glomerular filtration rate
†EAA = essential amino acids
‡At least 50% of allowance supplied as EAA
Based on data from Kopple and Blumenkrantz,[82] Harvey et al,[84] and Kopple.[85]

TABLE 10-10
Modified Glucose System for Renal Failure Patients
for Whom Dialysis is Undesirable or Contraindicated*

Preparation of 750 ml Unit†	
70% Glucose	500 ml
5.4% Essential amino acids‡	250 ml

Nutrients Provided Per Unit	
Non-protein calories	1190 kcal
Caloric density	1.6 kcal/ml
Glucose	350 gm
Nitrogen	1.6 gm
Essential Amino Acids	14 gm
Percent EAA§	100%

*Volume of solution prescribed depends on calorie and protein requirements and fluid status.
†Additives including vitamins and electrolytes discussed in text. Requirements for trace elements undetermined (see pp 70–72).
‡As Nephramine, includes histidine; similar solution available as Aminosyn-RF.
§EAA = essential amino acids.

TABLE 10-11
Modified Glucose System for Renal Failure Patients Receiving Dialysis or
for Whom Dialysis is not Contraindicated*

Preparation of 750 ml Unit†	
70% Glucose	500 ml
8.5% Amino Acids	250 ml

Nutrients Provided Per Unit	
Non-Protein calories	1190 kcal
Caloric density	1.6 kcal/ml
Glucose	350 gm
Nitrogen‡	3.25 gm
Total Amino Acids‡	22.8 gm
Essential Amino Acids§	12.6 gm
Non-essential Amino Acids	10.2 gm
Percent EAA§	55.3%

*Volume prescribed depends on calorie and protein requirements and fluid status.
†Additives including vitamins and electrolytes discussed in text.
 Requirements for trace elements undetermined (see pp 70–72).
‡Based on use of FreAmine III.
§Includes histidine as an essential amino acid (EAA).

tional protein, such as Isocal HCN and Magnacal, may be of value for those patients undergoing dialysis or for whom dialysis is not contraindicated. However, these products contain potassium and other electrolytes which may limit or preclude their use in some patients (see Table 4-2).

Chronic Renal Failure

Patients with chronic renal failure who develop an intercurrent disease which precludes adequate oral intake may be managed with the same enteral and parenteral feeding formulations used in patients with acute renal failure. Protein restriction is usually unnecessary when the glomerular filtration rate (GFR) exceeds 25 ml/min. Patients with chronic uremia with glomerular filtration rates between 4 and 10 ml/min may not require dialysis; protein intake for such persons should be about 40 gm/day. Patients on dialysis require additional protein to account for losses associated with this therapy. Protein-restricted patients should receive at least 50 percent of their protein intake as essential amino acids (Table 10-9).

Recent clinical investigations have suggested that α-keto-analogues of the essential amino acids may be effective as dietary supplements in chronic renal failure. The rationale for their use is that these compounds reduce urea production by diverting the nitrogen of urea precursors toward protein synthesis.[87] Favorable results have been reported, including improved nitrogen balance.[87-91] However, these substances are not yet commercially available, and their utility in clinical practice remains to be confirmed.

In summary, patients with acute or chronic renal failure with concomitant conditions requiring enteral or parenteral nutrition may benefit from nutrient formulations providing a high proportion of essential amino acids, reduced total protein content, and adequate nonprotein calories. The aim of such therapy is to maintain or improve nutritional status without aggravating and perhaps favorably affecting the course of renal failure and its metabolic abnormalities. The salutary effects may include stabilizing or reducing the levels of blood urea nitrogen, potassium, phosphorous, and magnesium and enhancing recovery from acute renal failure. These aims have been met in some series of patients but not in others. The inconsistent findings may reflect the heterogenous concurrent conditions present in the various series.

CANCER

Malnutrition is a frequent accompaniment of malignant disease, and when it occurs, prognosis is adversely affected.[92,93] (Table 10-12). Many factors contribute to a deteriorating nutritional state, including the very antitumor thera-

TABLE 10-12
Effect of Weight Loss on Survival

Tumor Type	Median Survival (Weeks)		
	NO WEIGHT LOSS	WEIGHT LOSS*	P-VALUE†
Favorable non-Hodgkin's lymphoma	‡	138	<0.01
Breast	70	45	<0.01
Acute nonlymphocytic leukemia	8	4	NS§
Sarcoma	46	25	<0.01
Unfavorable non-Hodgkin's lymphoma	107	55	<0.01
Colon	43	21	<0.01
Prostate	46	24	<0.05
Lung, small cell	34	27	<0.05
Lung, nonsmall cell	20	14	<0.01
Pancreas	14	12	NS
Nonmeasurable gastric	41	27	<0.05
Measurable gastric	18	16	NS

*All categories of weight loss (0–5 percent, 5–10 percent, and 10 percent) have been combined.
†The P-values refer to a test of the hypothesis that the entire survival curves are identical, not merely a test of the medians. However, in all disease sites under study, the median is a representative indicator of the survival distribution, and consequently its use as a summary statistic is acceptable.
‡Only 20 of 199 patients had died at the time of this report, so median survival could not be estimated. However, the observed rate of failure predicted that the survival would be significantly longer than for the group with weight loss.
§NS = Not significant.
From DeWys WD, et al: Am J Med 69:491–497, 1980.

py necessary to control the underlying malignancy.[92,94,95] Factors which may contribute to malnutrition in patients with cancer include:

1. Mechanical impairment of nutrient ingestion (e.g., oral tumors).
2. Aversion to food.
3. Taste abnormalities.
4. Altered visceral sensing (e.g., early satiety).
5. Metabolic and hormonal abnormalities (e.g., lactic acidemia, insulin resistance).
6. Surgical procedures.
7. Chemotherapy.
8. Radiation therapy.
9. Nutritional demands of the tumor.
10. (?) Enteropathy of malignancy.[96]

Thus many cancer patients fall victim to a vicious circle in which progressive malnutrition with its attendant complications is associated with an advancing malignant disease, the therapy for which may further contribute to the deteriorating nutritional status. This common sequence of events gives rise to the hypothesis that intensive nutritional support should favorably affect the clinical course of patients with cancer who are malnourished or in whom nutritional deficits are anticipated. Studies designed to test this hypothesis have produced many data bearing on the clinical and metabolic effects of enteral and parenteral nutrition in patients with cancer.

Perioperative Parenteral Nutrition
Significantly malnourished patients undergoing elective surgical operations experience an increased incidence of postoperative morbidity and mortality[97,98] which, according to Mullen and associates, can be significantly reduced by a week or more of preoperative parenteral nutrition.[98] It is assumed that the same benefit would be observed in malnourished cancer patients with localized tumors amenable to surgical intervention, but specific data are limited and often conflicting. Holter and Fischer were unable to demonstrate any benefit from 72 hours of preoperative TPN.[97] In a randomized study of patients with cancer of the esophagus or stomach, Heatley and associates found that a reduction in the incidence of postoperative wound infection was the only significant benefit associated with 7 to 10 days of preoperative TPN. However, malnutrition was not a criterion for entrance into the study.[99]

Thompson and associates conducted a prospective randomized appraisal of perioperative parenteral nutrition in a small series of patients with tumors of the gastrointestinal tract.[100] Twelve patients who had lost 10 lb or more received TPN for a mean of 18 days, including at least 5 days preoperatively and 8 days postoperatively. Results observed in the treatment group were compared to those seen in a similar group of 9 patients who did not receive TPN and to a control group of 20 untreated patients who had lost less than 10 lb. Patients receiving TPN were significantly better able to maintain body weight than patients in the other two groups, but the rate of major postoperative complications and mortality was not altered by nutritional support. However, a 10 lb weight loss was apparently a poor index of nutritional status in this study. Thus both the TPN treated and untreated patients who had lost ten or more pounds had nearly normal serum albumin levels (3.5 mg/dl and 3.4 mg/dl, respectively), and skin test reactivity was similar among all patients, including those in the control group.

More recently, Muller and associates reported the results of a randomized trial designed to examine the influence of ten days of preoperative TPN on the postoperative complication rate in patients with carcinoma of the esophagus, stomach, colon, rectum, or pancreas.[101] The 59 control patients were offered a regular 2400 kcal hospital diet; the treatment group received a TPN solution providing 37 kcal/kg/day. About 40 percent of the patients in each group had a normal nutritional status when entered into the study. A significant reduction in the rate of postoperative mortality and major complications (defined as intraabdominal abscess, peritonitis, anastomotic leakage, and ileus) was observed in the TPN group. The investigators attributed these clinical results to the improvement in humoral and cellular immunocompetence and protein status that was observed in the TPN group and to the deterioration in these factors that occurred during the preoperative period in the control group.

Nutritional Status During Chemotherapy and Radiotherapy

Improved nutritional status and weight gain can be achieved in many patients with cancer, even those with advanced disease.[102–104] For example, Copeland and associates assessed the value of total parenteral nutrition used as an adjunct to chemotherapy in 58 nutritionally depleted patients.[103] Each patient had lost over 10 percent of ideal or usual body weight and had a serum albumin level below 3.0 gm/dl. TPN was usually begun 3 to 10 days before starting chemotherapy and was continued for about 5 days after completion of therapy; the 58 patients received TPN for an average of 25.9 days. Fifty-two patients gained an average of 6.8 lb, whereas 6 patients lost an average of 7 lb. These investigators concluded that parenteral nutrition enabled them to administer chemotherapeutic agents to a group of patients who would otherwise have been denied adequate antitumor therapy because of fear of complications from malnutrition and inanition.

Rickard and associates studied the effectiveness of nutritional support in a series of 28 children with Stage III and IV solid tumors or second relapse leukemia or lymphoma during intensive multimodal anticancer therapy.[104] All patients received cycles of cytotoxic drugs, causing nausea and vomiting; 20 patients also received radiation therapy, and 15 underwent surgery. Twenty-one patients were normally nourished at the onset of therapy and received a carefully supervised program of oral nutrition. Sixteen of these 21 patients had a dramatic weight loss, averaging 16 percent of prediagnosis weight, and caloric intake was only 48 percent of recommended daily allowances. Eighteen patients, 7 of whom were initially depleted and 11 of whom had failed the oral nutrition program, received TPN for an average of 24 days; caloric intake in this group averaged 90 percent of recommended daily allowances. These investigators found that short periods of TPN for 9 to 14 days did not satisfactorily replete weight or restore serum albumin levels; however, transferrin levels were increased significantly and there was a subjective improvement in the general well-being of the patients. In contrast, TPN administered over a longer interval (approximately 28 days,) supported weight gain and was associated with increased serum albumin and transferrin to normal concentrations and reversal of anergy in 7 of 11 patients retested.

In a randomized prospective trial of TPN in patients with Stage III metastic testicular cancer, Samuels and associates found that patients receiving TPN during chemotherapy with vincristine and bleomycin, with or without added cisplatin, experienced significantly less weight loss than the control patients, who received a regular hospital diet and supplemental glucose and saline infusions during the same chemotherapy program.[105] However, the administration of TPN was not associated with an improved complete tumor response rate, and an increased number of life-threatening infections were observed in the TPN-treated group. On the other hand, these investigators found that aggressive effective chemotherapy was made possible by the addition of TPN to the management of several of the control patients who had had a substantial weight loss after initial chemotherapy. Based on these data, the authors concluded that the administration of TPN to patients with testicular cancer receiving vincristine, bleomycin, and cisplatin should be restricted to those who present with significant weight loss or to those who fail to regain lost weight during rest periods between courses of chemotherapy.

Malnutrition occurring in patients undergoing radiation therapy may be a result of the underlying malignant disease but also may be associated with or aggravated by the treatment *per se.* Thus radiation therapy may be associated with loss of taste, anorexia, and dysphagia or nausea, vomiting, and diarrhea secondary to radiation enteritis.[106] Such patients may obtain marked relief of symptoms when they receive nutrients intravenously and refrain from oral intake. Copeland and associates studied 39 malnourished patients who received TPN as an adjunct to radiation therapy to the gastrointestinal tract.[107,108] The average weight gain during TPN was 7.8 lb. Responding patients gained significantly more weight (13.0 lb) than did those patients who did not respond to radiation therapy (4.9 lb). In addition, Copeland et al. suggested that when nutritional depletion is so severe as to contraindicate radiation therapy, pretreatment TPN may improve the patient's condition so that safe therapy is possible.[108] Parenteral feedings may also be of value in patients undergoing preoperative radiation therapy to reverse wasting, achieve positive nitrogen balance, and make the patient as ready as possible for operation.[109]

Toxicity of chemotherapy and nutritional factors. There is considerable interest in delineating the relationship between nutritional status and the toxicity of chemotherapeutic drugs. Moertel was unable to demonstrate any relationship between pretreatment nutritional status and the incidence of gastrointestinal or hematopoietic toxicity among patients receiving 5-fluorouracil either alone or in combination with a nitrosourea preparation.[110] However, assessing the issue from a different point of view, Steiger and associates demonstrated in rats that the anorexia and negative nitrogen balance produced by 5-fluorouracil was obviated by total parenteral nutrition and that positive nitrogen balance could be achieved.[111] Souchon and associates found that the mean survival of rats receiving 15 mg/kg/day of 5-fluorouracil was doubled when total parenteral nutrition and bowel rest were instituted.[112] Moreover, the villous necrosis seen with this drug was eliminated. A similar protective effect on the intestinal mucosa was observed in rats when nutrition was provided as an elemental diet.[113,114]

Souchon and associates reported the results of a pilot study showing that patients receiving total parenteral nutrition tolerated a total dose of 7 gm of 5-fluorouracil and gained weight, as compared to orally fed patients who tolerated a dose of only 3.75 gm and lost weight.[112] These authors concluded that bowel rest and total parenteral nutrition appear to increase tolerance to 5-fluorouracil.

Dudrick observed that in cyclic multidrug therapy, therapeutic courses could be scheduled closer together because of the reduced weight loss and more rapid recovery from gastrointestinal toxicity when total parenteral nutrition was given.[115] However, he also noted that total parenteral nutrition did not alter the hematopoietic toxicity.

Issell and associates were the first to suggest that nutritional support may protect patients from the myelosuppressive toxicity of chemotherapy.[116] These investigators conducted a prospective randomized trial comparing the addition of total parenteral nutrition to *Corynebacterium parvum*, isophosphamide, and adriamycin (CIA) chemoimmunotherapy in 26 patients with extensive squamous cell carcinoma of the lung. The 13 patients randomized to receive CIA plus TPN received the latter for 10 days prior to the first course of CIA, and TPN was continued up to the start of the second course of therapy for a total of 31 days. The major dose-limiting toxic effect of CIA was leukopenia. Less myelosuppression was observed in the patients receiving TPN. The difference between the two groups in the lowest recorded leukocyte and neutrophil counts was statistically significant. Other significant effects observed in the TPN group as compared to the non-TPN group included decreased nausea and vomiting with chemotherapy and increased body weight and arm circumference.

The mechanism by which nutrition therapy produces any observed protective effect during chemotherapy is uncertain. Nutrition therapy may prevent the complications of malnutrition which are aggravated by chemotherapy, or it may have a specific, perhaps nonnutritional benefit—for example, permitting "bowel rest" during chemotherapy. In addition, any protective effect is undoubtedly related to the chemotherapeutic agents under consideration. Copeland and Dudrick found that gastrointestinal symptoms secondary to administration of 5-fluorouracil were reduced, but that the severe stomatitis and gastroenteritis associated with vinblastine and bleomycin therapy were unaffected by total parenteral nutrition.[107]

Efficacy of chemotherapy and nutritional factors.   Many data suggest that malnutrition limits the response to chemotherapy. It logically follows but remains to be proven that nutritional repletion will enhance the effectiveness of antitumor therapy.

In an analysis of patients with advanced carcinoma of the colon and rectum or stomach treated with a combination of 5-fluorouracil and a nitrosourea preparation, Moertel found a striking and statistically significant relationship between nutritional status and therapeutic results.[110] Those patients with pretreatment nutritional symptoms, such as anorexia, nausea, and vomiting, or those with a pretreatment weight 10 percent or more below ideal weight had response rates which were essentially one-half of those recorded for patients in better nutritional condition.

In a study evaluating the prognostic effect of weight loss prior to chemotherapy in cancer patients, the Eastern Cooperative Oncology Group reported an association between pretreatment weight loss and a lower frequency of tumor regression after chemotherapy in patients with breast cancer, acute leukemia, colon cancer, and non-small cell lung cancer.[93] However, only in breast cancer did this difference reach statistical significance.

In a retrospective review, Lanzotti and associates found that among patients having non-oat cell bronchogenic carcinoma with more than 6.5 percent body weight loss, only those receiving total parenteral nutrition responded to cyclic bleomycin, cyclophosphamide, vincristine, methotrexate, and 5-fluorouracil.[117] A clinical response was observed in 5 of the 10 patients receiving TPN, but there were no responders to chemotherapy among the 12 patients not receiving TPN.

Issell and associates also reviewed patients with non-oat cell lung cancer and found that such patients treated with CIA chemoimmunotherapy had a significantly poorer response and survival when they had experienced a pretherapy weight loss exceeding 6 percent.[118] In a subsequent prospective study by Issell et al., patients who were randomized to receive TPN in addition to CIA therapy experienced less toxicity (*supra vide*), but no difference in therapeutic response was found.[116] The interpretation of the latter observation is confounded, since over one-third (9 of 26) of the patients included in the study group had a pretherapy weight loss of less than 6 percent. This group is a subset of patients in whom an enhanced response to nutrition therapy may not be anticipated.

Samuels and associates in their study of advanced testicular cancer treated with chemotherapy (*supra vide*) were unable to demonstrate an improved rate of complete tumor response in TPN-treated patients.[105] It should be noted, however, that only 23 percent of the randomized patients had significant weight loss, defined as a loss exceeding 6 percent of usual body weight, and only two patients were severely malnourished, with weight losses exceeding 12 percent. Both of the latter two patients were assigned to the TPN group.

Popp and associates conducted a prospective trial of TPN in patients with advanced diffuse lymphoma who were treated with multidrug cyclic chemotherapy.[119] No survival benefit was associated with TPN administration. Again malnutrition was not a criterion for entrance into the study. Thus 70 percent of the TPN-treated patients and only 52 percent of the control patients were considered malnourished, which was defined as a weight loss exceeding 6 percent of pre-illness weight or a serum albumin concentration of less than 3.6 gm/dl. However, when the small subsets of malnourished patients in the TPN and control groups were analyzed separately, again no survival benefit was observed. It is possible that the definition of malnutrition was insufficiently stringent to identify the malnourished patients who would benefit from malnutritional repletion.

Thus, in each of the prospective studies conducted by Issell et al,[116] Samuels et al[105] and Popp et al[109] well-nourished patients were included in the randomization thereby potentially obscuring any benefit that might accrue to severely malnourished patients.

Nutrition and Immunocompetence

The relationship between immunologic reactivity, cancer, and nutrition is an area of current investigation. It is known that individuals who are immunologically depressed develop neoplasms with greater frequency than normal persons, and loss of immunocompetence after the development of malignant disease has an adverse effect on prognosis.[92,120,121] Patients with protein–calorie malnutrition exhibit impaired immunologic reactivity involving both the T- and B-cell systems; such impairment may be reversed following nutritional repletion.[122,123] The foregoing observations give rise to the hypothesis that the immunodepression seen in cancer patients may be partly due to nutritional deficits, that these deficits can be reversed with nutritional repletion, and, when they are reversed, response to therapy, and hence prognosis, should be improved.

Daly and associates analyzed sequential delayed hypersensitivity skin test reactivity in 160 malnourished cancer patients undergoing chemotherapy, surgery, radiotherapy, or supportive care prior to future therapy (Table 10-13).[124] Nutrition therapy with TPN for an average of 16 days was associated with restored skin test reactivity in 51 percent of the 90 initially anergic patients. The rate of conversion to reactivity was significantly lower among the radiotherapy patients. In addition, there was a significant increase in the morbidity and mortality of the surgical patients whose skin test reactions remained negative or converted from positive to negative when compared to those patients whose skin tests were positive after the course of TPN. No oth-

TABLE 10-13
Sequential Skin Test Reactivity in Cancer Patients Receiving
Total Parenteral Nutrition

	Chemo-therapy Group	Surgery Group	Radiation Therapy Group	Supportive Care Group
No. of patients	76	49	20	15
Days of TPN	28	25	26	18
Weight gain (lb)	7	7	6	6
Remained positive	25	23	6	?
Positive to negative	6	2	2	?
Remained negative	20	11	9	4
Negative to positive	25	13	3	5
Conversion to positive	25/45 (55%)	13/24 (54%)	3/12* (25%)	5/9 (55%)

Significantly different from surgery and chemotherapy groups.
From Daly JM, et al: Ann Surg 192:587–592, 1980.

er correlations could be drawn from the data concerning skin test reactivity and the outcome of antitumor therapy.

Haffejee and Angorn studied 20 patients with unresectable carcinoma of the esophagus who were malnourished.[125] The only therapy for the lesion was palliative esophageal intubation; tumor bulk remained unchanged. Reversal of negative nitrogen balance by an oral diet providing 3700 kcal/day was associated with a significant increase in total lymphocytes as well as in the T-cell fraction and a significant increase in the mitogenic response to phytohemagglutinin. However, skin test reactivity to dinitrochlorobenzene remained negative.

Thus available data suggest that nutrition therapy is effective in reversing immune deficits due to malnutrition and that when reversal occurs, the risk of surgery appears to be reduced. However, whether the course of the underlying malignancy is favorably affected by this improvement in immunocompetence remains to be proven.

Tumor Growth and Nutrition

Tumor growth stimulation during intensive nutritional repletion of cancer patients is a theoretic consideration which may have an adverse or perhaps salutary effect on the course of a malignant disease and the response to therapy. To date, tumor growth stimulation has not been observed during clinical assessment of patients receiving parenteral nutrition.[107,126,127] Recently, Mullen and associates analyzed tumor protein synthesis in a series of patients with gastrointestinal tumors who received either TPN or an oral diet.[128] Tumor protein synthesis was not enhanced in the TPN-treated group, but no direct inference regarding net tumor growth can be made without data on tumor protein catabolism. In fact, precise quantitative data on tumor growth in relation to nutrition therapy in humans are limited, since the methods useful in evaluating tumor growth in experimental animals are often not applicable to the study of human subjects. Thus much of the available information concerning the effect of dietary manipulation on tumor kinetics comes from the animal laboratory.

Steiger and associates studied the growth of mammary tumors in rats.[111] Tumor growth was greatly enhanced in the group of animals receiving TPN as compared to a group receiving only an infusion of 5 percent glucose. However, significant tumor growth stimulation was also observed in a third group of animals receiving only an infusion of 5 percent amino acids despite the fact that this diet was associated with a great loss of nontumor carcass weight. These latter findings emphasize that tumors are extremely adaptable parasites capable of sequestering nutrient substances and energy sources from the host even during dietary deprivation.[126] Subsequently, Cameron and Pavlat demonstrated that parenteral feedings stimulated tumor growth in hepatoma-bearing rats even when compared with animals fed a normal oral diet.[129] In addition, the tumor from the parenterally fed rats had higher mitotic activity. Daly and associates found that feeding a protein-free diet to rats with Walker-256 carcinosarcomas resulted in host carcass weight loss and tumor growth retardation.[126] However, nutritional repletion accelerated both host and tumor growth within 48 hours and within 6 days resulted in a tumor growth pattern similar to that observed in well nourished tumor-bearing rats.

Buzby and associates studied rats with mammary tumors and found that the tumor stimulation observed with a glucose-based system of TPN was obviated when all nonprotein calories were supplied as lipid even though nutritional repletion of the hosts was comparable with both systems.[130] Decreased stimulatory effect on tumor growth was not observed when glucose and lipid each provided half of the nonprotein calories. The basis for these observations is not clear.

Reports of tumor growth stimulation and increased mitotic activity with TPN lead to the hypothesis that the antitumor activity of chemotherapeutic agents that inhibit DNA synthesis may be enhanced during early nutritional repletion, when tumor growth and cell division are maximal. In fact, Daly and associates found that methotrexate was significantly more effective in a group of tumor-bearing rats during nutritional repletion than in a similar group of malnourished rats continued on a protein-free diet.[126] Cameron and Rogers examined tumor regression in hepatoma-bearing rats receiving hydroxyurea and total parenteral nutrition.[131] Their data indicated significantly greater tumor regression in rats that had TPN than in rats offered a liquid diet. However, survival time was shorter in the rats receiving TPN and hydroxyurea.

It should be emphasized that these findings in animals are not directly applicable to humans. The effect of nutritional manipulation in animals is undoubtedly magnified and perhaps otherwise altered by the more rapid doubling times of laboratory tumor systems when compared to human cancer.[107,126]

Conclusions

The link between malnutrition, nutritional repletion, and the efficacy and complications of primary antitumor therapy is complex and poorly defined.

TABLE 10-14
Intensive Nutrition Therapy in Cancer Patients:
Summary of Current Concepts

Primary Antitumor Therapy	Nutritional Status	Rationale for Nutritional Support	Present Indications for Adjuvant Enteral or Parenteral Nutrition
Surgery	Well nourished	To sustain nutrition when oral intake is precluded or contraindicated	Usual indications apply (e.g., postoperative fistula)
	Malnourished	To restore nutritional status and decrease postoperative morbidity and mortality	Preoperative nutritional repletion for 7–10 days
Chemotherapy	Well nourished	To prevent toxicity of chemotherapeutic agents, provide bowel rest, maintain nutrition	Indicated if oral intake is inadequate during chemotherapy
	Malnourished	To restore nutrition and thereby increase margin of safety of antitumor therapy, improve immune reactivity, (?) increase efficacy of cytotoxic agents	Pretherapy nutritional repletion
Radiotherapy	Well nourished	Reduce symptoms of radiation enteritis, maintain nutrition	Indicated if oral feedings are inadequate
	Malnourished	Increase margin of safety of radiotherapy	Pretherapy nutritional repletion

Published data are often inconsistent, and when correlations are observed, the cause and effect relationships often remain obscure. However, there are sufficient data to conclude that malnutrition is an unfavorable accompaniment of malignant disease and, consequently, that nutritional repletion is a logical adjuvant to primary oncologic therapy. Special nutrition therapy, however, is not recommended for patients with terminal disease for whom no primary palliative antitumor therapy is available. Current concepts and recommendations are summarized in Table 10-14.

PANCREATITIS

The rationale for intensive nutritional support in patients with severe protracted pancreatitis is primarily based on the observation that these patients nearly uniformly demonstrate a marked degree of nutritional depletion.[132,133] Since stimulating the inflamed pancreas is presumed to be undesirable, medical management of acute pancreatitis is directed in part to minimizing stimuli to pancreatic exocrine function. Consequently, the choice of the optimal feeding regimen is influenced by the comparative stimulatory effects of the available nutrient formulations. Additional considerations include the functional state of the gastrointestinal tract and the relative morbidity of the various feeding methods.

Current information indicates that nutrition therapies stimulate pancreatic exocrine secretions in the following descending order of magnitude: oral solid diets, oral elemental diets, intraduodenal elemental diets, intrajejunal elemental diets, total parenteral nutrition, and fasting (see pp. 96–98, and 193). Thus, in the early acute phase of severe pancreatitis, parenteral feedings are generally prescribed, because paralytic ileus frequently precludes use of the gastrointestinal tract and because intravenous feedings are least provocative to the pancreas. This hyposecretory effect has led to speculation that treatment with parenteral feedings, in addition to restoring nutrition, may exert a salutary effect on the clinical course of pancreatitis itself. Nevertheless, many authors advocate enteral feedings which can be used effectively to achieve nutritional repletion once bowel function has returned.[132-134] Liquid feeding preparations can be given through nasogastric or nasoduodenal feeding tubes or through a standard tube jejunostomy created during operation for pancreatitis. However, leakage and fistulization have been described following the latter procedure, so that tube jejunostomies may be unwarranted.[135] The value and safety of needle catheter jejunostomy have not been evaluated specifically in patients with acute pancreatitis.

Goodgame and Fischer reviewed the course of 44 patients with severe acute pancreatitis who received the glucose system of TPN for an average of 28 days.[136] Nutritional support was possible for periods of up to 3 months, but no direct benefit on the course of pancreatitis was observed. In addition, these authors reported a 17 percent incidence of catheter-related sepsis. Similar nutritional benefits were observed by Copeland and Dudrick but without an elevated incidence of catheter sepsis.[107]

Because of the etiologic association of hyperlipemia and acute pancreatitis, Eisenberg and associates evaluated the safety and efficacy of the lipid system of TPN in a group of pancreatitis patients not known to have underlying abnormalities of lipid metabolism.[137] Nutritional repletion was satisfactory, hyperlipemia did not develop, and none of the patients experienced an exacerbation of disease.

In summary, intensive nutritional support can ameliorate the nutritional consequences of severe pancreatitis, but a favorable effect on the natural course of the disease has not been documented.

FLUID-RESTRICTED PATIENTS

Various patients requiring parenteral nutrition have conditions in which fluid restriction is desirable and yet calorie and protein requirements are unaltered.

In patients requiring only modest fluid restriction, the standard glucose system is chosen over the standard lipid system. For patients requiring marked fluid restriction, a modified glucose system can be prepared in which nutrients are further concentrated to increase the protein content and the caloric density (Table 10-15). Candidates for this protocol may include elderly patients with cardiovascular disease; patients with congestive heart failure,

TABLE 10-15
Modified Glucose System for Fluid-Restricted Patients

Preparation of One Liter *	
70% Glucose	500 ml
10% Amino Acids	500 ml
Nutrients Provided Per Liter	
Non-protein calories	1190 kcal
Caloric density	1.2 kcal/ml
Glucose	350 gm
Nitrogen†	7.9 gm
Protein Equivalent	49.3 gm
Calorie‡/Nitrogen Ratio	151:1

Additives recommended for standard glucose system (Table 6-1) may need to be modified in accordance with disease state. For example, sodium may be omitted in patients with congestive heart failure.
†*Based on nitrogen content of Aminosyn 10 percent.*
‡*Non-protein kcal.*

NUTRITION THERAPY: CLINICAL APPLICATIONS

TABLE 10-16
Modified Lipid System for Fluid-Restricted
Patients Who Are Glucose Intolerant

Preparation of 750 ml Unit	
Bottle A	
20 percent Fat Emulsion	250 ml
Bottle B	
8.5 percent Amino Acids	350 ml
50 percent Glucose	100 ml
Additives* and Sterile Water	50 ml
Nutrients Provided Per Unit	
Non-protein calories	670 kcal
Caloric density	0.89 kcal/ml
Nitrogen†	4.6 gm.
Protein Equivalent	28.4 gm.
Calorie‡/Nitrogen ratio	146:1

*Additives recommended for standard lipid system (Table 7-1) may need to be modified in accordance with disease state.
†Based on nitrogen content of FreAmine III
‡Non-protein kcal
Note: This modified lipid system must be infused into a central vein.

edema, or respiratory distress syndrome; or certain patients following intracranial injury or surgery. Patients requiring fluid restriction who in addition are markedly glucose intolerant may receive the modified lipid system outlined in Table 10-16. In this system, 250 ml of 20 percent fat emulsion are substituted for the usual 500 ml of 10 percent fat emulsion comprising Bottle A. In this way a 750 ml nutritional unit is prepared which has an increased caloric density and protein concentration, but a concomitant increase in osmolarity precludes peripheral venous administration.

These modified parenteral nutrient solutions are generally not appropriate for patients who are protein-intolerant, as in renal or hepatic failure.

Fluid-restricted patients who are candidates for enteral feedings may receive one of the high caloric density products listed in Tables 4-1 and 4-2.

PERIOPERATIVE MALNUTRITION

A substantial body of information attests to a significant association between malnutrition and postoperative morbidity and mortality. In 1936, Studley observed a 10-fold increase in postoperative mortality among patients with intractable peptic ulcer disease who had sustained a preoperative weight loss of

20 percent or more.[138] In 1955, Rhoads and Alexander demonstrated an association between postoperative infections and poor nutritional status and depressed serum albumin levels.[139] The effects of protein deficiency on wound healing and the relationship between skin test reactivity and prognosis in surgical patients have already been discussed (see pp. 12, 42–43).

More recently, the prognostic nutritional index (PNI) of Mullen and associates has been used to quantify the probability that various deficits in putative nutritional indices will have an adverse effect on postoperative outcome (see pp. 43–45).[140,141] These investigators found that patients prospectively identified to be at high risk for postoperative complications (PNI $\geq$ 50 percent) actually experienced a 6-fold increase in complications, a 9-fold increase in major sepsis (pneumonia, intraabdominal sepsis, septicemia), and an 11-fold increase in mortality when compared to those patients thought to be at low risk (PNI $<$ 40 percent) (see Table 2-16).[141,142]

These various studies relating nutritional status and postoperative prognosis have led to the logical supposition that perioperative nutritional repletion will ameliorate the adverse effects associated with nutritional deficits. This view is widely accepted on the basis of clinical experience, but data from controlled trials are limited. As previously discussed, Holter and Fischer[97] and Thompson and associates[100] were unable to demonstrate that perioperative parenteral nutrition had a favorable effect on the postoperative course of cancer patients. However, both studies indicated that nutritional indices can be maintained or improved by intensive nutrition therapy. Thus preservation or increase of body weight,[97,100,143–146] increased serum albumin levels,[97] and positive nitrogen balance[144,147,148] can be achieved following major surgery in patients receiving perioperative enteral[143–146] or parenteral[97,100,147,148] nutrition.

Muller and associates observed a significant reduction in postoperative mortality and major complications in cancer patients who had received 10 days of preoperative TPN.[101] Convincing data supporting the concept that nutritional repletion has a salutary effect on postoperative outcome have also been presented by Mullen and associates.[98] These authors analyzed the postoperative course of a series of 145 patients who had undergone a major elective abdominal or thoracic operation. The course of 50 patients who had received at least 7 days of total parenteral nutrition prior to operation was compared to that of 90 patients who had had no preoperative nutritional support (Table 10-17). Nearly all of the patients (93 percent) received TPN in the postoperative period. The effect of preoperative TPN was correlated with admission nutritional status by stratifying the patients retrospectively according to their prognostic nutritional index. Significantly improved clinical outcome was observed only in the group of patients identified as "high risk" (PNI $\geq$ 50 percent). In this group, preoperative nutritional support was associated with a 2.4-fold reduction in all complications, a nearly 7-fold reduction in major sepsis, and a 5-fold reduction in mortality.

TABLE 10-17

Effect of Preoperative Total Parenteral Nutrition on Postoperative Morbidity and Mortality

Patient Group	Number of Patients	Total Complications	Septic Complications	Major Septic Complications	Deaths
Low-risk patients (PNI <40%)					
Control	32	4 (13%)	3 (9%)	2 (6%)	2 (6%)
TPN	18	2 (11%)	1 (6%)	1 (6%)	0 (0%)
P-value*	—	NS†	NS	NS	NS
Intermediate-risk patients (PNI = 40–49%)					
Control	18	8 (44%)	3 (17%)	3 (17%)	4 (22%)
TPN	10	2 (20%)	2 (20%)	0 (0%)	0 (0%)
P-value*	—	NS	NS	NS	NS
High-risk patients (PNI ≥ 50%)					
Control	45	25 (56%)	16 (36%)	15 (33%)	21 (47%)
TPN	22	5 (23%)	3 (14%)	1 (5%)	2 (9%)
P-value*	—	<0.01	NS	<0.05	<0.01
All patients					
Control	95	37 (39%)	22 (23%)	20 (21%)	27 (28%)
TPN	50	9 (18%)	6 (12%)	2 (4%)	2 (4%)
P-value*	—	<0.01	NS	<0.01	<0.005

*Probability by chi-square analysis that a real difference exists between patients who received TPN and those who did not (controls).
†NS = not significant.
Adapted from Mullen JL, et al: Ann Surg 192:604–613, 1980.

Preoperative nutritional support can often be provided satisfactorily either enterally or parenterally, but parenteral nutrition has generally been recommended in the period immediately following abdominal surgery. However, various investigators have reported successful enteral feeding in the immediate postoperative period using the technique of needle catheter jejunostomy.[143,144,149] This procedure involves the insertion of a small-diameter polyethylene catheter into the proximal jejunum at the termination of an abdominal operation (Fig. 10-5 A–D). The apparatus required is a 14 gauge needle and a 24 to 36 inch 16 gauge catheter. These materials are available in the Intracath central venous catheter placement unit (Deseret Pharmaceutical Company, Sandy, Utah) or in the Vivonex jejunostomy kit (Norwich–Eaton, Norwich, NY). The needle is inserted into the submucosal layer of the antimesenteric border of a jejunal segment just distal to the ligament of Treitz. A lengthy intramural tunnel is created by telescoping the intestine over the needle before the needle enters the lumen. Then an 18 inch segment of the catheter is advanced into the lumen and its proximal end is brought out through the abdominal wall.[144,149,150] Prior to feeding, the intraluminal position of the catheter is confirmed radiographically using a water-soluble contrast medium.[150]

Early postoperative jejunal feedings with an elemental diet, often begun in the recovery room, are possible because small bowel motility and absorptive capacity apparently are little affected by celiotomy if they are normal at the time of operation.[149] In contrast, immediate oral feedings are precluded by impaired gastric and colonic motility usually lasting at least several days.[143,150]

After considerable clinical experience, Page and associates have recommended needle catheter jejunostomy for patients undergoing extensive emergency and elective operations on the upper gastrointestinal or pancreaticobiliary tracts, for patients with intraabdominal malignancies when adjunctive radiotherapy or chemotherapy or both are contemplated, and for patients with multiple injuries who undergo abdominal exploration.[149] Early postoperative enteral feeding is not necessary for normally nourished patients who will be able to eat within a week of undergoing an uncomplicated operation. In addition, immediate enteral feeding is usually contraindicated in patients with generalized peritonitis, small bowel obstruction, extensive small bowel adhesions, intrinsic small bowel disease, or extensive retroperitoneal resection, because these conditions can affect the function of the small bowel.[144]

The elemental diet administered with this technique is initially provided diluted in small volumes. Volume and concentration are subsequently increased gradually, as described in Chapter 4. Abdominal distention and diarrhea may occur, as with other methods of enteral feeding, but major complications associated with needle catheter jejunostomy appear to be unusual. Catheter dislodgement with interperitoneal leakage or infusion of the feeding solution has been described, but this should be rare if proper location of the catheter is confirmed radiographically before use and the jejunum adjacent to the catheter exit site is sutured to the parietal peritoneum.

Page and associates reviewed their experience treating 199 patients with needle catheter jejunostomy.[149] Intraperitoneal leakage, occurring in two patients, was the only major complication during 7238 patient-days of catheter exposure.

Dunn and associates used this method of early postoperative feeding in eight patients who had sustained massive intraabdominal injuries involving the liver, pancreas, and upper gastrointestinal tract.[143] The patients were receiving 2200 to 2400 kcal/day within 2 days of operation and were maintained at this level for an average of 11 days. Body weight, lean muscle mass, serum albumin and transferrin levels, and total lymphocyte count were maintained during this period of nutritional support.

Hoover and associates observed positive nitrogen balance and preservation of body weight among 26 patients undergoing extensive upper gastrointestinal operation who received an elemental diet via a catheter jejunostomy.[144] Moderate diarrhea occurred in 9 of the 26 patients.

Catheter jejunostomy has the advantage that nutritional support can be resumed or initiated immediately following operation, obviating the need for intravenous feedings and their potential complications. In addition, enteral feedings can be continued on an outpatient basis with little difficulty. Furthermore, catheter jejunostomy feedings are cost-effective, since this technique is much less expensive than parenteral nutrition. The advocates of immediate postoperative enteral feedings have suggested that this method is equivalent in its effectiveness to parenteral nutrition, but this impression has not been subjected to a controlled clinical trial.

MINOR CATABOLIC STATES

Blackburn and associates introduced the concept of intravenous "protein-sparing therapy" to preserve body cell mass in normally nourished or mildly malnourished noncritically ill patients unable to eat for brief periods.[151] Such therapy consists of peripheral venous infusions of amino acids in a 3 to 5 percent solution providing 1 to 1.5 gm/kg/day.

Many investigators have observed a significant reduction in net nitrogen losses in fasting patients who receive these hypocaloric amino acid infusions in place of the traditional 5 percent solution of glucose,[151-155] but nitrogen balance generally remains slightly negative[156] and significant anabolism is rarely achieved. Skillman and associates, however, observed that a 3.5 percent amino acid infusion providing 75 gm/day improved albumin synthesis in postoperative patients, as compared to 5 percent glucose.[157] The addition of 150 gm of glucose or 50 gm of lipids per day to the amino acid regimen has no signifi-

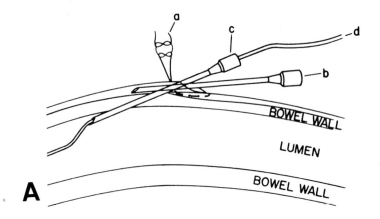

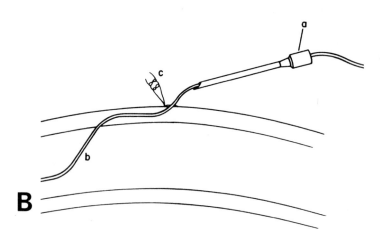

Figure 10-5. Technique of needle jejunostomy *(From Page CP, et al: Am J Surg 138:939–945, 1979)* **A:** Through a seromuscular pursestring suture (a), a 14 gauge needle is inserted for a distance within the wall of the bowel (b). The needle is then pushed into the lumen of the bowel (c) and the plastic catheter (d) is threaded through the needle.

B: The needle is withdrawn from the lumen of the bowel (a) and the catheter is threaded approximately 18 inches down the lumen of the bowel (b). The pursestring suture (c) is then secured.

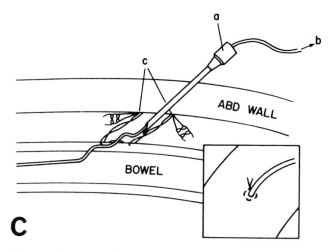

C: The guide wire is removed and the hub of the catheter (Intracath) is amputated. The needle is removed from the operative field and a similar clean needle is passed percutaneously back into the peritoneal cavity (a). The catheter which exits the bowel wall is then passed out of the abdomen through the tract created by the needle (b). The site of catheter exit from the bowel wall is then attached to the abdominal (ABD) wall with two seromuscular sutures of No. 2-0 silk (c). A larger diagram of the pursestring suture is shown in the inset.

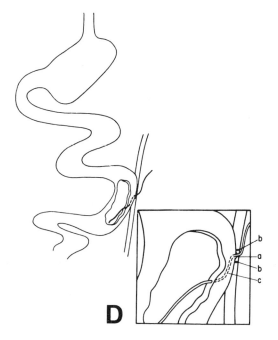

D: A diagram of the completed needle catheter jejunostomy emphasizing the presence of the pursestring suture (in the inset) (a); the attachment of the bowel wall to the abdomenal wall (b); and the antireflux submucosal tunnel (c).

cant additional effect on nitrogen economy.[153] These latter findings evidently disprove the mechanism of protein-sparing suggested by Blackburn and associates.[151] These investigators postulated that withholding glucose in favor of amino acids alone would improve nitrogen balance because the associated decrease in serum insulin levels would allow greater endogenous fat mobilization and utilization, thereby sparing lean body mass.

Greenberg and Jeejeebhoy studied the effect of similar hypocaloric regimens but provided increased amounts of amino acids.[158] They observed positive nitrogen balance (1.54 gm nitrogen/day) in moderately ill patients receiving 1.83 gm/kg/day of amino acids. However, acutely injured and postoperative patients were excluded from the study group. It is presumed that patients receiving amino acid infusions derive nonprotein calories from endogenous adipose reserves, and therefore, this therapy is only applicable in patients with adequate fat stores.

Although some improvement in nitrogen balance is observed, the clinical benefits, if any, of protein-sparing therapy have not been established.[152,156] This is not surprising, since brief periods of catabolism in previously normal individuals (for example, following uncomplicated elective surgery) are probably inconsequential and are unlikely to have an adverse clinical effect.[159,160] Since protein-sparing therapy was conceived as a method by which the potential complications of central venous nutrition could be avoided, the advent of effective methods of providing all required nutrients by peripheral vein, as in the lipid system, further weakens the rationale for hypocaloric amino acid infusions. In addition, it is clear that amino acid therapy does not approach the metabolic requirements of seriously ill patients.

Thus brief catabolic episodes in previously well patients do not require special nutrition therapy; the modest protein-sparing effect of 5 percent glucose infusions remains cost-effective. More seriously ill patients or those unable to eat for longer periods (exceeding a week) are optimally managed with total parenteral nutrition.

LIVER DISEASE

Patients with liver disease are frequently malnourished,[161] and yet adequate nutritional repletion is often precluded when hepatic failure supervenes because of the accompanying protein intolerance manifest as lethargy, encephalopathy, and, finally, coma.

Many patients with modest hepatic insufficiency and even mild encephalopathy will tolerate the standard amino acid formulations, provided administration is limited to 50 to 60 gm of amino acids per day.[162] The nutrient solution outlined in Table 10-18 may be suitable for some of these patients.

Two units (1500 ml) of this solution will provide nearly 2400 nonprotein

TABLE 10-18
Modified Glucose System for Mild Hepatic Insufficiency*

Preparation of 750 ml Unit†	
70% Glucose	500 ml
10% Amino Acids	250 ml
Nutrients Provided Per Unit	
Non-Protein calories	1190 kcal
Glucose	350 gm
Amino Acids	25 gm

*Volume prescribed depends on protein and fluid tolerance.
†Additives depend on clinical status. Patients may require less sodium and more potassium than usually provided in glucose system.

kcal and about 50 gm of amino acids. Further protein restriction is necessary for patients who remain or become encephalopathic on this program. Another approach to parenteral nutrition is to provide the protein source exclusively as essential amino acids.[163,164] This can be accomplished using a protocol previously described in this chapter for patients with acute renal failure (Table 10-10). However, the efficacy of essential amino acids in liver failure has not been evaluated.

Thus providing adequate nutritional support to patients with severe hepatic failure with encephalopathy remains an unsolved problem. Fischer and his associates have pursued an experimental approach to nourishing these patients in which an intravenous nutrient formulation greatly enriched in branched-chain amino acids has been developed which appears to have a salutary effect not only on nutritional status but on the course of hepatic encephalopathy as well.[165–168]

Patients with chronic liver disease often have elevations in plasma levels of aromatic amino acids, including tyrosine, phenylalanine, and tryptophan, as well as methionine, glutamate, aspartate, and ornithine. In contrast, the branched-chain amino acids—leucine, isoleucine, and valine—are usually depressed.[169] These observations have led to the suggestion that the depressed ratio of branched-chain to aromatic amino acids may have etiologic importance in hepatic coma.[166,170,171] According to this hypothesis, the high circulating insulin levels occurring in liver failure promote skeletal muscle uptake of the branched-chain amino acids. The resultant depressed plasma levels of branched-chain amino acids facilitate development of high levels of aromatic amino acids in the brain since these two amino acid groups compete at the blood–brain barrier for entry into the central nervous system. High levels of brain phenylalanine are thought to inhibit tyrosine decarboxylase activity, thus interfering with normal tyrosine metabolism to catecholamines, which

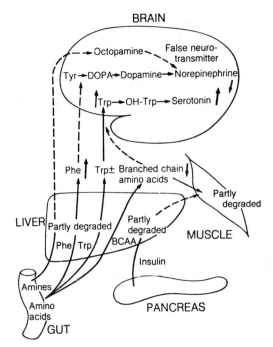

Figure 10-6. Suggested role of branched-chain amino acids in hepatic coma. Owing to unrestricted passage of insulin into the general circulation in hepatic coma, branched-chain amino acids are removed excessively by muscle. In consequence of this lowering of plasma branched-chain amino acids, there is less competition with aromatic amino acids for entry into the brain. In the brain, false neurotransmitters, lowered catecholamines, and increased serotonin are thought to be responsible for hepatic coma. *(From Crim MC, Munro HN: In Shils ME (ed): Defined-Formula Diets for Medical Purposes. Chicago, American Medical Association, 1977)*

are important in brain neurotransmitter function. The resulting excess tyrosine is shunted to octopamine, a presumed false neurotransmitter which may also be derived from tyramine, an amine produced by bacterial action in the gut and entering the general circulation in cases of hepatic failure.[170] The combination of false neurotransmitters, excess serotonin (derived from increased brain tryptophan), and low levels of brain catecholamines is thought to contribute to the development of hepatic coma (Fig. 10-6).[169,170,172] A corollary of this hypothesis is that restoration of the normal branched-chain: aromatic amino acid ratio should not only provide specific treatment for hepatic encephalopathy but should also allow administration of enough amino acids to attain nitrogen balance without precipitating hepatic coma.[169]

Experimental data supporting this hypothesis comes largely from Fischer's laboratory. When encephalopathic dogs and monkeys were treated with a solution providing 23 percent glucose and enriched in branched-chain amino acids and low in phenylalanine, tryptophan, and methionine (F080, Table 10-19) the animals awoke from coma. The arousal from hepatic encephalopathy coincided with normalization of both plasma and cerebral spinal fluid amino acids and neurotransmitters patterns.[167,168]

Preliminary data from humans with encephalopathy on the basis of an acute exacerbation of chronic cirrhosis indicate that infusion of F080 results

TABLE 10-19
Experimental Amino Acid Solution Used in Severe Liver Failure (F080)

	Grams/Liter
ESSENTIAL AMINO ACIDS	
L-isoleucine	4.50
L-leucine	5.50
L-lysine HCl	3.80
L-methionine	0.50
L-phenylalanine	0.50
L-threonine	2.25
L-tryptophan	0.38
L-valine	4.20
NON-ESSENTIAL AMINO ACIDS	
L-alanine	3.75
L-arginine	3.00
L-histidine	1.20
L-proline	4.00
L-serine	2.50
Glycine	4.50
L-cysteine-HCl-H$_2$O	0.20
TOTAL NITROGEN	6.25
PROTEIN EQUIVALENT	40
GLUCOSE	230

From: Fischer JE, et al: Surgery 80:77–91, 1976.

in awakening from or improvement in hepatic encephalopathy, normalization of the amino acid pattern, and, in most of the patients, maintenance of nitrogen equilibrium or positive nitrogen balance with the infusion of up to 120 gm/24 hr of amino acids.[166,167] Recently, similar favorable effects have been reported in a patient receiving a liquid feeding product, Hepatic-Aid, which is enriched in branched-chain amino acids (see Table 4-3).[167] Limited data suggest that the favorable effects of branched-chain amino acid therapy seen in encephalopathic cirrhotic patients are not usually achieved in patients with acute fulminant hepatitis.[166]

Despite these experimental results, the false neurotransmitter hypothesis requires further study. Whether a decline in branched-chain amino acids facilitates transfer of aromatic amino acids across the blood–brain barrier in encephalopathic humans, as in the case of animal models, is uncertain.[169] In addition, doubt has been cast on the role of octopamine by an experiment in which the infusion of this substance directly into the brain of rats, raising tissue octopamine levels 20,000-fold and greatly reducing catecholamine levels, failed to provoke hepatic coma.[173] Finally, tryptophan and phenylalanine, although elevated in the plasma of encephalopathic patients, cannot be shown directly to produce the coma state.

Thus nutritional management of patients with severe liver insufficiency remains problematic. Protein restriction using available formulations is recommended at present, but recent advances in the laboratory may result in a special formulation of amino acids, allowing adequate nutritional repletion as well as symptomatic improvement of the liver disease.

Finally, the specific liver abnormalities associated with intestinal bypass surgery for morbid obesity have been ameliorated in several patients by treatment with the standard glucose system of parenteral nutrition[174] or by a calorie-free, 4.25 percent amino acid infusion.[175] Both forms of treatment reversed fatty infiltration of the liver.

REFERENCES

1. Edmunds LH Jr, Williams GM, Welch CE: External fistulas arising from the gastrointestinal tract. Ann Surg 152:445–471, 1960.
2. Chapman R, Foran R, Dunphy JE: Management of intestinal fistulas. Am J Surg 108:157–164, 1964.
3. Sheldon GF, Gardiner BN, Way LW, Dunphy JE: Management of gastrointestinal fistulas. Surg Gynecol Obstet 133:385–389, 1971.
4. Rocchio MA, Mocha CJ, Haas KF, Randall HT: Use of chemically defined diets in the management of patients with high output gastrointestinal cutaneous fistulas. Am J Surg 127:148–156, 1974.
5. Voitk AJ, Echave V, Brown RA, et al: Elemental diet in the treatment of fistulas of the alimentary tract. Surg Gynecol Obstet 137:68–72, 1973.
6. MacFadyen BV Jr, Dudrick SJ, Ruberg RL: Management of gastrointestinal fistulas with parenteral hyperalimentation. Surgery 74:100–105, 1973.
7. Himal HS, Allard Jr, Nadeau JE, et al: The importance of adequate nutrition in closure of small intestinal fistulas. Br J Surg 61:724–726, 1974.
8. Dietel M: Nutritional management of external gastrointestinal fistulas. Can J Surg 19:505–511, 1976.
9. Graham JA: Conservative treatment of gastrointestinal fistulas. Surg Gynecol Obstet 144:512–514, 1977.
10. Reber HA, Roberts C, Way LN, Dunphy JE: Management of external gastrointestinal fistulas. Ann Surg 188:460–467, 1978.
11. Soeters PB, Ebeid AM, Fischer JE: Review of 404 patients with gastrointestinal fistulas. Ann Surg 190:189–202, 1979.
12. Silberman H, Granson M, Fong G, et al: Management of external gastrointestinal fistulas with glucose and lipids. Surg Gynecol Obstet 150:856–858, 1980.
13. Thomas RJS: The response of patients with fistulas of the gastrointestinal tract to parenteral nutrition. Surg Gynecol Obstet 153:77–80, 1981.

14. Fischer JE: Nutritional support in the seriously ill patient. Curr Probl Surg 17:465–532, 1980.
15. Wolfe BM, Keltner RM, William VL: Intestinal fistula output in regular, elemental, and intravenous alimentation. Am J Surg 124:803–806, 1972.
16. Schrock TR: Short bowel syndrome, in Dunphy JE, Way LW (eds): Current Surgical Diagnosis and Treatment, ed 5. Los Altos, CA, Lange Medical Publications, 1981, pp 552–554.
17. Weser E. Fletcher JT, Urban E: Short bowel syndrome. Gastroenterology 77:575–579, 1979.
18. Tilson MD: Pathophysiology and treatment of the short bowel syndrome. Surg Clin North Am 60:1273–1284, 1980.
19. Sheldon GF: Role of parenteral nutrition in patients with short bowel syndrome. Am J Med 67:1021–1029, 1979.
20. Weser E: The management of patients after small bowel resection. Gastroenterology 71:146–150, 1976.
21. Williamson RCN: Intestinal adaption. N Engl J Med 298:1393–1402, 1444–1450, 1978.
22. Feldman EJ, Dowling RH, McNaughton J, Peters TJ: Effects of oral versus intravenous nutrition on intestinal adaption after small bowel resection in the dog. Gastroenterology 70:712–719, 1976.
23. Levine GM, Deren JJ: Dietary and non-dietary factors mediating hyperplasia of residual gut mucosa after small bowel resection in the rat. Clin Res 22:363A, 1974.
24. Driscoll RH Jr, Rosenberg IH: Total parenteral nutrition in inflammatory bowel disease. Med Clin North Am 62:185–201, 1978.
25. Hill GL, Blackett RL, Pickford IR, Bradley JA: A survey of protein nutrition in patients with inflammatory bowel disease: A rational basis for nutritional therapy. Br J Surg 64:894–896, 1977.
26. Axelsson C, Jarnum S: Assessment of the therapeutic value of an elemental diet in chronic inflammatory bowel disease. Scand J Gastroenterol 12:89–95, 1977.
27. Goode A, Feggetter JGW, Hawkins T, Johnston IDA: Use of an elemental diet for long-term nutritional support in Crohn's disease. Lancet 1:122–124, 1976.
28. Rocchio MA, Mo Cha C, Haas KF, Randall HT: Use of chemically defined diets in the management of patients with acute inflammatory bowel disease. Am J Surg 127:469–475, 1974.
29. Voitk AJ, Echave V, Feller JH, et al: Experience with elemental diet in the treatment of inflammatory bowel disease. Arch Surg 107:329–333, 1973.
30. Anderson DL, Boyce HW: Use of parenteral nutrition in treatment of advanced regional enteritis. Am J Dig Dis 18:633–640, 1973.
31. Cohen MI, Boley SJ, Daum F, et al: The role and effect of parenteral nutrition on the liver and its use in chronic inflammatory bowel disease in childhood. Adv Exp Med Biol 46:214–224, 1974.
32. Franklin FA, Grand RJ: Parenteral nutrition for inflammatory bowel disease in childhood and adolescence. Proceedings of the International Congress on Parenteral Nutrition, University of Montpelier, France, 1974, pp 583–589.
33. Marshall F II: Hyperalimentation as a treatment of Crohn's disease. Am J Surg 128:652–653, 1974.

34. Vogel CM, Corwin TR, Baue AE: Intravenous hyperalimentation in the treatment of inflammatory diseases of the bowel. Arch Surg 108:460–467, 1974.
35. Reilly J, Ryan JA, Strole W, Fischer JE: Hyperalimentation in inflammatory bowel disease. Am J Surg 131:192–200, 1976.
36. Elson CO, Layden TJ, Nemchausky BA, et al: An evaluation of total parenteral nutrition in the management of inflammatory bowel disease. Dig Dis Sci 25:42–48, 1980.
37. Stanchev P: Parenteral nutrition in the treatment of ulcerohaemorrhagic colitis. Proceedings of the International Congress on Parenteral Nutrition, University of Montpelier, France, 1974, pp 501–507.
38. Mullen JL, Hargrove WC, Dudrick SJ, et al: Ten years experience with intravenous hyperalimentation and inflammatory bowel disease. Ann Surg 187:523–529, 1978.
39. Rombeau JL, Barot LR, Williamson CE, Mullen, JL: Preoperative total parenteral nutrition and surgical outcome in patients with inflammatory bowel disease. Am J Surg 143:139–143, 1982.
40. Layden T. Rosenberg J. Nemchausky B, et al: Reversal of growth arrest in adolescents with Crohn's disease after parenteral alimentation. Gastroenterology 70:1017–1021, 1976.
41. Strobel CT, Byrne WJ, Ament ME: Home parenteral nutrition in children with Crohn's disease: An effective management alternative. Gastroenterology 77:272–279, 1979.
42. Eisenberg HW, Turnbull RB, Weakley FL: Hyperalimentation as preparation for surgery in transmural colitis (Crohn's disease). Dis Colon Rectum 17:469–475, 1974.
43. Dudrick SJ, MacFadyen BV Jr, Daly JM: Management of inflammatory bowel disease with parenteral hyperalimentation, in Clearfield HR, Dinoso VP Jr (eds): Gastrointestinal Emergencies. New York, Grune and Stratton, 1976, pp 193–199.
44. Dickinson RJ, Ashton MG, Axon ATR, et al: Controlled trial of intravenous hyperalimentation and total bowel rest as an adjunct to the routine therapy of acute colitis. Gastroenterology 79:1199–1204, 1980.
45. Rault RMJ, Scribner BH: Treatment of Crohn's disease with home parenteral nutrition. Gastroenterology 72:1249–1252, 1977.
46. Pruitt BA Jr: Postburn hypermetabolism and nutrition of the burn patient, in Ballinger WF, Collins JA, Dudricker WR, et al (eds): Manual of Surgical Nutrition. Philadelphia, WB Saunders, 1975, pp 396–412.
47. Wilmore DW: Nutrition and metabolism following thermal injury. Clin Plast Surg 1:603–619, 1974.
48. Bartlett RH, Allyn PA, Medley T, Wetmore N: Nutritional therapy based on positive caloric balance in burn patients. Arch Surg 112:974–980, 1977.
49. Curreri PW, Luterman A: Nutritional support of the burned patient. Surg Clin North Am 58:1151–1156, 1978.
50. Wilmore DW, Pruitt BA Jr: Parenteral nutrition in burn patients, in Fischer JE (ed): Total Parenteral Nutrition. Boston, Little, Brown and Co, 1976, pp 231–252.
51. Curreri PW: Nutritional support of burn patients. World J Surg 2:215–222, 1978.

52. Alexander JW, MacMillan BG, Stinnett JD, et al: Beneficial effects of aggressive protein feeding in severely burned children. Ann Surg 192:505–517, 1980.
53. Wilmore DW, Moylan JA, Helmkamp GM, Pruitt BA Jr: Clinical evaluation of a 10% intravenous fat emulsion for parenteral nutrition in thermally injured patients. Ann Surg 178:503–513, 1973.
54. Pruitt BA Jr, McManus WF, Kim SH, Treat RC: Diagnosis and treatment of cannula-related intravenous sepsis in burn patients. Ann Surg 191:554, 1980.
55. Warden GD, Wilmore DW, Pruitt BA Jr: Central venous thrombosis: A hazard of medical progress. J Trauma 13:620–626, 1973.
56. Larkin JM, Moylan JA: Complete enteral support of thermally injured patients. Am J Surg 131:722–724, 1976.
57. Choctaw WT, Fujita C, Zawacki BE: Prevention of upper gastrointestinal bleeding in burn patients: A role for elemental diet. Arch Surg 115:1073–1076, 1980.
58. Hiebert JM, McGough M, Rodeheaver G, et al: The influence of catabolism on immunocompetence in burned patients. Surgery 86:242–247, 1979.
59. Giordano C: Use of exogenous and endogenous urea for protein synthesis in normal and uremic subjects. J Lab Clin Med 62:231–246, 1963.
60. Giovannetti S, Maggiore Q: A low nitrogen diet with proteins of high biological value for severe chronic uremia. Lancet 1:1000–1003, 1964.
61. Rose WC, Dekker EE: Urea as a source of nitrogen for the biosynthesis of amino acids. J Biol Chem 223:107–121, 1956.
62. Richards P. Nutritional potential of nitrogen recycling in man. Am J Clin Nutr 25:615–625, 1972.
63. Mitch WE: Effects of intestinal flora on nitrogen metabolism in patients with chronic renal failure. Am J Clin Nutr 31:1594–1600, 1978.
64. Varcoe R, Halliday D, Carson ER, et al: Efficiency of utilization of urea nitrogen for albumin synthesis by chronically uraemic and normal man. Clin Sci Mol Med 48:379–390, 1975.
65. Varcoe AR, Halliday D, Carson ER, et al: Anabolic role of urea in renal failure. Am J Clin Nutr 31:1601–1607, 1978.
66. Walser M: Urea metabolism in chronic renal failure. J Clin Invest 53:1385–1392, 1974.
67. Fischer JE: Nutritional support in the seriously ill patient. Curr Probl Surg 17:465–532, 1980.
68. Wilmore DW, Dudrick SJ: Treatment of acute renal failure with intravenous essential L-amino acids. Arch Surg 99:669–673, 1969.
69. Dudrick SJ, Steiger E, Long J: Renal failure in surgical patients: Treatment with intravenous essential amino acids and hypertonic glucose. Surgery 68:180–186, 1970.
70. Abel RM, Abbott WM, Beck CH Jr, et al: Essential L-amino acids for hyperalimentation in patients with disordered nitrogen metabolism. Am J Surg 128:317–323, 1974.
71. Abel RM, Abbott WM, Fischer JE: Intravenous essential L-amino acids and hypertonic dextrose in patients with acute renal failure: Effects on serum potassium, phosphate, and magnesium. Am J Surg 123:632–638, 1972.
72. Abel RM, Beck CH Jr, Abbott WM, et al: Improved survival from acute renal failure after treatment with intravenous essential L-amino acids and glucose: Results of a prospective, double-blind study. N Engl J Med 288:695–699, 1973.

73. Abel RM, Shih VE, Abbott WM, et al: Amino acid metabolism in acute renal failure: Influence of intravenous essential L-amino acid hyperalimentation therapy. Ann Surg 180:350–355, 1974.
74. Abbott WM, Abel RM, Fischer JE: Treatment of acute renal insufficiency after aortoiliac surgery. Arch Surg 103:590–594, 1971.
75. Leonard CD, Luke RG, Siegel RR: Parenteral essential amino acids in acute renal failure. Urology 6:154–157, 1975.
76. Baek S. Makabali GG, Bryan-Brown CW, et al: The influence of parenteral nutrition on the course of acute renal failure. Surg Gynecol Obstet 141:405–408, 1975.
77. Sofio C, Nicora R: High calorie essential amino acid parenteral therapy in acute renal failure. Acta Chir Scand 466: [Suppl] 98–99, 1976.
78. Feinstein EI, Blumenkrantz MJ, Healy M, et al: Clinical and metabolic responses to parenteral nutrition in acute renal failure: A controlled double blind study. Medicine (Baltimore) 60:124–137, 1981.
79. Toback FG: Amino acid enhancement of renal regeneration after acute tubular necrosis. Kidney Int 12:193–198, 1977.
80. Kopple JD, Swendseid ME: Evidence that histidine is an essential amino acid in normal and chronically uremic man. J Clin Invest 55:881–891, 1975.
81. Blumenkrantz MJ, Kopple JD, Koffler A, et al: Total parenteral nutrition in the management of acute renal failure. Am J Clin Nutr 31:1831–1840, 1978.
82. Kopple JD, Blumenkrantz MJ: Total parenteral nutrition and parenteral fluid therapy, in Maxwell MH, Kleeman CR (eds): Clinical Disorders of Fluid and Electrolyte Metabolism, ed 3. New York, McGraw–Hill Book Co, 1980, pp 413–498.
83. Lee HA, Sharpstone P, Ames AC: Parenteral nutrition in renal failure. Postgrad Med J 43:81–91, (February) 1967.
84. Harvey KB, Blumenkrantz MJ, Levine SE, Blackburn GL: Nutritional assessment and treatment of chronic renal failure. Am J Clin Nutr 33:1586–1597, 1980.
85. Kopple JD: Nutritional management of chronic renal failure. Postgrad Med 64:135–144, (November) 1978.
86. Meng HC: Commentary: Treatment of chronic uremia, in Shils ME (ed): Defined-Formula Diets for Medical Purposes. Chicago, American Medical Association, 1977, pp 123–124.
87. Walser M: Principles of keto acid therapy in uremia. Am J Clin Nutr 31:1756–1760, 1978.
88. Bergstrom J, Ahlberg M, Alvestrand A, Furst P: Metabolic studies with keto acids in uremia. Am J Clin Nutr 31:1761–1766, 1978.
89. Walser M: Keto acids in the treatment of uremia. Clin Nephrol 6:180–186, 1975.
90. Walser M, Coulter AW, Dighe S, Crantz FR: The effect of keto-analogues of essential amino acids in severe chronic uremia. J Clin Invest 52:678–690, 1973.
91. Zimmermann EW, Meisinger E, Weinel B, Strauch M: Essential amino acid/ketoanalogue supplementation: An alternative to unrestricted protein intake in uremia. Clin Nephrol 11:71–78, 1979.
92. Costa G, Donaldson SS: Effects of cancer and cancer treatment on the nutrition of the host. N Engl J Med 300:1471–1474, 1979.

93. DeWys WD, Begg C, Lavin PT, et al: Prognostic effect of weight loss prior to chemotherapy in cancer patients. Am J Med 69:491–497, 1980.
94. DeWys WD: Nutritional care of the cancer patient. JAMA 244:374–376, 1980.
95. DeWys WD, Kisner D: Maintaining caloric needs in the cancer patient. Contemp Surg 15:25–32, 1979.
96. Dymock IW: Enteropathy in malignant disease. Br J Cancer 20:236–238, 1966.
97. Holter AR, Fischer JE: The effects of perioperative hyperalimentation on complications in patients with carcinoma and weight loss. J Surg Res 23:31–34, 1977.
98. Mullen JL, Buzby GP, Mathews DG, et al: Reduction of operative morbidity and mortality by combined preoperative and postoperative nutritional support. Ann Surg 192:604–613 1980.
99. Heatley RV, Williams RHP, Lewis MH: Pre-operative intravenous feeding—a controlled trial. Postgrad Med J 55:541–545, 1979.
100. Thompson BR, Julian TB, Stremple JF: Perioperative parenteral nutrition in patients with gastrointestinal cancer. J Surg Res 30:497–500, 1981.
101. Muller JM, Dienst C, Brenner U, Pichlmaier H: Preoperative parenteral feeding in patients with gastrointestinal carcinoma. Lancet 1:68–71, 1982.
102. Daly JM, Dudrick SJ, Copeland EM III: Parenteral nutrition in patients with head and neck cancer: Techniques and results. Otolaryngol Head Neck Surg 88:707–713, 1980.
103. Copeland EM III, MacFadyen BV Jr, Lanzotti VJ, Dudrick SJ: Intravenous hyperalimentation as an adjunct to cancer chemotherapy. Am J Surg 129:167–173, 1975.
104. Rickard KA, Grosfeld JL, Kirksey A, et al: Reversal of protein–energy malnutrition in children during treatment of advanced neoplastic disease. Ann Surg 190:771–781, 1979.
105. Samuels ML, Selig DE, Ogden S, et al: IV hyperalimentation and chemotherapy for Stage III testicular cancer: A randomized trial. Cancer Treat Rep 65:615–627, 1981.
106. Donaldson SS: Nutritional consequences of radiotherapy. Cancer Res 37:2407–2413, 1977.
107. Copeland EM III, Dudrick SJ: Intravenous hyperalimentation in inflammatory bowel disease, pancreatitis, and cancer. Surg Annu 12:83–101, 1980.
108. Copeland EM III, Souchon EA, MacFadyen BV Jr, et al: Intravenous hyperalimentation as an adjunct to radiation therapy. Cancer 39:609–616, 1977.
109. Ruberg RL, Dudrick SJ: Intravenous hyperalimentation in head and neck tumor surgery: Indications and precautions. Br J Plast Surg 30:151–153, 1977.
110. Moertel CG: Nutrition and chemotherapy of cancer. Proceedings of the Workshop on Diet and Nutrition in the Therapy and Rehabilitation of the Cancer Patient, National Institutes of Health, Bethesda, Maryland, March 26, 1975, pp 65–71.
111. Steiger E, Oram-Smith J, Miller E, et al: Effects of nutrition on tumor growth and tolerance to chemotherapy. J Surg Res 18:445–461, 1975.
112. Souchon EA, Copeland EM, Watson P, Dudrick SJ: Intravenous hyperalimentation as an adjunct to cancer chemotherapy with 5-fluorouracil. J Surg Res 18:451–454, 1975.
113. Bounous G, Hugon J, Gentile JM: Elemental diet in the management of the in-

testinal lesion produced by 5-fluorouracil in the rat. Can J Surg 14:298–311, 1971.

114. Miller JM, Valbuena RM, Remigo MR: Protection by an elemental diet against the toxic intestinal changes of 5-fluorouracil in rats. J Abdom Surg 19:25–27, 1977.

115. Dudrick SJ: Artificial feeding techniques. Proceedings of the Workshop on Diet and Nutrition in the Therapy and Rehabilitation of the Cancer Patient, National Institutes of Health, Bethesda, Maryland, March 26, 1975, pp 29–35.

116. Issell BF, Valdivieso M, Zaren HA, et al: Protection against chemotherapy toxicity by IV hyperalimentation. Cancer Treat Rep 62:1139–1143, 1978.

117. Lanzotti VJ, Copeland EM, George SL, et al: Cancer chemotherapeutic response and intravenous hyperalimentation. Cancer Chem Rep (Part I) 59:437–439, 1975.

118. Issell BF, Valdivieso M, Hersh EM, et al: Combination chemoimmunotherapy for extensive non-oat cell lung cancer. Cancer Treat Rep 62:1059–1063, 1978.

119. Popp MB, Fisher RI, Wesley R, et al: A prospective randomized study of adjuvant parenteral nutrition in the treatment of advanced diffuse lymphoma: Influence on survival. Surgery 90:195–203, 1981.

120. Eilber FR, Morton DC: Impaired immunologic reactivity and recurrence following cancer surgery. Cancer 25:362–365, 1970.

121. Hersh EM, Marligit GM, Gutterman JV: Immunological evaluation of malignant disease. JAMA 236:1739–1742, 1976.

122. Bistrian BR, Blackburn GL, Scrimshaw NS, Flatt NP: Cellular immunity in semistarved states in hospitalized adults. Am J Clin Nutr 28:1148–1155, 1975.

123. Law DK, Dudrick SI, Abdou NI: Immunocompetence of patients with protein–calorie malnutrition. Ann Intern Med 79:545–550, 1973.

124. Daly JM, Dudrick SJ, Copeland EM III: Intravenous hyperalimentation: Effect on delayed cutaneous hypersensitivity in cancer patients. Ann Surg 192:587–592, 1980.

125. Haffejee AA, Angorn IB: Nutritional status and nonspecific cellular and humoral immune response in esophageal carcinoma. Ann Surg 189:475–479, 1979.

126. Daly JM, Reynolds HM, Rowland BJ, et al: Tumor growth in experimental animals: Nutritional manipulation and chemotherapeutic response in the rat. Ann Surg 191:316–322, 1980.

127. Copeland EM, MacFadyen BV, Dudrick SJ: Intravenous hyperalimentation in cancer patients. J Surg Res 16:241–274, 1974.

128. Mullen JL, Buzby GP, Gertner MH, et al: Protein synthesis dynamics in human gastrointestinal malignancies. Surgery 87:331–338, 1980.

129. Cameron IL, Pavlat WA: Stimulation of growth of a transplantable hepatoma in rats by parenteral nutrition. J Natl Cancer Inst 56:597–601, 1976.

130. Buzby GP, Mullen JL, Stein TP, et al: Host–tumor interaction and nutrient supply. Cancer 45:2940–2948, 1980.

131. Cameron IL, Rogers W: Total intravenous hyperalimentation and hydroxyurea chemotherapy in hepatoma-bearing rats. J Surg Res 23:279–288, 1977.

132. Blackburn GL, Williams LF, Bistrian BR, et al: New approaches to the management of severe pancreatitis. Am J Surg 131:114–124, 1976.

133. Feller JH, Brown RA, Toussaint GPM, Thompson AG: Changing methods in the treatment of severe pancreatitis. Am J Surg 127:196–201, 1974.

134. Voitk A, Brown RA, Echave V, et al: Use of an elemental diet in the treatment of complicated pancreatitis. Am J Surg 125:223–227, 1973.
135. Holden JL, Berne TV, Rosoff L Sr: Pancreatic abscess following acute pancreatitis. Arch Surg 111:858–861, 1976.
136. Goodgame JT, Fischer JE: Parenteral nutrition in the treatment of acute pancreatitis: Effect on complications and mortality. Ann Surg 186:651–658, 1977.
137. Eisenberg D, Dixon NP, Silberman H: Safety and efficacy of lipid infusions in pancreatitis. JPEN 4:599, 1980.
138. Studley HO: Percentage of weight loss: A basic indicator of surgical risk in patients with chronic peptic ulcer. JAMA 106:458–460, 1936.
139. Rhoads JE, Alexander CE: Nutritional problems of surgical patients. Ann NY Acad Sci 63:268–275, 1955.
140. Mullen JL, Buzby GP, Waldman MT, et al: Prediction of operative morbidity and mortality by preoperative nutritional assessment. Surg Forum 30:80–82, 1979.
141. Mullen JL: Consequences of malnutrition in the surgical patient. Surg Clin North Am 61:465–487, 1981.
142. Buzby GP, Mullen JL, Matthews DC, et al: Prognostic nutritional index in gastrointestinal surgery. Am J Surg 139:160–167, 1980.
143. Dunn EL, Moore EE, Bohus RW: Immediate postoperative feeding following massive abdominal trauma: The catheter jejunostomy. JPEN 4:393–395, 1980.
144. Hoover HC Jr, Ryan JA, Anderson EJ, Fischer JE: Nutritional benefits of immediate postoperative jejunal feeding of an elemental diet. Am J Surg 139: 153–159, 1980.
145. Sagar S, Harland P, Shields R: Early postoperative feeding with elemental diet. Br Med J 1:293–295, 1979.
146. Yeung CK, Young GA, Hackett AF, Hill GL: Fine needle catheter jejunostomy: An assessment of a new method of nutritional support after major gastrointestinal surgery. Br J Surg 66:727–732, 1979.
147. Rush BF, Richardson JD, Griffen WO: Positive nitrogen balance immediately after abdominal operations. Am J Surg 119:70–76, 1970.
148. Van Way CW III, Meng HC, Sandstead HH: Nitrogen balance in postoperative patients receiving parenteral nutrition. Arch Surg 110:272–276, 1975.
149. Page CP, Carlton PK, Andrassy RJ, et al: Safe, cost-effective postoperative nutrition: Defined formula diet via needle–catheter jejunostomy. Am J Surg 138:939–945, 1979.
150. Page CP, Ryan JA Jr, Haff RC: Continual catheter administration of an elemental diet. Surg Gynecol Obstet 142:184–188, 1976.
151. Blackburn GL, Flatt JP, Clowes GHA, O'Donnell TE: Peripheral intravenous feeding with isotonic amino acid solutions. Am J Surg 125:447–454, 1973.
152. Freeman JB, Stegink LD, Meyer PD, et al: Metabolic effects of amino acid vs. dextrose infusion in surgical patients. Arch Surg 110:916–921, 1975.
153. Greenberg GR, Marliss EB, Anderson GH, et al: Protein-sparing therapy in postoperative patients: Effects of added hypocaloric glucose or lipid. N Engl J Med 294:1411–1416, 1976.
154. Hoover HC Jr, Grant JP, Gorschboth C, Ketcham AS: Nitrogen-sparing intravenous fluids in postoperative patients. N Engl J Med 293:172–175, 1975.
155. Schulte WJ, Condon RE, Kraus MA: Positive nitrogen balance using isotonic

crystalline amino acid solution. Arch Surg 110:914–915, 1975.

156. Watters JM, Freeman JB: Parenteral nutrition by peripheral vein. Surg Clin North Am 61:593–604, 1981.

157. Skillman JJ, Rosenoer VM, Smith PC, Fang MS: Improved albumin synthesis in postoperative patients by amino acid infusion. N Engl J Med 295:1037–1040, 1976.

158. Greenberg GR, Jeejeebhoy KN: Intravenous protein-sparing therapy in patients with gastrointestinal disease. JPEN 3:427–432, 1979.

159. Moore FD, Brennan MR: Intravenous amino acids. N Engl J Med 293:194–195, 1975.

160. Felig P: Intravenous nutrition: Fact and fancy. N Engl J Med 294:1455–1456, 1976.

161. O'Keefe SJ, Carraher TE, El-Zayadi AR, et al: Malnutrition and immunocompetence in patients with liver disease. Lancet 2:615–617, 1980.

162. Fischer JE, Bower RH: Nutritional support in liver disease. Surg Clin North Am 61:653–660, 1981.

163. Abel RM, Abbott WM, Beck CH Jr, et al: Essential L-amino acids for hyperalimentation in patients with disordered nitrogen metabolism. Am J Surg 128:317–323, 1974.

164. Fischer JE, Yoshimura N, Aguirre A, et al: Plasma amino acid patterns with hepatic encephalopathy: Effects of amino acid infusions. Am J Surg 127:40–47, 1974.

165. Fischer JE, Funovics JM, Aguirre A, et al: The role of plasma amino acids in hepatic encephalopathy. Surgery 78:276–290, 1975.

166. Fischer JE, Rosen HM, Ebeid AM, et al: The effect of normalization of plasma amino acids on hepatic encephalopathy in man. Surgery 80:77–91, 1976.

167. Freund H, Yoshimura N. Fischer JE: Chronic hepatic encephalopathy: Long term therapy with a branched chain amino-acid-enriched elemental diet. JAMA 242:347–349, 1979.

168. Smith AR, Rossi-Fanelli F, Ziparo V, et al: Alterations in plasma and CSF amino acids, amines and metabolites in hepatic coma. Ann Surg 187:343–350, 1978.

169. Baker AL: Amino acids in liver disease: A cause of hepatic encephalopathy? JAMA 242:355–356, 1979.

170. Munro HN, Fernstrom JD, Wurtman RJ: Insulin, plasma amino acid imbalance, and hepatic coma. Lancet 1:722–724, 1975.

171. Soeters PB, Fischer JE: Insulin, glucagon, amino-acid imbalance, and hepatic encephalopathy. Lancet 2:880–882, 1976.

172. Crim MC, Munro HN: Protein and amino acid requirements and metabolism in relation to defined-formula diets, in Shils ME (ed): Defined-Formula Diets for Medical Purposes. Chicago, American Medical Association, 1977, pp 5–15.

173. Zieve L, Olsen RL: Can hepatic coma be caused by a reduction of brain noradrenaline or dopamine? Gut 18:688–691, 1977.

174. Ames FC, Copeland EM, Leeb DC, et al: Liver dysfunction following small-bowel bypass for obesity: Nonoperative treatment of fatty metamorphosis with parenteral hyperalimentation. JAMA 235:1249–1252, 1976.

175. Heimburger SL, Steiger E, LoGerfo P, et al: Reversal of severe fatty hepatic infiltration after intestinal bypass for morbid obesity by calorie-free amino acid infusion. Am J Surg 129:229–235, 1975.

INDEX

F

False neurotransmitter hypothesis, 276–278
Fasting
  glycogen stores and, 12
  losses of protein from organs and tissues after, 1–2, 4
Fat administration, protein-sparing effect as not observed with, 218
Fat emulsions
  cottonseed oil, 122, 125
  formulas for, 124
  pulmonary diffusion capacity and, 196–198
  safe for intravenous infusion, 182–189
  safflower oil (Liposyn), 125, 182–183
  soybean oil (Intralipid), *see* Soybean emulsion
Fat metabolism, endogenous, and gram-negative sepsis, 224–225
"Fat overload syndrome" with cottonseed emulsion in infants or children, 125
Fat-soluble vitamins (A, D, E, and K)
  as adequately stored, 206
  dietary supplements of calcium and, in short bowel syndrome, 238
Fatty acids, essential, *see* Essential fatty acids
Feeding program, oral, in burn wounds, 244–245
Fluid and electrolyte balance in parenteral nutrition, 134–135
  gastrointestinal fistulas and, 234
Fluid and electrolyte disturbances in short bowel syndrome, nutritional therapy and, 235–238
Fluid restriction, glucose system and, 226
  nutritional therapy and, 266–267

5-Fluorouracil, anorexia and negative nitrogen balance, and, 259
Folate deficiency and TPN, 207
Food blender, electric, 79
Foods, specific dynamic action (SDA) of, 53
Fructose in parenteral nutrition, 120–121
Fuel composition of normal man, 24
Feul utilization and glucose system in injured and septic patients, 225
Fuels, body, caloric and oxygen and carbon dioxide equivalents of, 57
Fungal species causing TPN-related sepsis, 174
Fungi and bacteria, growth of, in TPN solutions, 169, 170

G

Gastric acid secretion
  amino acids and, 191–192
  elemental diets and, 93
  glucose system and, 191
Gastric acidity and malnutrition, 8–9
Gastric emptying
  elemental diets and, 93
  of solid food, glucose system and, 192
Gastric secretory function, chronic TPN and, 192
Gastrointestinal disorders or dysfunction
  bleeding, elemental diet and, 93–94
  enteral nutrition and, 79–80
  fistulas, nutritional therapy and, 230–235
    closure rate and mortality in, 232–233
  TPN and, 118
Gastrointestinal symptoms of dumping syndrome, 109–110
Gastrointestinal tract and malnutrition, 8–9